T0383787

# The Resident's Guide to Shoulder and Elbow Surgery

Caroline M. Chebli · Anand M. Murthi
Editors

# The Resident's Guide to Shoulder and Elbow Surgery

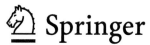
Springer

*Editors*
Caroline M. Chebli
James A. Haley Medical Center
Tampa, FL, USA

Anand M. Murthi
MedStar Union Memorial Hospital
Baltimore, MD, USA

ISBN 978-3-031-12254-5      ISBN 978-3-031-12255-2   (eBook)
https://doi.org/10.1007/978-3-031-12255-2

This Springer imprint is published by the registered company Springer Nature Switzerland AG
The registered company address is: Gewerbestrasse 11, 6330 Cham, Switzerland

*To our ACESS (Association of Clinical Elbow and Shoulder Surgeons) family who are the authors of this guidebook. They don't understand the concept of an actual deadline unless there is a party and then they are always on time!! But we love them anyway and thank them for their time and commitment to education.*

# Preface

The field of Shoulder and Elbow Surgery has grown tremendously in the recent past. When we were applying for fellowship, there were only a few positions available. Today, it is a highly competitive Accreditation Council for Graduate Medical Education and/or American Shoulder and Elbow Surgeons approved fellowship within the match. This popularity is partly due to the incredible advances that have been made over the last 20 or so years. New technology and innovation have allowed us to improve our diagnostics and patient care. To that end, it is difficult to decipher the best practices within this rapidly growing field. As physicians who are actively involved in the education of medical students, residents, and fellows, we sought to create a reference guide for best practices. We gathered some of the most prolific thinkers in the field and paired them with residents and fellows to create this book. Many of the authors are fellowship directors, residency directors, chairman, team physicians, and national and international educators. The book is meant to be a quick guide for medical students, residents, and fellows. It is organized in outline form for easy reference. As anyone who has ever been in the "hot-seat" during rounds or in the operating room, you will recognize the value in having a quick reference to the most asked questions. References are included to validate the information and for a more in-depth review of the topic. We hope this guide will aid in medical education and illuminate each topic so that the salient information is readily accessible.

Tampa, FL, USA                                                                 Caroline M. Chebli
Baltimore, MD, USA                                                              Anand M. Murthi

# Contents

# Glenohumeral Osteoarthritis

**1**

Blake C. Meza ⓘ, Joshua I. Mathew ⓘ,
and Lawrence V. Gulotta ⓘ

## Introduction

Primary glenohumeral osteoarthritis is a chronic degenerative disorder of the articular cartilage of the shoulder, defined by damage to the articular cartilage as a result of chronic stresses, overuse, repetitive microtrauma, and structural anomalies in joint and cartilage composition.

## Epidemiology

- Occurs in a bimodal distribution.
  - Men in their 50s
  - Men and women in their 70s and 80s
- Recent estimates suggest that nearly one-third of the global population over age 60 suffer from glenohumeral osteoarthritis [1].
- The rate of radiographic evidence of glenohumeral arthritis is even higher, but the presence of arthritic changes on X-ray does not necessarily correlate with symptomatic disease.
- Like other diseases of the elderly, the global disease burden of glenohumeral osteoarthritis, as well as the future potential need for surgical intervention, will continue to increase as the population ages [2].
- Risk factors:
  - Several factors are associated with an increased risk of developing glenohumeral osteoarthritis, including age, sex, obesity, genetics, previous injuries, and certain occupations or sports [3, 4].

B. C. Meza · J. I. Mathew · L. V. Gulotta (✉)
Shoulder and Elbow Division, Sports Medicine Institute, Hospital for Special Surgery,
New York, NY, USA
e-mail: GulottaL@hss.edu

© The Author(s), under exclusive license to Springer Nature Switzerland AG 2022
C. M. Chebli, A. M. Murthi (eds.), *The Resident's Guide to Shoulder and Elbow Surgery*, https://doi.org/10.1007/978-3-031-12255-2_1

- BMI greater than 24 has been associated with an increased risk of glenohumeral arthritis, whereas BMI greater than 30 has been associated with increased odds of requiring shoulder arthroplasty.
- Caucasian patients of Northern European descent are believed to be at increased risk for degenerative arthritis of the shoulder [5].

1. **History**
   - Patients with glenohumeral osteoarthritis will typically report having shoulder pain with activity but not at rest, shoulder stiffness, crepitus, or "catching" with shoulder motion.
   - Obtain a thorough history from the patient in order to differentiate other possible etiologies of their shoulder pain.

   (a) *Description of Pain*
       - Onset, location, descriptive characteristics
         - How long has the patient had pain? Is it progressively getting worse?
         - Where is the pain located?
         - Is it sharp? Is it more like an aching cramp? Does it radiate down the arm or into the neck?
       - Alleviating or aggravating factors
         - Osteoarthritic pain occurs with side-to-side movement of the shoulder
         - Have they found holding the arm in certain positions or performing specific activities is more difficult?
         - What have they taken for the pain? Has it helped their pain?
       - Severity
         - As the disease progresses, patients will commonly have difficulty with sleeping on the arthritic shoulder and other activities of daily living.
         - Does the pain interfere with work, getting dressed, or sleeping?
         - Is their dominant or nondominant arm affected?
       - Other symptoms
         - Is their shoulder stiff? Do they feel like their shoulder "gets caught"?
         - Are any other joints affected?
         - Are they having any systemic symptoms, like fevers, chills, etc.?
   (b) *Other Etiologies to Consider*
       - Differential diagnosis for shoulder pain: rotator cuff injury, adhesive capsulitis, fracture, other types of arthritis (posttraumatic arthritis, inflammatory arthropathy, and rotator cuff arthropathy)
         - Any history of recent or remote trauma to the shoulder?
         - Is there a personal or family history of autoimmune disorders (i.e., rheumatoid arthritis) or endocrinopathies (i.e., diabetes, hypothyroidism)?
       - Prior treatments
         - Physical therapy, corticosteroid injections, and over-the-counter anti-inflammatories may all play a role in the nonoperative management.
         - Has the patient tried any of these? If so, did they experience any improvement in symptoms? For how long?

- Medical and social history
  - An in-depth evaluation of medical and social comorbidities that could impact surgical outcomes should be completed.
  - Does the patient use tobacco or alcohol? If so, how much and for how long?
  - Is the patient dependent on narcotics for analgesia? How many pills are they taking? How are they obtaining them? Have they tried to cut back?
  - For medically complex patients, preoperative medical clearance should be obtained, and chronic conditions such as hypertension, diabetes, and cardiac disease should be optimized.
- Potential postoperative considerations
  - Factors that impact the postoperative course and rehabilitation of patients should also be discussed prior to surgery.
  - What kind of work does a patient do?
  - Do they have the necessary family or friend support system to aid their recovery? What is their baseline functional status and what activities are they hoping to return after surgery?
  - Open communication about each of these will help set expectations for both surgeon and patient.

2. **Physical Examination**
   - The initial physical examination of the arthritic shoulder does not deviate from a standard shoulder exam.

   (a) *Inspection/Palpation*
   - Are there prior incisions? Are they healed? Are there any rashes or skin lesions over where a future incision may be required?
   - Is there an effusion or superficial swelling?
   - Do you notice any erythema or warmth or other sign of infection?
   - The acromioclavicular joint, clavicle, biceps tendon, footprint of the rotator cuff, and posterior glenohumeral joint line should all be palpated to assess for tenderness or step-off.

   (b) *Range of Motion*
   - Active and passive motion of the shoulder should also be assessed.
     - Evaluate forward flexion, abduction, internal rotation (IR), and external rotation (ER) at the side and in abduction.
   - As a result of contraction of the anterior glenohumeral capsule that occurs with posterior humeral head subluxation, external rotation is usually lost first.
     - Followed later by forward flexion and internal rotation.
   - Stability of the glenohumeral joint should be assessed by raising the arm in the scapular plane or moving it actively from 90° of abduction to 90° of flexion.
     - Posterior humeral head subluxation with either of these movements is suggestive of glenohumeral instability.

(c) *Strength Testing*
- A thorough neurovascular exam of the upper extremity must be performed, paying particular attention to the strength of the deltoid and rotator cuff musculature.

(d) *Directed Tests*
- Although concomitant ipsilateral rotator cuff injuries are rare in patients with glenohumeral osteoarthritis, the integrity of each muscle should be evaluated with the appropriate provocative maneuver.
  - Jobe's empty can test (supraspinatus)
  - Belly press or lift off (subscapularis)
  - Resisted external rotation with 90° of flexion (teres minor)
  - Resisted external rotation with arm at side (infraspinatus)
- If there is any suspicion of neck pain or possible cervical etiology, Spurling maneuver should be performed.

3. **Imaging**
   (a) *X-Rays*
   - Despite advances in imaging technology, plain radiographs of the shoulder remain the gold standard for the initial evaluation and diagnosis of glenohumeral osteoarthritis.
   - A true AP (Grashey) and axillary views should be obtained on initial presentation to fully assess glenohumeral joint for signs of arthritis.
     - When performed correctly, these combined views show the hallmarks of glenohumeral osteoarthritis: joint space narrowing, loss of articular cartilage, reactive subchondral sclerosis and cysts, osteophytes, and glenoid wear.
       Osteophytes most frequently occur in the inferior aspect of the humeral head and contribute to the biomechanical changes of the shoulder.
       Results in posterior humeral head subluxation and flattening and progressive glenoid bone loss.
         Progressive cycle as the joint reactive forces are spread across a smaller articular contact area over time, leading to more posterior wear.
       "Bad arthritic triad": glenoid biconcavity, posterior humeral head subluxation, and glenoid retroversion [6].
       Anterior glenoid cartilage remains unaffected due to the relative positioning and posterior-directed forces of the humeral head on the glenoid.
     - Grashey view is an AP radiograph taken in the scapular plane to allow optimal visualization of the glenohumeral joint.
       Obtained by angling the beam 30° medial to the sagittal plane and aiming at the coracoid process, with the cassette placed parallel to the plane of the scapula.
     - Equally important is the axillary view as this can be obtained with the arm elevated in the scapular plane, placing it in more of a functional position.

Demonstrates posterior subluxation of the humeral head, joint space narrowing, and the central loss of articular cartilage.

Sometimes referred to as the "truth view" for glenohumeral osteoarthritis as it allows for visualization of the earliest stages of degenerative changes of the joint [5].

(b) *CT Scan*

- CT scans are particularly helpful for preoperative templating and surgical planning.
- The pattern of glenoid wear can also be classified from axial CT slices.
  – Walch Classification [7] with recent modifications (Fig. 1.1)
    Type A glenoids: Concentric glenoid wear with a well-centered humeral head

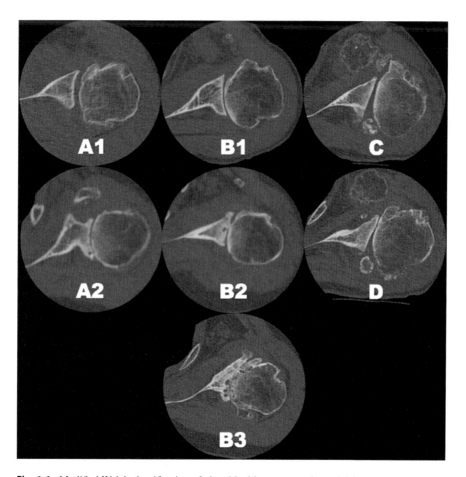

**Fig. 1.1** Modified Walch classification of glenoid with representative axial CT images. (**A1**) centered humeral head with minor erosion. (**A2**) centered humeral head with major central erosion. (**B1**) posterior subluxated head without bony erosion. (**B2**) posterior subluxated head, biconcave glenoid. (**B3**) Monoconcavity with >15° retroversion. (**C**), dysplastic glenoid (>25° retroversion). (**D**), glenoid anteversion and/or anterior subluxation

A1: Only minor central erosion

A2: More severe central erosion

Type B glenoids: Eccentric posterior glenoid wear and posterior "arthrogenic subluxation" of the humeral head

B1: Posterior wear with degenerative changes

B2: "Biconcave" posterior wear

B3: Monoconcave posterior wear with humeral head subluxation or retroversion >15°

Type C glenoids: Dysplastic and >25° of retroversion

Type D glenoids: Glenoid anteversion or anterior humeral head subluxation

- Three-dimensional reconstructions have been shown to be beneficial in evaluating glenoid morphology [8, 9].
  - Helps to determine how much reaming of the glenoid is necessary to neutralize its retroversion

(c) *MRI*
  - MRIs are indicated as part of the preoperative workup when rotator cuff insufficiency or another diagnosis is being considered.
  - Patients with inflammatory arthropathies should obtain an MRI given the relatively high rate of rotator cuff pathology in this population.

(d) *Ultrasound*
  - There is little role for ultrasound in the workup of glenohumeral arthritis.

4. **Treatment Algorithm**

(a) *Nonoperative Management*
  - There are several approaches to conservative management of glenohumeral osteoarthritis, which should be explored prior to moving forward with operative intervention.
  - In general, these strategies cannot reverse the degenerative process; however, they can address the resultant symptoms, particularly pain and stiffness.
  - Potential nonoperative treatments include activity modification, physical therapy, corticosteroid injections, anti-inflammatories, and other oral medications, such as glucosamine.
  - Activity modification.
    - Avoid activities that worsen pain, especially axial loading.
  - Physical therapy.
    - Focus on range of motion and shoulder strength.
    - May help alleviate stiffness that occurs due to contracture of the joint capsule.
  - Anti-inflammatories.
    - Naproxen or meloxicam typically used.
    - Caution patients about side effects including GI bleeds, hepatic injury.
  - Corticosteroid injections [10].
    - Can be done independently or with ultrasound guidance.
    - Help to confirm if symptoms are coming from intra-articular process.

- Avoid surgery for 3 months after corticosteroid injection due to risk of infection of hardware.
  - Viscosupplement injections (e.g., hyaluronic acid) may provide temporary relief for patients with early to moderate arthritis but are typically not effective for patients with severe arthritis [11, 12]. There can be issues with reimbursement in that most major formulations are not FDA approved for use in the shoulder.
(b) *Operative Treatment*
  - Generally, operative treatment for glenohumeral is indicated when nonoperative management fails to sufficiently address the patient's symptoms.
    - The appropriate duration of a trial of nonoperative management is not well defined.
  - Goals of operative intervention are to decrease pain and stiffness, increase function and independence, and, possibly, permit return to work.
  - Stability and mobility of the joint are the outcome of interest, not restoration of "normal" joint structure.
  - *Options for surgical treatment* of shoulder arthritis include arthroscopy, total shoulder arthroplasty, reverse total shoulder arthroplasty, and, less commonly, hemiarthroplasty (Table 1.1).
  - Arthroscopic surgical debridement of the arthritic shoulder is not effective nor indicated. Arthroscopic interventions can be considered in the following situations:
    - Loose body removal is indicated in patients with mechanical symptoms related to the loose body.
    - Biceps tenodesis can be indicated in patients that get symptomatic relief from a cortisone injection into the long head of the biceps tendon sheath.

**Table 1.1** Comparison of indications, implants, complications of surgical techniques for shoulder arthroplasty for glenohumeral osteoarthritis (GH OA)

| Procedure | Indications | Implants | Complications |
| --- | --- | --- | --- |
| Total shoulder arthroplasty (TSA) | GH OA with intact rotator cuff, adequate glenoid bone stock | Humeral head ("ball") and glenoid ("socket") resurfacing | Glenoid loosening, component wear, instability (anterior > posterior), rotator cuff injury, infection |
| Reverse total shoulder arthroplasty (rTSA) | GH OA with intact deltoid, rotator cuff insufficiency | Convex glenoid component ("ball") and concave humeral articulating cup ("socket") | Scapular notching, acromial and scapular spine stress fractures, baseplate failure, dislocation, infection |
| Hemiarthroplasty | Rare; young patient (>55 years) with active lifestyle, intact rotator cuff, adequate glenoid bone stock | Humeral head resurfacing with stem into proximal humerus; no glenoid component | High revision rate, infection |

- Capsular release and removal of the inferior humeral osteophyte can be indicated for patients with minimal pain in which lack of motion is their primary complaint.
- *Surgical Approach*
  - Regardless of planned procedure, the anterior or deltopectoral approach is the standard approach for shoulder arthroplasty.
  - Patient should be placed in beach chair position or supine with ipsilateral scapular bump.
  - Internervous plane: axillary nerve (deltoid) and medial and lateral pectoral nerves (pectoralis major).
  - May need to release 1–2 cm of pectoralis tendon for better exposure.
  - Dangers: cephalic vein, musculocutaneous nerve, axillary nerve.
  - Though less common, the anterosuperior approach to the shoulder may also be utilized. Through this approach, the surgeon reflects the anterior deltoid from the acromion, exposing the glenohumeral joint.
    Total Shoulder Arthroplasty (TSA)
      Anatomic replacement of the glenohumeral joint with humeral head ("ball") and glenoid ("socket") resurfacing
      Indications
        Debilitating glenohumeral osteoarthritis with intact rotator cuff
      Contraindications
        Rotator cuff deficiency or arthropathy
          TSA shown to help pain relief, not function in these patients [13]
        Insufficient or poor glenoid bone stock
        Deltoid dysfunction
        Active infection
      Outcomes
        Good to excellent satisfaction and pain relief in >90% of cases [14]
        Patient-reported outcomes slightly worse in younger (<65 years old) patients [15]
        Failure rate ~1% per year
      Techniques
        Keys to success
          Visualization of glenoid.
            Release all subacromial/subdeltoid adhesions
            Adequate release of inferior capsule off humerus after taking down subscapularis
              Must protect axillary nerve as this is done
            Adequate humeral head cut
              Along the anatomic neck, directly up to the supraspinatus insertion
            Complete removal of osteophytes

Management of subscapularis.

Subscapularis peel, tenotomy, or lesser tuberosity oste-otomy (LTO) are all feasible options [11, 16, 17].

LTO is biomechanically stronger than tenotomy, allows for better healing, and results in longer surgical times [18, 19].

The goal is to place the glenoid implant in 10° or less of retroversion.

Glenoid version can be corrected by reaming the "high side."

In cases of severe retroversion (>20°, i.e., Walch B3 or C), it can augment with bone graft.

Implants

Glenoid component is typically an all-polyethylene cemented peg or keel [20, 21].

Metal-backed glenoid components are rare in the USA due to a high failure rate [22–24].

Humeral stem should be placed in 25–45° of retroversion.

There are many new types of humeral implants (short stem, long stem, stemless, and resurfacing); however, no head-to-head comparisons exist [11].

Unclear impact on survivorship, patient outcomes, pain relief.

Postoperative protocol

The goal is to protect the subscapularis, regardless of tenotomy or osteotomy, and then slowly strengthen it [25].

An example of a postoperative protocol is:

0–2 weeks: Sling, pendulums, distal ROM of wrist, digits

2–6 weeks: Sling, passive gentle ROM—limit active/passive ER and active IR

6–12 weeks: Discontinue sling, aggressive ROM

>12 weeks: Strengthen shoulder

6 months: Return to full activities

Little evidence exists for superiority of home program versus standard physical therapy program [26].

Complications

Polyethylene wear and glenoid component loosening [27, 28]

Average time to revision: 8 years [29, 30].

Polyethylene wear may be more common with metal-backed glenoids [31].

Humeral component failure

Related to malpositioning (version, varus/valgus) or loosening

Less common than glenoid component failure

Glenohumeral instability

Anterior due to subscapularis weakness

May also be related to anterior deltoid weakness, capsular failure, inappropriate anteversion of glenoid or humeral component [5, 32]

Posterior

Due to excessive retroversion of either component, posterior glenoid bony deficiency or inappropriate soft tissue tensioning posteriorly

Superior/inferior

Associated with rotator cuff deficiency or fracture

Infection (*C. acnes*, coagulase negative staphylococci)

Occurs in 0–4% of cases.

*C. acnes* often results in false-negative aspiration results.

Nerve injury

Axillary, musculocutaneous, radial, median, ulnar, and suprascapular nerves all at risk

Highlights importance of physical exam for each nerve pre- and postoperatively

Rotator cuff tear [33].

Rates around 15% at 5 years, higher at 20 years [33]

Multifactorial

Patients who have GH OA are of similar age to those with RTC tears.

Arthroplasty alters biomechanics of previously abnormal joint, resulting in new forces across formerly less utilized muscles.

When cutting the humeral head, the rotator cuff or greater tuberosity may be inadvertently violated.

Periprosthetic fracture

Stiffness

Reverse Total Shoulder Arthroplasty

Non-anatomic replacement of glenohumeral joint with convex glenoid component ("ball") and concave humeral articulating cup ("socket")

Indications

Debilitating glenohumeral osteoarthritis with rotator cuff tear or arthropathy

"Pseudoparalysis" due to inability to actively abduct shoulder to 90°

Contraindications

Deltoid insufficiency

Active infection

Outcomes

Due to loss of rotator cuff, patients are limited in ER/IR

Techniques

rTSA works by medializing and displacing the center of rotation of the joint inferiorly

Converts glenoid joint reactive forces that occur with elevation into compressive forces

Distalizes deltoid insertion, resulting in better tension to work as an abductor more effectively

Coronal plane alignment of glenoid is crucial.

Glenoid baseplate needs to be neutral or slightly inferior tilted.

Reduces risk of scapular notching.

Complications

Typically, mechanical failures occur early on and functional failures occur later.

Overall, complication rates higher than TSA (10–20%) [34, 35].

Component loosening or baseplate failure.

Glenosphere and baseplate can dissociate.

Humeral stem and cup can dissociate.

Scapular notching [36, 37].

Impingement of humeral component and inferior glenoid.

Can cause polyethylene wear and osteolysis.

Incidence decreasing with baseplate lateralization.

Acromial stress or scapular spine fracture [38, 39].

Due to excessive tension of deltoid or related to screw placement

Nonoperative management preferred.

Dislocation [40].

Occurs in 2–3.4% of cases.

Rates have decreased with implementation of new implants and increasing surgeon familiarity with rTSA.

Infection (*C. acnes*, coagulase negative staphylococci).

Generally accepted higher rate than TSA, as many rTSAs are performed as revision cases.

Higher risk in those less than 65 years old and revision cases [41].

Glenohumeral instability, periprosthetic fractures, nerve injury similar to TSA.

Hemiarthroplasty

Resurfacing of the humeral head only.

Can be done with cemented or uncemented press fit prosthesis

High revision rate due to frequency of conversion of hemiarthroplasty to TSA [42].

Limited role for hemiarthroplasty in patients—possibly younger patients (<55 years old) with limited glenoid disease and active lifestyle (i.e., manual labor or heavy lifting).

Recent AAOS Clinical Practice Guidelines [11] recommend TSA over hemiarthroplasty due to better outcomes with regard to pain relief, stiffness, patient satisfaction, and complication rates.

## References

1. Singh JA, Sperling J, Buchbinder R, McMaken K. Surgery for shoulder osteoarthritis. Cochrane Database Syst Rev. 2010;(10):CD008089.
2. Day JS, Lau E, Ong KL, Williams GR, Ramsey ML, Kurtz SM. Prevalence and projections of total shoulder and elbow arthroplasty in the United States to 2015. J Shoulder Elb Surg. 2010;19(8):1115–20.
3. Wall KC, Politzer CS, Chahla J, Garrigues GE. Obesity is associated with an increased prevalence of glenohumeral osteoarthritis and arthroplasty: a cohort study. Orthop Clin North Am. 2020;51(2):259–64.
4. De Martino I, Gulotta LV. The effect of obesity in shoulder arthroplasty outcomes and complications. Orthop Clin North Am. 2018;49(3):353–60.
5. Matsen FA III, Lippitt S, Rockwood C, Wirth M. The shoulder. In: Rockwood and Matsen's. 5th ed. Philadelphia, PA: Elsevier; 2016. p. 831–1042.
6. Matsen FA III, Warme WJ, Jackins SE. Can the ream and run procedure improve glenohumeral relationships and function for shoulders with the arthritic triad? Clin Orthop Relat Res. 2015;473(6):2088–96.
7. Walch G, Boulahia A, Boileau P, Kempf JF. Primary glenohumeral osteoarthritis: clinical and radiographic classification. The Aequalis Group. Acta Orthop Belg. 1998;64(Suppl 2):46–52.
8. Hoenecke HR Jr, Hermida JC, Flores-Hernandez C, D'Lima DD. Accuracy of CT-based measurements of glenoid version for total shoulder arthroplasty. J Shoulder Elbow Surg. 2010;19(2):166–71. https://doi.org/10.1016/j.jse.2009.08.009. Epub 2009 Dec 2. PMID: 19959378.
9. Lewis GS, Armstrong AD. Glenoid spherical orientation and version. J Shoulder Elbow Surg. 2011;20(1):3–11. https://doi.org/10.1016/j.jse.2010.05.012. Epub 2010 Oct 8. PMID: 20932782.
10. Stitik TP, Kumar A, Foye PM. Corticosteroid injections for osteoarthritis. Am J Phys Med Rehabil. 2006;85(11 Suppl):S51–65; quiz S66–8.
11. Khazzam MS, Pearl ML. AAOS Clinical Practice Guideline: management of glenohumeral joint osteoarthritis. J Am Acad Orthop Surg. 2020;28(19):790–4.
12. Kwon YW, Eisenberg G, Zuckerman JD. Sodium hyaluronate for the treatment of chronic shoulder pain associated with glenohumeral osteoarthritis: a multicenter, randomized, double-blind, placebo-controlled trial. J Shoulder Elb Surg. 2013;22(5):584–94.
13. Neer CS II, Watson KC, Stanton FJ. Recent experience in total shoulder replacement. J Bone Joint Surg Am. 1982;64(3):319–37.
14. Simovitch RW, Friedman RJ, Cheung EV, Flurin P-H, Wright T, Zuckerman JD, et al. Rate of improvement in clinical outcomes with anatomic and reverse total shoulder arthroplasty. J Bone Joint Surg Am. 2017;99(21):1801–11.

15. Roberson TA, Bentley JC, Griscom JT, Kissenberth MJ, Tolan SJ, Hawkins RJ, et al. Outcomes of total shoulder arthroplasty in patients younger than 65 years: a systematic review. J Shoulder Elb Surg. 2017;26(7):1298–306.

16. Louie PK, Levy DM, Bach BRJ, Nicholson GP, Romeo AA. Subscapularis tenotomy versus lesser tuberosity osteotomy for total shoulder arthroplasty: a systematic review. Am J Orthop. 2017;46(2):E131–8.

17. Aibinder WR, Bicknell RT, Bartsch S, Scheibel M, Athwal GS. Subscapularis management in stemless total shoulder arthroplasty: tenotomy versus peel versus lesser tuberosity osteotomy. J Shoulder Elb Surg. 2019;28(10):1942–7.

18. Schrock JB, Kraeutler MJ, Houck DA, Provenzano GG, McCarty EC, Bravman JT. Lesser tuberosity osteotomy and subscapularis tenotomy repair techniques during total shoulder arthroplasty: a meta-analysis of cadaveric studies. Clin Biomech. 2016;40:33–6.

19. Levine WN, Munoz J, Hsu S, Byram IR, Bigliani LU, Ahmad CS, et al. Subscapularis tenotomy versus lesser tuberosity osteotomy during total shoulder arthroplasty for primary osteoarthritis: a prospective, randomized controlled trial. J Shoulder Elb Surg. 2019;28(3):407–14.

20. Rahme H, Mattsson P, Wikblad L, Nowak J, Larsson S. Stability of cemented in-line pegged glenoid compared with keeled glenoid components in total shoulder arthroplasty. J Bone Joint Surg Am. 2009;91(8):1965–72.

21. Welsher A, Gohal C, Madden K, Miller B, Bedi A, Alolabi B, et al. A comparison of pegged vs. keeled glenoid components regarding functional and radiographic outcomes in anatomic total shoulder arthroplasty: a systematic review and meta-analysis. JSES Open Access. 2019;3(3):136–144.e1.

22. Taunton MJ, McIntosh AL, Sperling JW, Cofield RH. Total shoulder arthroplasty with a metal-backed, bone-ingrowth glenoid component. Medium to long-term results. J Bone Joint Surg Am. 2008;90(10):2180–8.

23. Tammachote N, Sperling JW, Vathana T, Cofield RH, Harmsen WS, Schleck CD. Long-term results of cemented metal-backed glenoid components for osteoarthritis of the shoulder. J Bone Joint Surg Am. 2009;91(1):160–6.

24. Watson ST, Gudger GKJ, Long CD, Tokish JM, Tolan SJ. Outcomes of Trabecular Metal-backed glenoid components in anatomic total shoulder arthroplasty. J Shoulder Elb Surg. 2018;27(3):493–8.

25. Kennedy JS, Garrigues GE, Pozzi F, Zens MJ, Gaunt B, Phillips B, et al. The American Society of Shoulder and Elbow Therapists' consensus statement on rehabilitation for anatomic total shoulder arthroplasty. J Shoulder Elb Surg. 2020;29(10):2149–62.

26. Mulieri PJ, Holcomb JO, Dunning P, Pliner M, Bogle RK, Pupello D, et al. Is a formal physical therapy program necessary after total shoulder arthroplasty for osteoarthritis? J Shoulder Elb Surg. 2010;19(4):570–9.

27. Franta AK, Lenters TR, Mounce D, Neradilek B, Matsen FA III. The complex characteristics of 282 unsatisfactory shoulder arthroplasties. J Shoulder Elb Surg. 2007;16(5):555–62.

28. Matsen FA III, Clinton J, Lynch J, Bertelsen A, Richardson ML. Glenoid component failure in total shoulder arthroplasty. J Bone Joint Surg Am. 2008;90(4):885–96.

29. Deshmukh AV, Koris M, Zurakowski D, Thornhill TS. Total shoulder arthroplasty: long-term survivorship, functional outcome, and quality of life. J Shoulder Elb Surg. 2005;14(5):471–9.

30. Raiss P, Schmitt M, Bruckner T, Kasten P, Pape G, Loew M, et al. Results of cemented total shoulder replacement with a minimum follow-up of ten years. J Bone Joint Surg Am. 2012;94(23):e1711–0.

31. Papadonikolakis A, Matsen FA III. Metal-backed glenoid components have a higher rate of failure and fail by different modes in comparison with all-polyethylene components: a systematic review. J Bone Joint Surg Am. 2014;96(12):1041–7.

32. Miller BS, Joseph TA, Noonan TJ, Horan MP, Hawkins RJ. Rupture of the subscapularis tendon after shoulder arthroplasty: diagnosis, treatment, and outcome. J Shoulder Elb Surg. 2005;14(5):492–6.

33. Levy DM, Abrams GD, Harris JD, Bach BRJ, Nicholson GP, Romeo AA. Rotator cuff tears after total shoulder arthroplasty in primary osteoarthritis: a systematic review. Int J Shoulder Surg. 2016;10(2):78–84.

34. Frankle M, Levy JC, Pupello D, Siegal S, Saleem A, Mighell M, et al. The reverse shoulder prosthesis for glenohumeral arthritis associated with severe rotator cuff deficiency. A minimum two-year follow-up study of sixty patients surgical technique. J Bone Joint Surg Am. 2006;88(Suppl 1):178–90.

35. Guery J, Favard L, Sirveaux F, Oudet D, Mole D, Walch G. Reverse total shoulder arthroplasty. Survivorship analysis of eighty replacements followed for five to ten years. J Bone Joint Surg Am. 2006;88(8):1742–7.

36. Simovitch RW, Zumstein MA, Lohri E, Helmy N, Gerber C. Predictors of scapular notching in patients managed with the Delta III reverse total shoulder replacement. J Bone Joint Surg Am. 2007;89(3):588–600.

37. Friedman RJ, Barcel DA, Eichinger JK. Scapular notching in reverse total shoulder arthroplasty. J Am Acad Orthop Surg. 2019;27(6):200–9.

38. Crosby LA, Hamilton A, Twiss T. Scapula fractures after reverse total shoulder arthroplasty: classification and treatment. Clin Orthop Relat Res. 2011;469(9):2544–9.

39. Teusink MJ, Otto RJ, Cottrell BJ, Frankle MA. What is the effect of postoperative scapular fracture on outcomes of reverse shoulder arthroplasty? J Shoulder Elb Surg. 2014;23(6):782–90.

40. Chalmers PN, Rahman Z, Romeo AA, Nicholson GP. Early dislocation after reverse total shoulder arthroplasty. J Shoulder Elb Surg. 2014;23(5):737–44.

41. Morris BJ, O'Connor DP, Torres D, Elkousy HA, Gartsman GM, Edwards TB. Risk factors for periprosthetic infection after reverse shoulder arthroplasty. J Shoulder Elb Surg. 2015;24(2):161–6.

42. Bryant D, Litchfield R, Sandow M, Gartsman GM, Guyatt G, Kirkley A. A comparison of pain, strength, range of motion, and functional outcomes after hemiarthroplasty and total shoulder arthroplasty in patients with osteoarthritis of the shoulder. A systematic review and meta-analysis. J Bone Joint Surg Am. 2005;87(9):1947–56.

# Rotator Cuff Tear Arthropathy

**2**

Kevin J. Cronin, Christopher D. Joyce,
and Joseph A. Abboud

## Introduction

Rotator cuff tear arthropathy is a specific pattern of shoulder pathology resulting from rotator cuff muscle insufficiency which leads to diminished acromiohumeral space, loss of joint congruence, and glenohumeral joint wear. The first-line treatment includes nonsurgical options to control symptoms, and surgical intervention is considered when nonoperative modalities fail.

1. **History (How to Ask Directed Questions)**
   (a) Prevalence
   - First described by Neer in 1983 and thought to be a rare phenomenon resulting from chronic rotator cuff insufficiency [1].
   - More common in females and elderly patients [2].
   - While the diagnosis of rotator cuff tear arthropathy (CTA) is becoming more frequent, the pathology and clinical presentation between patients can be extremely different. Thus, a detailed history and understanding of the patient's complaints and goals is extremely important in making treatment decisions.

K. J. Cronin (✉)
Rothman Institute at Thomas Jefferson University, Philadelphia, PA, USA

Florida Orthopaedic Institute, Tampa, FL, USA
e-mail: KCronin@floridaortho.com

C. D. Joyce
Department of Orthopaedics, University of Utah, Salt Late City, UT, USA

J. A. Abboud
Rothman Institute at Thomas Jefferson University, Philadelphia, PA, USA
e-mail: Joseph.Abboud@rothmanortho.com

© The Author(s), under exclusive license to Springer Nature Switzerland AG 2022
C. M. Chebli, A. M. Murthi (eds.), *The Resident's Guide to Shoulder and Elbow Surgery*, https://doi.org/10.1007/978-3-031-12255-2_2

- CTA is a chronic, degenerative condition beginning with tearing of the superior rotator cuff, followed by loss of cartilage and bony erosion. The rotator cuff provides a concavity-compression effect, stabilizing the humeral head within the glenoid. When this is lost, the humeral head migrates proximally. This proximal humeral migration leads to superior glenoid erosion and shortening of the deltoid. This shortening inhibits the deltoid's ability to function as a flexor and abductor of the shoulder. As disease progresses, the humeral head continues to migrate proximally and articulates with the acromion and coracoacromial arch. This leads to classic findings of "femoralization" of the humeral head and "acetabularization" of the acromion.

(b) What is the primary complaint?
  - Pain.
  - Loss of motion.
  - Weakness.
  - Inability to perform activities of daily living.
  - Understanding a patient's goals is necessary for determination of appropriate treatment. For example, a patient with end-stage radiographic findings may have minimal pain and preserved range of motion and thus is treated with conservative measures.

(c) What is the patient's baseline activity level?
  - Hand dominance
    – More commonly occurs in dominant arm [3].
    – Dysfunction in the dominant arm will be more noticeable and debilitating in most patients.
  - Ambulatory status
  - Medical comorbidities
  - Contralateral arm function
    – This is particularly important in upper extremity pathology and when considering possible surgical intervention. Profound dysfunction in the contralateral limb will make certain activities exceedingly difficult.
  - Goals
  - Age
  - Profession
  - Hobbies

(d) Characteristics of pain
  - Chronicity
    – Patients presenting with cuff tear arthropathy typically have symptoms for years and possibly decades.
    – Acute symptom onset may represent increasing rotator cuff tear size or an acute synovitis flare.
  - When is the pain the worst?
    – Nighttime (classic)
    – With certain activities (reaching away from body, behind the back)
  - What alleviates pain? By how much?
  - Radiation
  - Severity

(e) Prior treatments
- Oral medications
  - NSAIDS
  - Acetaminophen
- Physical therapy
- Injections
  - How many and how recent?
  - Effectiveness?
  - Corticosteroids vs. ketorolac.
  - Location of injection?
      It is important to attempt to identify the anatomic location of any prior injections. While the subacromial and glenohumeral spaces are likely confluent in rotator cuff tear arthropathy, the location of a prior injection may explain why it did or did not work.
- Surgery
  - Prior open or arthroscopic rotator cuff repairs.
  - Evaluate deltoid function.

2. **Physical Exam (Which Correlate to the Complaint)**
   (a) The one basic requirement in all cases of rotator cuff tear arthropathy is tear and insufficiency of the rotator cuff. The physical exam will typically be consistent with rotator cuff pathology. As the disease process accelerates, additional exam findings may become present as well.
   (b) As with all shoulder examinations, a detailed examination of the cervical spine must also be performed. This includes range of motion, palpation, strength, reflexes, and assessment for myelopathy or radiculopathy.
   (c) Inspection/palpation.
   - Large joint effusion is commonly present.
   - Extra-articular extravasation of synovial fluid may occur.
     - Subacromial space. Bogginess or fullness around the shoulder.
     - Geyser sign. Cyst formation in the superior shoulder soft tissue resulting from synovial fluid escape through the AC joint in the setting of underlying rotator cuff tear.
   - Atrophy of the supraspinatus and infraspinatus is common. Exam should include a detailed evaluation of the patient in a surgical gown or with shirt removed to assess for atrophic changes. Atrophy of the deltoid is also important to evaluate for especially if considering surgical intervention.
   - Long head biceps rupture common.
   - Palpation: Special attention should be given to palpating the acromion as advanced stage rotator cuff tear arthropathy may be associated with acromial insufficiency or fractures [4].
   (d) ROM.
   - Important to assess both active and passive range of motion.
   - ROM in all planes:
     - Forward elevation
     - Abduction
     - External rotation (arm at side and at 90° abduction)
     - Internal rotation (arm at side and at 90° abduction)

- Early in the disease process, prior to glenohumeral deformity, range of motion may be normal actively and passively. As rotator cuff tear size increases, loss of active motion with preserved passive motion is typical. However, as the glenohumeral joint begins to degrade secondary to chronic imbalance in the shoulder joint dynamics, loss of passive motion ensues.

   (e) Strength testing.
   - Individual rotator cuff muscle testing.
      - Supraspinatus: "Empty can test." Arm held in a forward elevated and abducted position with the thumb pointing towards the floor. Upward pressure from the patient against the examiner will elicit weakness and/or pain in supraspinatus tears.
      - Infraspinatus: External rotation with arm at the side.
      - Teres minor: Hornblower's sign. Inability to externally rotate the shoulder with the arm at 90° abduction causing the hand to drop.
      - Subscapularis: Lift off test, belly press test, and bear hug test all require active internal rotation of the arm in various positions and usually cannot be performed with a fully torn subscapularis.

   (f) Directed tests based on history or mechanism of injury.
   - Anterosuperior escape/pseudoparalytic shoulder.
   - Elevation of shoulder girdle to compensate for insufficient rotator cuff.
   - External rotation or internal rotation lag signs.

3. **Imaging**
   (a) X-rays:
   - Standard anteroposterior (AP).
   - True AP (Grashey).
   - Scapular Y (lateral).
   - Axillary.
   - Plain X-rays are the primary method of diagnosis and classification in rotator cuff tear arthropathy. While advanced imaging may be helpful for operative planning purposes, in most cases, several plain radiographic findings are indicative of cuff tear arthropathy.
      - Proximal humeral head migration (Fig. 2.1)

         Loss of force coupling in massive rotator cuff tears result in decentering of the humeral head. The deltoid pulls the humeral head proximally.

         Measured by the acromiohumeral interval. Measurement less than 7 mm is concerning for proximal head migration.

         Loss of integrity of Bani's line which is the arch formed by the medial proximal humerus and the lateral border of the scapula (Fig. 2.1).
      - Superior glenoid erosion

         Secondary to chronic proximal migration of the humeral head (Favard classification).

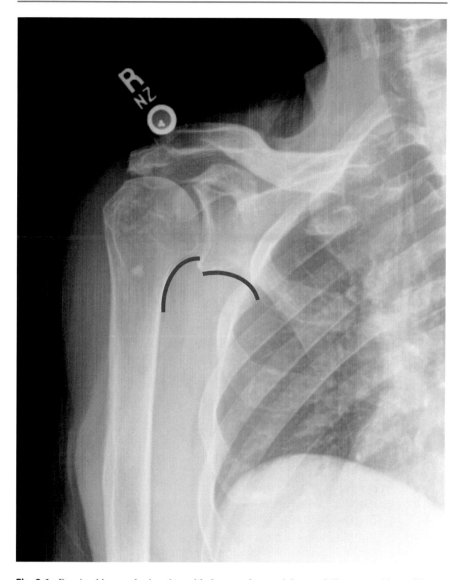

**Fig. 2.1** Proximal humeral migration with decreased acromiohumeral distance and loss of integrity of Bani's line

- Acromial changes
  Inferior acromial sclerosis (sourcil sign). Early finding, secondary to increased contact pressure from humeral head.
  Acromial acetabularization. Later finding, progressive thinning.
- Humeral head changes
  Early changes show femoralization.
  Late changes show humeral head destruction.

(b) Classifications
- Hamada [5] (Table 2.1)
- Seebauer [6] (Table 2.2)
- Favard [7] (Table 2.3)
  - Best for categorizing superior-inferior glenoid wear pattern
  - Particularly important in cuff tear arthropathy as chronic superior migration of the humeral head may result in superior glenoid wear

(c) MRI
- Can assess rotator cuff integrity in early cuff tear arthropathy cases.
- Assess for teres minor atrophy in massive tears with ER lag.
- If plain radiographic findings indicative of cuff tear arthropathy, MRI does not have much diagnostic utility.

(d) CT scan
- Useful for preoperative planning. Not typically required for diagnosis.
- Glenoid wear may be under-appreciated on plain radiographs. This is important to identify preoperatively as failure to do so may result in a higher risk of surgical failure.

**Table 2.1** Hamada classification. AHI, acromiohumeral interval; RCT, rotator cuff tear

| Grade | Acromion | Glenohumeral joint | Soft tissues |
|---|---|---|---|
| 1 | AHI ≥ 6 mm | No change | Massive RCT, biceps intact |
| 2 | AHI ≤ 5 mm | No change | Massive RCT, biceps torn |
| 3 | Acetabularization | No change | Massive RCT, biceps torn |
| 4 | Acetabularization | Narrowed joint space | Massive RCT, biceps torn |
| 5 | Acetabularization | Humeral head collapse | Massive RCT, biceps torn |

**Table 2.2** Seebauer classification

| | Type I | | Type II | |
|---|---|---|---|---|
| | A | B | A | B |
| Superior migration | No | No | Yes | Yes |
| Humeral head | Femoralization | Femoralization | Femoralization | Anterosuperior escape |
| Glenoid/ acromion | Acetabularization | Medial glenoid erosion | Superior wear | No CA arch stabilization |
| Soft tissue | Intact anterior restraints | Compromised GH stability | Incompetent anterior restraints | Incompetent anterior restraints |

**Table 2.3** Favard glenoid classification

| Type | Characteristic |
|---|---|
| E0 | No glenoid erosion. Superior humeral head migration only |
| E1 | Concentric glenoid erosion |
| E2 | Superior glenoid erosion, biconcavity. Neoglenoid and paleoglenoid |
| E3 | Superior glenoid erosion, monoconcavity. Neoglenoid only |
| E4 | Inferior glenoid erosion |

4. **Treatment Algorithm Based on Diagnosis**
   (a) Treatment should be individualized to each patient. When discussing treatment options, the surgeon should consider the patient's pathology, physiological age, preoperative function, hand dominance, hobbies, function, and goals.
   (b) **Nonoperative treatment**
   - The first-line treatment for rotator cuff tear arthropathy consists of nonoperative modalities.
   - Symptoms usually consist of either pain, loss of function, or both. Understanding the difference between these two will help to guide treatment options.
   - Pain can be treated with over-the-counter nonsteroidal anti-inflammatory drugs (NSAIDs) [8]. Patients should be counseled on the risks of taking these medications long term including, but not limited to, gastric ulcers, renal dysfunction, and elevations in blood pressure. These medications are not benign. Narcotic pain medications should be avoided.
   - Disuse secondary to pain can result in stiffness of the glenohumeral joint along with weakness of the deltoid. Shoulder mechanics can often be enhanced with a home program of gentle range of motion and strengthening exercises. We recommend the deltoid strengthening program popularized by Levy and the Reading Shoulder Unit [9].
   - Subacromial corticosteroid injections can also be used for pain relief. These should be used sparingly due to their known effect on tissue quality and risk of infection if future surgery is considered [10]. The risk of infection is rare but does occur [11]. Diabetic patients should also be counseled regarding the potential transient elevation in blood glucose levels after the injection.
   - NSAIDs and corticosteroid injections are helpful for temporarily relieving pain associated with rotator cuff tear arthropathy [8]. They will not improve range of motion or function, unless the decreased function is solely limited by pain.
   (c) **Operative treatment**
   - Operative treatment options may be considered when a patient has failed nonoperative modalities and continues to have significant interference with activities of daily living and quality of life.
   - **Surgical options**
     - **Arthroscopic debridement.** Arthroscopic debridement plays a limited role in cuff tear arthropathy. Potential pathology that can be addressed arthroscopically include removal of loose bodies, capsular release, or limited microfracture [12]. While beneficial results have been reported in the literature, the indications for intervention and procedures performed vary greatly, making it difficult to appropriately evaluate the literature [13]. A systematic review found insufficient evidence to support the routine use of arthroscopic debridement [14]. If performing arthroscopic debridement for cuff tear arthropathy, it is crucial to preserve the integrity of the coracoacromial ligament.

- **Hemiarthroplasty.** Historically, hemiarthroplasty was the treatment of choice for the rotator cuff deficient shoulder [15]. It can be used for pain relief and limited restoration of function. In the rotator cuff deficient patient, the hemiarthroplasty relies on the preserved coracoacromial arch and the anterior deltoid [16]. The indications for this continue to decline with the advent of improved treatment options.
- **Cuff tear arthropathy prosthesis.** The CTA prosthesis has an extended humeral head surface which fits within the coracoacromial arch and allows for articulation of the lateral aspect of the humeral head against the acromion [8]. This can be considered in patients with retained active motion and preserved integrity of the coracoacromial arch [17]. Benefits include preservation of glenoid bone stock.
- **Reverse shoulder arthroplasty.** Reverse shoulder arthroplasty (RSA) is the mainstay of treatment for rotator cuff arthropathy in the older individual. To compensate for a lack of rotator cuff, RSA lengthens the lever arm of the deltoid and increases its abduction power. The design of the prosthesis also prevents superior migration and instability seen with anatomic shoulder arthroplasty or hemiarthroplasty [8]. Significant improvements in both function and pain relief are seen in the appropriately selected patients [18, 19].
- **Surgical approaches**
  - **Deltopectoral approach.** The deltopectoral approach is the workhorse of the shoulder and familiar to many shoulder surgeons. It allows access to the glenohumeral joint and is extensile both proximal and distal [20]. The approach utilizes the internervous plane between the pectoralis major (medial and lateral pectoral nerves) and the deltoid (axillary nerve). This interval is commonly marked by the cephalic vein, which should be protected [21].
  - **Superior approach.** The glenohumeral joint can also be accessed by splitting the deltoid laterally, most commonly between the anterior and middle heads. The advantage of this approach is the direct visualization of the glenoid during arthroplasty as well as limited retraction on the anterior head of the deltoid compared with the deltopectoral approach [21]. Disadvantages include decreased exposure of the humerus and risk to the axillary nerve [22].
- **Risks and complications**
  - Complications and failure of surgical treatment for rotator cuff arthropathy, most notably reverse shoulder arthroplasty, are not uncommon. While the procedure generally results in acceptable functional outcomes and pain relief, complications do occur. In long-term studies, the 10-year survival rate was shown to be 93% [19].

    **Instability.** Instability can be seen after RSA, most commonly due to inappropriate soft tissue tensioning or component malposition [23]. Treatment can include attempted closed reduction or, with recurrent instability, revision arthroplasty [24].

**Infection.** Infection can be a devastating complication after shoulder arthroplasty. Given the low virulence organisms typically implicated in infected shoulder arthroplasty, such as *Cutibacterium acnes*, diagnosis can prove difficult [24]. Treatment options include irrigation and debridement, modular component exchange, single-stage revision, two-stage revision, antibiotic spacer, or resection arthroplasty [25].

**Fracture.** Fracture can occur both intraoperatively or postoperatively during reverse shoulder arthroplasty. If components are stable, they can generally be treated nonoperatively [24]. Any instability or loose components should be treated with open reduction internal fixation or reverse arthroplasty [26].

**Nerve injury.** There are multiple nerves at risk during RSA, most notably the axillary and musculocutaneous nerves [21]. The axillary nerve should be identified and protected throughout the procedure. The musculocutaneous nerve is less often directly encountered during primary procedures. Additionally, distalizing the humerus during component placement may put the brachial plexus on stretch [27].

**Acromial and scapular spine stress fracture.** Acromial and scapular spine stress fractures are a complication unique to RSA. They occur at a rate of 1–4% and can lead to significant pain and dysfunction if they lead to non-union. Consensus regarding the potential risk factors and optimal treatment is lacking [28].

**Scapular notching.** Scapular notching is unique to RSA and risk factors include humeral medialization and positioning the glenoid baseplate too high on the glenoid. This phenomenon occurs due to impingement of the polyethylene tray against the inferior glenoid neck leading to inferior glenoid bone loss and asymmetric polyethylene wear. While once controversial, recent data supports worse functional outcomes and early glenoid loosening in those with significant scapular notching [29].

## References

1. Neer CS II, Craig EV, Fukuda H. Cuff-tear arthropathy. J Bone Joint Surg Am. 1983;65(9):1232–44.
2. Zeman CA, Arcand MA, Cantrell JS, Skedros JG, Burkhead WZ Jr. The rotator cuff-deficient arthritic shoulder: diagnosis and surgical management. J Am Acad Orthop Surg. 1998;6(6):337–48.
3. Jensen KL, Williams GR Jr, Russell IJ, Rockwood CA Jr. Rotator cuff tear arthropathy. J Bone Joint Surg Am. 1999;81(9):1312–24.
4. Dennis DA, Ferlic DC, Clayton ML. Acromial stress fractures associated with cuff-tear arthropathy. A report of three cases. J Bone Joint Surg Am. 1986;68(6):937–40.

5. Hamada K, Fukuda H, Mikasa M, Kobayashi Y. Roentgenographic findings in massive rotator cuff tears. A long-term observation. Clin Orthop Relat Res. 1990;254:92–6.

6. Visotsky JL, Basamania C, Seebauer L, Rockwood CA, Jensen KL. Cuff tear arthropathy: pathogenesis, classification, and algorithm for treatment. J Bone Joint Surg Am. 2004;86-A(Suppl 2):35–40.

7. Sirveaux F, Favard L, Oudet D, Huquet D, Walch G, Mole D. Grammont inverted total shoulder arthroplasty in the treatment of glenohumeral osteoarthritis with massive rupture of the cuff. Results of a multicentre study of 80 shoulders. J Bone Joint Surg (Br). 2004;86(3):388–95.

8. Ecklund KJ, Lee TQ, Tibone J, Gupta R. Rotator cuff tear arthropathy. J Am Acad Orthop Surg. 2007;15(6):340–9.

9. Levy O, Mullett H, Roberts S, Copeland S. The role of anterior deltoid reeducation in patients with massive irreparable degenerative rotator cuff tears. J Shoulder Elb Surg. 2008;17(6):863–70.

10. Izquierdo R, Voloshin I, Edwards S, Freehill MQ, Stanwood W, Wiater JM, et al. Treatment of glenohumeral osteoarthritis. J Am Acad Orthop Surg. 2010;18(6):375–82.

11. Rhee YG, Cho NS, Kim BH, Ha JH. Injection-induced pyogenic arthritis of the shoulder joint. J Shoulder Elb Surg. 2008;17(1):63–7.

12. Millett PJ, Fritz EM, Frangiamore SJ, Mannava S. Arthroscopic management of glenohumeral arthritis: a joint preservation approach. J Am Acad Orthop Surg. 2018;26(21):745–52.

13. Williams BT, Beletsky A, Kunze KN, Polce EM, Cole BJ, Verma NN, et al. Outcomes and survivorship after arthroscopic treatment of glenohumeral arthritis: a systematic review. Arthroscopy. 2020;36(7):2010–21.

14. Namdari S, Skelley N, Keener JD, Galatz LM, Yamaguchi K. What is the role of arthroscopic debridement for glenohumeral arthritis? A critical examination of the literature. Arthroscopy. 2013;29(8):1392–8.

15. Williams GR Jr, Rockwood CA Jr. Hemiarthroplasty in rotator cuff-deficient shoulders. J Shoulder Elb Surg. 1996;5(5):362–7.

16. Keener JD, Chalmers PN, Yamaguchi K. The humeral implant in shoulder arthroplasty. J Am Acad Orthop Surg. 2017;25(6):427–38.

17. Matsen FA III, Somerson JS, Hsu JE, Lippitt SB, Russ SM, Neradilek MB. Clinical effectiveness and safety of the extended humeral head arthroplasty for selected patients with rotator cuff tear arthropathy. J Shoulder Elb Surg. 2019;28(3):483–95.

18. Poondla RK, Sheth MM, Heldt BL, Laughlin MS, Morris BJ, Elkousy HA, et al. Anatomic and reverse shoulder arthroplasty in patients 70 years of age and older: a comparison cohort at early to mid-term follow up. J Shoulder Elb Surg. 2021;30:1336.

19. Bacle G, Nove-Josserand L, Garaud P, Walch G. Long-term outcomes of reverse total shoulder arthroplasty: a follow-up of a previous study. J Bone Joint Surg Am. 2017;99(6):454–61.

20. Bohsali KI, Bois AJ, Wirth MA. Fractures of the proximal humerus. In: Rockwood CA, Matsen FA, Wirth MA, Lippitt SB, Fehringer EV, Sperling JW, editors. Rockwood and Matsen's the shoulder. Philadelphia, PA: Elsevier; 2018.

21. Chalmers PN, Van Thiel GS, Trenhaile SW. Surgical exposures of the shoulder. J Am Acad Orthop Surg. 2016;24(4):250–8.

22. Gupta R, Patel NA, Mazzocca AD, Romeo A. Understanding and treating iatrogenic nerve injuries in shoulder surgery. J Am Acad Orthop Surg. 2020;28(5):e185–e92.

23. Kohan EM, Chalmers PN, Salazar D, Keener JD, Yamaguchi K, Chamberlain AM. Dislocation following reverse total shoulder arthroplasty. J Shoulder Elb Surg. 2017;26(7):1238–45.

24. Chalmers PN, Boileau P, Romeo AA, Tashjian RZ. Revision reverse shoulder arthroplasty. J Am Acad Orthop Surg. 2019;27(12):426–36.

25. Cronin KJ, Hayes CB, Sajadi KR. Antibiotic cement spacer retention for chronic shoulder infection after minimum 2-year follow-up. J Shoulder Elb Surg. 2020;29(9):e325–e9.

26. Brusalis CM, Taylor SA. Periprosthetic fractures in reverse total shoulder arthroplasty: current concepts and advances in management. Curr Rev Musculoskelet Med. 2020;13(4):509–19.

27. Kim HJ, Kwon TY, Jeon YS, Kang SG, Rhee YG, Rhee SM. Neurologic deficit after reverse total shoulder arthroplasty: correlation with distalization. J Shoulder Elb Surg. 2020;29(6):1096–103.
28. Routman HD, Simovitch RW, Wright TW, Flurin PH, Zuckerman JD, Roche CP. Acromial and scapular fractures after reverse total shoulder arthroplasty with a medialized glenoid and lateralized humeral implant: an analysis of outcomes and risk factors. J Bone Joint Surg Am. 2020;102(19):1724–33.
29. Friedman RJ, Barcel DA, Eichinger JK. Scapular notching in reverse total shoulder arthroplasty. J Am Acad Orthop Surg. 2019;27(6):200–9.

# Inflammatory Arthritis

# 3

Ian D. Engler and Andrew Jawa

## Introduction

- Inflammatory arthritis of the shoulder and elbow encompasses a number of diagnoses and presents different challenges than the more common osteoarthritis, owing to systemic illness alongside greater joint and soft tissue destruction.
- Rheumatoid arthritis (RA) is the most frequent inflammatory arthritis managed by orthopedic surgeons and will be the primary focus of this chapter.
- Historically, inflammatory arthritis was very commonly seen by the upper extremity surgeon. Since the drastic improvement in medical management of autoimmune disorders in recent decades, the severity of disease has greatly decreased, leading to many fewer surgical candidates.

1. History
   (a) Inflammatory arthritis encompasses multiple different diagnoses, each of which are autoimmune disorders and systemic illnesses. Therefore, the entirety of the patient much be considered, not just the joint of interest.
      - Underlying diagnoses associated with inflammatory arthritis:
         – Rheumatoid arthritis
            Primarily upper extremity involvement, polyarticular [1].

I. D. Engler (✉)
Department of Orthopaedic Surgery, Tufts Medical Center, Boston, MA, USA

Central Maine Healthcare Orthopedics, Central Maine Medical Center, Lewiston, USA

A. Jawa
Department of Orthopaedic Surgery, Tufts Medical Center, Boston, MA, USA

Harvard Shoulder and Elbow Fellowship, Boston Sports and Shoulder Center, New England Baptist Hospital, Tufts Medical School, Boston, MA, USA
e-mail: ajawa@nebh.org

Historically, 55% of RA patients develop erosion of the glenohumeral joint, of whom 73% have bilateral disease and almost 50% have severe erosion [2].

Historically, 20–50% of RA patients develop elbow involvement, generally within 5 years of onset of disease. When the elbow is involved, 90% also have hand/wrist involvement, and 80% also have shoulder involvement [3]. The contralateral elbow is commonly involved [4].

- Psoriatic arthritis

  Initially oligoarticular and mild disease, but severe and disabling in 20% of patients [5]. In 20% of patients with psoriasis [6]. More asymmetric than RA.

- Crystalline arthropathies: Gout, pseudogout (i.e., calcium pyrophosphate crystal deposition [CPPD])

- Others: Reactive arthritis (post-infectious), inflammatory bowel disease arthritis, lupus, ankylosing spondylitis, Lyme disease

  Less common; more often managed by a rheumatologist than an orthopedic surgeon; more often lower extremity involvement

(b) Pathology of inflammatory arthritis: The synovitic reaction is often much more pronounced than in osteoarthritis. This leads to increased pain, stiffness (in part from the patient immobilizing the joint to prevent pain), and tissue destruction. Beyond cartilage damage, the disease can compromise bone, joint capsule, ligaments, and tendons.

(c) Patients may present with a known diagnosis of inflammatory arthritis. For those who do not have a known diagnosis, the orthopedic surgeon must be on the lookout for the below signs and symptoms of inflammatory arthritis to differentiate it from the much more common osteoarthritis.

(d) Joint-specific questions to ask:

- Do you have pain, swelling, redness, or stiffness? Evaluate exact location, duration, exacerbating and alleviating factors.

- How impairing are your symptoms? Are you most limited by pain, stiffness, weakness, or otherwise? This can help guide treatment options.

- What treatment(s) to the joint have you had in the past?

(e) Systemic questions to ask:

- Do you have a known diagnosis of inflammatory arthritis? If so, elucidate the manifestations and treatment to date.

  - Any family history of inflammatory arthritis or autoimmune diseases?

- How long have you had symptoms? Duration is important in severity and progression of the disease.

- What symptoms do you have outside of your shoulder/elbow? These include fevers/chills, pain/swelling/redness/stiffness of other joints, and the below symptoms more specific to individual diseases:

  - Any recent infection or symptoms thereof (e.g., dysuria in a urinary tract infection, cough/wheezing/sore throat in an upper respiratory illness)? Seen in reactive arthritis.

  - Any recent tick bite or bulls eye rash? Seen in Lyme arthritis.

  - Any psoriasis (silver flaking skin, especially on extensor surfaces)? Seen in psoriatic arthritis.

- Any abdominal pain, diarrhea, or blood/mucus in the stool? Seen in inflammatory bowel disease arthritis.
- Any back pain, heel pain, tendinopathy, or eye irritation (uveitis)? Seen in spondyloarthritis.
- Any Raynaud symptoms in the fingers, alopecia, cutaneous eruptions, or mucosal ulcers? Seen in systemic rheumatic diseases such as lupus.

2. Physical Exam
   (a) Though a detailed physical exam of the joint in question is vital, the physician must examine more broadly to evaluate for manifestations of systemic disease. These include:
   - Other joints (including spine)—pain, swelling, redness, stiffness
     - Key to evaluate the entire ipsilateral extremity given the frequent concomitant pathology in adjacent joints and the fact that adjacent joints help compensate for limitation in the joint of interest
   - Skin findings—rashes (e.g., erythema migrans of Lyme, butterfly rash of lupus), psoriasis, nail lesions
   (b) Inspection/palpation
   - Evaluate for joint swelling and redness, pain with palpation or range of motion, skin findings or masses around the joint (rashes as above, rheumatoid nodules, gouty tophi), quality of the skin
   (c) Range of motion
   - Evaluate full active and passive ROM of the joint in each plane of motion to assess stiffness. Stiffness is common in inflammatory arthritis given the degree of inflammation and subsequent scar tissue formation in and around the joint.
   (d) Strength testing
   - Evaluate strength in each plane of motion of the joint. Be sure to differentiate weakness from pain limiting the motion, in part by asking the patient for their limiting factor. Pain is more often the limiting factor in inflammatory arthritis.

3. Imaging
   (a) Imaging can help differentiate inflammatory arthritis from osteoarthritis based on the inflammatory response and level of erosions of the joint and soft tissues. This is truer and more present in advanced disease. Imaging may aid in diagnosis, complete assessment of pathology, and treatment planning.
   (b) X-rays: Standard shoulder and/or elbow series are obtained at the first visit and at intervals of several months thereafter. These may show wide-ranging degrees of bony changes, ranging from bone erosion (most common; in more advanced disease; a hallmark of RA) to osteophytes (most common in ankylosing spondylitis) or a combination (notably in psoriatic arthritis).
   - Four radiographic signs of arthritis: Joint space narrowing, marginal osteophytes, subchondral cysts, subchondral sclerosis
     - Subchondral sclerosis is less common in inflammatory arthritis than it is in osteoarthritis.
   - Larsen Grading Scale of rheumatoid joints [7] (Fig. 3.1)
     - Grade 0: No radiographic abnormalities
     - Grade I: Slight joint space narrowing, soft tissue swelling, periarticular osteoporosis

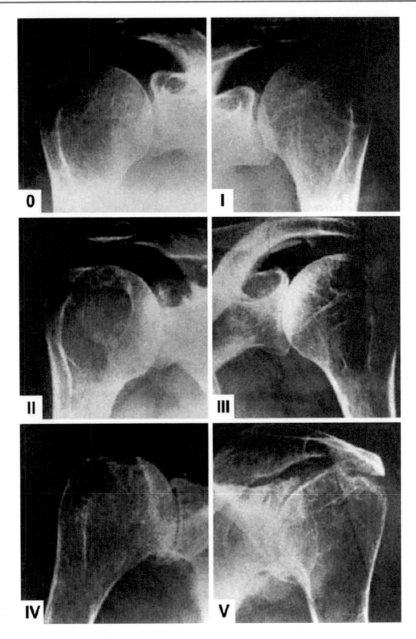

**Fig. 3.1** Larsen classification of the rheumatoid shoulder. Grade 0: No radiographic abnormalities. Grade I: Slight joint space narrowing, soft tissue swelling, periarticular osteoporosis. Grade II: One or more small erosions (diameter <1 mm). Grade III: Medium destruction, marked erosions. Grade IV: Severe abnormality and erosions, minimal joint space, original bony outlines partly preserved. Grade V: Mutilating changes, destruction of original bony outlines. (Reproduced from Thomas et al. The rheumatoid shoulder: current consensus on diagnosis and treatment. Joint Bone Spine 2006; 73(2):139–143. © Elsevier Masson SAS. All rights reserved)

- – Grade II: One or more small erosions (diameter <1 mm)
- – Grade III: Medium destruction, marked erosions
- – Grade IV: Severe abnormality and erosions, minimal joint space, original bony outlines partly preserved
- – Grade V: Mutilating changes, destruction of original bony outlines
- Mayo Clinic classification of the rheumatoid elbow [8]
  - – Grade I: No radiographic abnormalities except periarticular osteopenia with soft tissue swelling
  - – Grade II: Mild to moderate joint space narrowing, minimal or no architectural distortion
  - – Grade III: Variable joint space narrowing with or without subchondral cysts, architectural alteration (e.g., thinning of olecranon, resorption of trochlea)
    - IIIA (bone loss of one humeral column) vs. IIIB (both columns)
  - – Grade IV: Extensive articular damage, loss of subchondral bone, subluxation or ankylosis of joint
- Walch classification of glenoid erosion [9]
  - – A: Centered humeral head, central wear
    - A1: Minor erosion
    - A2: Major erosion
    - (i)  Common in RA when the rotator cuff remains intact
  - – B: Posteriorly subluxated head, posterior wear
    - B1: No erosion
    - B2: Posterior erosion, biconcavity
    - B3: Posterior erosion, monoconcavity (>15° retroversion)
  - – C: Dysplastic, >25° retroversion
  - – D: Anteriorly subluxated head, glenoid anteversion
- Favard classification of superior glenoid wear [10]
  - – E0: Superior humeral migration without glenoid erosion
  - – E1: Concentric erosion of the glenoid
  - – E2: Superior glenoid erosion
    - Common in RA due to inflammatory destruction of the rotator cuff and subsequent superior migration of the humeral head
  - – E3: Glenoid erosion extends to the inferior aspect of the glenoid
- (c) CT scan: Useful given erosion and subsequent bone loss from the inflammatory process. Can demonstrate the bony stability of a joint, the bone stock available for surgical intervention (i.e., shoulder or elbow arthroplasty), and loose bodies.
- (d) MRI: Particularly helpful in inflammatory arthritis given the frequent soft tissue destruction (e.g., cartilage, joint capsule, ligaments, and tendons) by the inflammatory process. Unlike osteoarthritis, which is confined to the bone and cartilage, periarticular soft tissues are often damaged in inflammatory arthritis.
- (e) Ultrasound: Can be used to assess for ligament and tendon compromise given the soft tissue damage in inflammatory arthritis, though it is less commonly used than MRI.

4. Treatment
    (a) Nonoperative treatment:
        • Medical management: The mainstay of treatment of inflammatory arthritis of all severities. Medical management has the ability to address all involved joints and organs and suppress the disease, limiting symptoms and ongoing joint destruction. Without adequate medical management, surgical options should not be considered because they will be at increased risk of failure.
            – Close relationship with rheumatology is important.
            – Early diagnosis and initiation of treatment is key to minimize joint destruction.
            – Common medications:
                Disease-modifying anti-inflammatory drugs (DMARDs): Methotrexate (MTX), sulfasalazine, hydroxychloroquine, leflunomide
                Common anti-inflammatories: Non-steroidal anti-inflammatory drugs (NSAIDs), glucocorticoids
                Biologic agents (often TNF-alpha antagonists): Etanercept, adalimumab, infliximab, anakinra (IL-1 antagonist), rituximab
        • Physical therapy: Allows patients to keep or regain range of motion and strength despite joint inflammation. Focus on pain-relieving strategies, such as heat/ice, avoiding painful activities, and rest.
            – Bracing: Hinged elbow braces can provide structural support, especially in the setting of medial and lateral ligament compromise. Dynamic splints can increase range of motion in the setting of contracture.
        • Glucocorticoid injection: Targeted means to reduce intra-articular or subacromial inflammation. They are a key nonoperative treatment modality that have been shown to reduce pain and inflammation in the affected joint.
            – Indications: Moderate disease, symptoms unrelieved by above measures, not yet a candidate for surgery.
            – Judicious use is important given the risk of infection and soft tissue damage from multiple injections over time.
            – Betamethasone injections in early RA patients (alongside the initiation of DMARD treatment): No relapse in 62% of joints at 1 year and 56% at 2 years (50% of shoulders and 50% of elbows at 2 years) [11].
        • Biologics injections: Less routine and performed by rheumatologist, but good outcomes.
            – RCT of corticosteroid injections vs. TNF-alpha inhibitor: Significant 20% increase in efficacy of biologics over corticosteroids through 24 weeks [12].
        • Crystalline arthropathies (gout and pseudogout): Generally successfully treated with medical management.
            – Acute flare: NSAIDs, corticosteroids, colchicine.

> If poor response, intraarticular steroid injection or less commonly surgical irrigation and debridement may be considered.

– Chronic prevention: Allopurinol (gout), colchicine or NSAIDs (pseudogout)

> In the rare case of joint destruction, operative management may be pursued similar to the management of RA.

(b) Operative treatment—factors to consider:

- In these commonly polyarticular diseases, the most symptomatic joints should be addressed first. If the shoulder and elbow are equivalent, Neer argues to operate on the shoulder first [13] (a pain-free mobile shoulder can reduce stress on the elbow), though other authors argue to choose the elbow first (finding greater functional improvement of the upper limb with doing so) [14].
- Stopping anti-inflammatory medication prior to surgery: This is an important consideration in this population. See Table 3.1 for details.
- In the setting of RA, surgeons should always order preoperative flexion-extension cervical spine X-rays to evaluate for instability from cervical rheumatoid spondylitis, which includes atlantoaxial subluxation, cranial settling (or basilar invagination), and subaxial subluxation. Any instability must be more closely evaluated, and fusion may be indicated. Undiagnosed instability can cause neurologic damage in the perioperative period due to manipulation of the cervical spine. Up to 61% of RA patients screened preoperatively have been found to have radiographic evidence of cervical instability [17].
- Rheumatoid arthritis is by far the most common diagnosis among the inflammatory arthropathies treated by orthopedic surgeons and will be discussed below. Other arthritides may warrant surgical intervention if the joint destruction is severe enough, using an algorithm similar to that described below, but more frequently they are managed with medical intervention by a rheumatologist.

**Table 3.1** When to stop anti-inflammatory medication prior to surgery. (DMARDs = Disease-modifying anti-inflammatory drugs. NSAIDs = non-steroidal anti-inflammatory drugs.) [15, 16]

| Medication class | Medication(s) within class | When to stop before surgery |
|---|---|---|
| DMARDs | Methotrexate, sulfasalazine, hydroxychloroquine, and leflunomide | May continue through surgery |
| NSAIDs | Ibuprofen, naproxen, piroxicam | 5 half-lives before surgery depending on bleeding risk |
| Steroids | Prednisone | Varies based on dose and the stress of surgery |
| Biologics | Etanercept, adalimumab, infliximab, anakinra (IL-1 antagonist), rituximab | Minor procedures: May continue through surgery |
| | | Major procedures: Schedule surgery for the end of the dosing cycle (except etanercept, which should be stopped 2 weeks before surgery). Resume 2 weeks after surgery |

(c) Operative treatment—shoulder:
- • Early-to-mid-stage inflammatory arthritis
    - – Arthroscopic shoulder debridement
        Purpose: Allows for synovectomy, removal of loose bodies, sub-acromial bursal debridement, acromioplasty, intra-articular debridement, capsular release
        Indications: Failure of nonoperative management, younger patients in whom arthroplasty is not preferred, milder disease, contractures
        Outcomes:
        Synovectomy: At mean 5.5 years post-op, reliable pain relief with less effect on ROM, with 19% unsatisfactory results. Consistent radiographic progression of disease [18].
        Subacromial debridement combined with other procedures as needed: At mean 2 years, 82% of patients were satisfied. Worse outcomes with advanced glenohumeral chondral damage [19].
        Capsular release: At 5 years post-op, active flexion improved from 69° to 126°, and ER improved from 1° to 32°. There was greater improvement with less severe disease [20].
- • End-stage inflammatory arthritis
    - – Shoulder arthroplasty
        Purpose: Arthroplasty is a proven technique to decrease pain and increase function in the setting of inflammatory arthritis.
        Indications: Failure of nonoperative management, severe disease and functional limitation.
        Contraindications: Very high activity level, poor patient compliance, young patient (relative).
        Approach: deltopectoral.
        Risks: Infection, dislocation, axillary nerve injury, aseptic loosening, fracture.
        Pre-op planning: Must consider the challenges of deficient rotator cuff, glenoid bone deficiency, internal rotation deformity.
        Deficient rotator cuff:
        Full thickness tear in 19–47% of RA patients at the time of arthroplasty [21].
        Rotator cuff compromise and upward migration of the humeral head is inevitable in the rheumatoid shoulder; generally occurs between Larsen grades 3 and 4 [22].
        Glenoid bone deficiency: Erosions may necessitate the use of an augmented baseplate or allograft to achieve adequate fixation and version.
    - – Anatomic total shoulder arthroplasty (TSA)
        Indications: Intact rotator cuff
        Limited due to frequent rotator cuff pathology
        Commonly performed in the 1980s prior to the Grammont prosthesis
        Outcomes:
        Survival: 97% at 5 years, 97% at 10 years, 89% at 20 years [23]

Reoperation: 3–36% [23, 24]

Patient-reported outcomes (PROs): At 8 years, good pain relief in 90% [25]

TSA better than hemiarthroplasty when rotator cuff intact (improved pain/abduction, lower risk of revision) [24]

ROM: At 8 years, increase in forward elevation from 44° to 75° [25]

Proximal humeral head migration: At 8 years, 55% (rTSA was not an option) [25]

Radiographic lucencies: 50–80% of cemented glenoids [24, 25], 32% of humeri at 12 years [24]

Glenoid loosening: 30–50% [25]

Can revise to hemiarthroplasty if loose glenoid

Glenohumeral subluxation: At 12 years, 82% [24]

- Reverse total shoulder arthroplasty (rTSA) (Fig. 3.2)

Purpose: Design allows for a deficient rotator cuff (commonly compromised in inflammatory arthropathy)

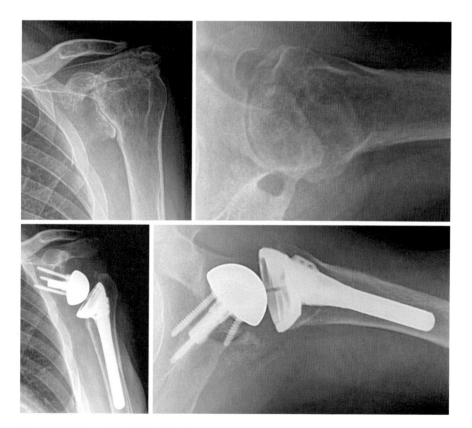

**Fig. 3.2** Radiographs of the left shoulder of a 55-year-old man with rheumatoid arthritis. Preoperative radiographs show a Favard E2 glenoid. Postoperative radiographs show a reverse total shoulder arthroplasty with a superiorly augmented baseplate due to the superior glenoid erosion

Indications: Deficient rotator cuff

Outcomes:

Survival: 5-year revision-free survival of 99% and operation-free survival of 97% [26]

Reoperation: 9% at mean 4 years [27], 9.1% at 4.5 years [28], 14% at 1 year [21]

PROs: 92% satisfaction, decreased pain [26]. ASES scores from 28 pre-op to 82 at 3 years post-op, VAS pain from 7 to 1 [21]

Worse outcomes with more advanced disease

ROM: Substantial increase, elevation increased from 52° pre-op to 126° [21]

Aseptic glenoid loosening: 0% at mean 4 years, [27] 5% at mean 3 years, [21] 25% with severe RA and rotator cuff tear [29]

Notching: 0% at mean 3 years, [21] 35% at mean 4.5 years, [28] 52% at mean 4 years [27]

Infection: 9.5–25% [21, 29, 30]

Vs 1–3% of rTSA in the general population [21]

(d) Operative treatment—elbow

• Early-to-mid-stage arthritis

– Elbow arthroscopy

Purpose: Allows for debridement, synovectomy, removal of loose bodies, excision of osteophytes, and contracture release. Allows greater visualization of the entire joint than an open procedure.

Indications: Pain and/or stiffness refractory to nonoperative management in the setting of mild chondral damage or less on X-ray or MRI (Mayo grades 1 and 2), loose bodies, symptomatic osteophytes, contractures, younger patients with severe chondral damage in whom arthroplasty is not preferred.

Contraindications: Moderate or severe chondral damage (Mayo grade 3).

Though can consider if not a candidate for arthroplasty (just shown to have worse outcomes with more advanced disease).

Approach: Standard, but be very cautious of nerves given deformity.

Risks: Significantly increased risk of transient nerve palsy compared to elbow arthroscopy for osteoarthritis (likely due to greater contractures, deformity, and capsular thinning), increased risk of infection.

Nerve palsy: 9.3% in RA elbow arthroscopy vs. 0.8% in non-RA elbow arthroscopy [31].

Infection: Inflammatory arthritis has an odds ratio of 2.81 for infection in elbow arthroscopy [32].

Outcomes: Good in milder disease, worse with more chondral damage.

PROs: Increased Mayo elbow performance score from 48 pre-op to 78 at 2 years and 70 at mean of 9 years [33].

24% had clinically apparent recurrent synovitis.

Conversion to TEA: 10% at mean 9 years [33].

Pre-op planning:

In contracture, evaluate whether there is a soft endpoint (consistent with soft tissue etiology, necessitating capsular release) or firm endpoint (consistent with osseous etiology, necessitating resection of osteophytes or radial head).

If articular deformity limits rotation, and the medial collateral ligament is intact, radial head excision may be indicated. This has somewhat fallen out of favor due to the risk of instability; see below.

Test the elbow in varus and valgus to evaluate stability of the collateral ligaments given the possibility of ligament attenuation.

- Late-stage arthritis.
  - Open synovectomy ± radial head excision

    Purpose: Decrease pain, may increase forearm rotation and decrease impingement with the capitellum

    Indication: Arthroscopy deemed to be too difficult given pathology or surgeon comfort; radial head impingement (for excision)

    More common historically, less common with the rise of elbow arthroscopy given improved visualization with arthroscopy

    Contraindication to radial head excision: Elbow instability

    Approach:

    Lateral: Most commonly used, allows visualization of most synovium (except olecranon fossa and medial recess)

    Kaplan (ECRB-EDC), EDC split, Kocher (ECU-anconeus)

    Posterior: Allows for later arthroplasty through same incision, more morbid so rarely used unless TEA is planned

    Bryan-Morrey (posterior, triceps-reflecting)

    Risk: Subsequent valgus instability, more difficult later arthroplasty

    Alternatively may reshape the radial head to prevent this risk

    Radial head arthroplasty has shown poor outcomes with silicone implants but not been studied with a metal implant.

    Outcomes: Documented improved outcomes in multiple studies, though effect wanes over time [4]

  - Total elbow arthroplasty (TEA) (Fig. 3.3)

    Purpose: Remove cartilage and deformed bone to decrease associated pain and stiffness

    Indications: Failure of prior less invasive procedures, end-stage chondral damage, older age (preferably 65 years and older), low activity level

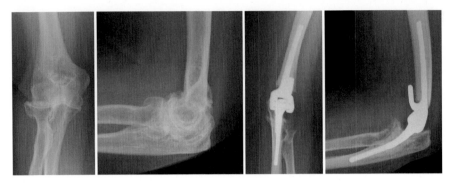

**Fig. 3.3** Radiographs of the left elbow of a 39-year-old woman with rheumatoid arthritis. Preoperative and postoperative radiographs following semiconstrained total elbow arthroplasty

Contraindications: Young patient, mild-moderate chondral damage, massive bone loss, high activity level (postop 5 lb lifting restriction for life)

Nonconstrained design: contraindicated given risk of instability (especially medially)

Approach: Posterior

Bryan-Morrey: Triceps reflected laterally off ulna

Triceps splitting

Risks: Ulnar nerve injury, instability (especially with unconstrained implants), aseptic loosening (especially with constrained implants), infection, triceps weakness, bushing wear (more often a radiographic issue than a clinical one)

Outcomes:

PROs: Post-op Mayo elbow performance scores of 87–94 [34]

Semiconstrained in RA:

Survival: 97% at 5 years, 85–92% at 10 years, 83% at 15 years, 68% at 20 years [35, 36]

PROs: 86% good or excellent results at minimum 10 years post-op [35] and 90% at mean 7 years post-op [36]

Semiconstrained in more advanced RA:

Survival: 80% at 5 years in the primary group and 58% in the revision group [34]; 92% at 10 years, 83% at 15 years, 68% at 20 years [37]

PROs: Excellent pain relief and good functional return [34]

Nonconstrained:

Instability: 7–19% [38]

– Soft tissue interposition arthroplasty

Indications: Young patients wanting to avoid TEA, salvage procedure after infection, irretrievable prosthesis

Outcomes: Improved pain, relatively high patient satisfaction, worse functional outcomes than TEA, often extensive subsequent bone loss [39, 40]

## References

1. Smolen JS. Undifferentiated early inflammatory arthritis in adults. UpToDate. 2018;
2. Lehtinen JT, Kaarela K, Belt EA, Kautiainen HJ, Kauppi MJ, Lehto M. Incidence of glenohumeral joint involvement in seropositive rheumatoid arthritis. A 15 year endpoint study. J Rheumatol. 2000;27:347.
3. Kauffman JI, Chen AL, Stuchin S, Di Cesare PE. Surgical management of the rheumatoid elbow. J Am Acad Orthop Surg. 2003;11:100–8.
4. Steinmann SP, King GJ, Savoie FH III. Arthroscopic treatment of the arthritic elbow. J Bone Joint Surg Am. 2005;87:2113–21.
5. Gladman D, Antoni C, Mease P, Clegg D, Nash P. Psoriatic arthritis: epidemiology, clinical features, course, and outcome. Ann Rheum Dis. 2005;64:ii14–7.
6. Alinaghi F, Calov M, Kristensen LE, Gladman DD, Coates LC, Jullien D, et al. Prevalence of psoriatic arthritis in patients with psoriasis: a systematic review and meta-analysis of observational and clinical studies. J Am Acad Dermatol. 2019;80:251–265.e219.
7. Larsen A, Dale K, Eek M. Radiographic evaluation of rheumatoid arthritis and related conditions by standard reference films. Acta Radiol Diagn. 1977;18:481–91.
8. Morrey B, Adams R. Semiconstrained arthroplasty for the treatment of rheumatoid arthritis of the elbow. J Bone Joint Surg Am. 1992;74:479–90.
9. Bercik MJ, Kruse K II, Yalizis M, Gauci M-O, Chaoui J, Walch G. A modification to the Walch classification of the glenoid in primary glenohumeral osteoarthritis using three-dimensional imaging. J Shoulder Elb Surg. 2016;25:1601–6.
10. Sirveaux F, Favard L, Oudet D, Huquet D, Walch G, Mole D. Grammont inverted total shoulder arthroplasty in the treatment of glenohumeral osteoarthritis with massive rupture of the cuff: results of a multicentre study of 80 shoulders. J Bone Jt Surg Br. 2004;86:388–95.
11. Hetland ML, Østergaard M, Ejbjerg B, Jacobsen S, Stengaard-Pedersen K, Junker P, et al. Short-and long-term efficacy of intra-articular injections with betamethasone as part of a treat-to-target strategy in early rheumatoid arthritis: impact of joint area, repeated injections, MRI findings, anti-CCP, IgM-RF and CRP. Ann Rheum Dis. 2012;71:851–6.
12. Carubbi F, Zugaro L, Cipriani P, Conchiglia A, Gregori L, Danniballe C, et al. Safety and efficacy of intra-articular anti-tumor necrosis factor α agents compared to corticosteroids in a treat-to-target strategy in patients with inflammatory arthritis and monoarthritis flare. Int J Immunopathol Pharmacol. 2016;29:252–66.
13. Neer C II, Watson K, Stanton F. Recent experience in total shoulder replacement. J Bone Joint Surg Am. 1982;64:319–37.
14. Friedman RJ, Ewald FC. Arthroplasty of the ipsilateral shoulder and elbow in patients who have rheumatoid arthritis. J Bone Jt Surg Am. 1987;69:661–6.
15. Goodman SM, Springer B, Guyatt G, Abdel MP, Dasa V, George M, et al. 2017 American College of Rheumatology/American Association of Hip and Knee Surgeons guideline for the perioperative management of antirheumatic medication in patients with rheumatic diseases undergoing elective total hip or total knee arthroplasty. J Arthroplast. 2017;32:2628–38.
16. Howe CR, Gardner GC, Kadel NJ. Perioperative medication management for the patient with rheumatoid arthritis. J Am Acad Orthop Surg. 2006;14:544–51.
17. Kwek T, Lew T, Thoo F. The role of preoperative cervical spine X-rays in rheumatoid arthritis. Anaesth Intensive Care. 1998;26:636–41.
18. Smith AM, Sperling JW, O'Driscoll SW, Cofield RH. Arthroscopic shoulder synovectomy in patients with rheumatoid arthritis. Arthroscopy. 2006;22:50–6.
19. Weber A, Bell S. Arthroscopic subacromial surgery in inflammatory arthritis of the shoulder. Rheumatology. 2001;40:384–6.
20. Kanbe K, Chiba J, Inoue Y, Taguchi M, Iwamatsu A. Analysis of clinical factors related to the efficacy of shoulder arthroscopic synovectomy plus capsular release in patients with rheumatoid arthritis. Eur J Orthop Surg Traumatol. 2015;25:451–5.

21. Holcomb JO, Hebert DJ, Mighell MA, Dunning PE, Pupello DR, Pliner MD, et al. Reverse shoulder arthroplasty in patients with rheumatoid arthritis. J Shoulder Elb Surg. 2010;19:1076–84.
22. Lehtinen JT, Belt EA, Lybäck CO, Kauppi MJ, Kaarela K, Kautiainen HJ, et al. Subacromial space in the rheumatoid shoulder: a radiographic 15-year follow-up study of 148 shoulders. J Shoulder Elb Surg. 2000;9:183–7.
23. Haleem A, Shanmugaraj A, Horner NS, Leroux T, Khan M, Alolabi B. Anatomic total shoulder arthroplasty in rheumatoid arthritis: a systematic review. Should Elb. 2022;14:142.
24. Sperling JW, Cofield RH, Schleck CD, Harmsen WS. Total shoulder arthroplasty versus hemiarthroplasty for rheumatoid arthritis of the shoulder: results of 303 consecutive cases. J Shoulder Elb Surg. 2007;16:683–90.
25. Søjbjerg JO, Frich LH, Johannsen HV, Sneppen O. Late results of total shoulder replacement in patients with rheumatoid arthritis. Clin Orthop Relat Res. 1999;366:39–45.
26. Mangold DR, Wagner ER, Cofield RH, Sanchez-Sotelo J, Sperling JW. Reverse shoulder arthroplasty for rheumatoid arthritis since the introduction of disease-modifying drugs. Int Orthop. 2019;43:2593–600.
27. Ekelund A, Nyberg R. Can reverse shoulder arthroplasty be used with few complications in rheumatoid arthritis? Clin Orthop Relat Res. 2011;469:2483–8.
28. Postacchini R, Carbone S, Canero G, Ripani M, Postacchini F. Reverse shoulder prosthesis in patients with rheumatoid arthritis: a systematic review. Int Orthop. 2016;40:965–73.
29. Rittmeister M, Kerschbaumer F. Grammont reverse total shoulder arthroplasty in patients with rheumatoid arthritis and nonreconstructible rotator cuff lesions. J Shoulder Elb Surg. 2001;10:17–22.
30. Guery J, Favard L, Sirveaux F, Oudet D, Mole D, Walch G. Reverse total shoulder arthroplasty: survivorship analysis of eighty replacements followed for five to ten years. J Bone Joint Surg Am. 2006;88:1742–7.
31. Kelly EW, Morrey BF, O'Driscoll SW. Complications of elbow arthroscopy. J Bone Joint Surg Am. 2001;83:25.
32. Camp CL, Cancienne JM, Degen RM, Dines JS, Altchek DW, Werner BC. Factors that increase the risk of infection after elbow arthroscopy: analysis of patient demographics, medical comorbidities, and steroid injections in 2,704 medicare patients. Arthroscopy. 2017;33:1175–9.
33. Horiuchi K, Momohara S, Tomatsu T, Inoue K, Toyama Y. Arthroscopic synovectomy of the elbow in rheumatoid arthritis. J Bone Joint Surg Am. 2002;84:342–7.
34. Shi LL, Zurakowski D, Jones DG, Koris MJ, Thornhill TS. Semiconstrained primary and revision total elbow arthroplasty with use of the Coonrad-Morrey prosthesis. J Bone Joint Surg Am. 2007;89:1467–75.
35. Gill DR, Morrey BF. The Coonrad-Morrey total elbow arthroplasty in patients who have rheumatoid arthritis. A ten to fifteen-year follow-up study. J Bone Jt Surg Am. 1998;80:1327–35.
36. Pham TT, Delclaux S, Huguet S, Wargny M, Bonnevialle N, Mansat P. Coonrad-Morrey total elbow arthroplasty for patients with rheumatoid arthritis: 54 prostheses reviewed at 7 years' average follow-up (maximum, 16 years). J Shoulder Elb Surg. 2018;27:398–403.
37. Sanchez-Sotelo J, Baghdadi YM, Morrey BF. Primary linked semiconstrained total elbow arthroplasty for rheumatoid arthritis: a single-institution experience with 461 elbows over three decades. J Bone Joint Surg Am. 2016;98:1741.
38. Gschwend N, Simmen BR, Matejovsky Z. Late complications in elbow arthroplasty. J Shoulder Elb Surg. 1996;5:86–96.
39. Larson AN, Morrey BF. Interposition arthroplasty with an Achilles tendon allograft as a salvage procedure for the elbow. J Bone Joint Surg Am. 2008;90:2714–23.
40. Ljung P, Jonsson K, Larsson K, Rydholm U. Interposition arthroplasty of the elbow with rheumatoid arthritis. J Shoulder Elb Surg. 1996;5:81–5.

# Rotator Cuff Tear

**4**

Noah Quinlan and Robert Z. Tashjian

## Introduction

Rotator cuff tears are common shoulder injuries, particularly as patients age. Thorough history taking, physical exam, and imaging review are essential in guiding treatment which includes both nonoperative and operative interventions depending on symptoms and tear characteristics.

1. History
   (a) Onset
   - When did you first notice something wrong with your shoulder?
   - Was this due to an acute injury or gradual progression?
     - Tears may be acute, chronic, or acute on chronic.
     - Acute traumatic injuries are generally more amenable to repair with better outcomes [1].
   - Since you first noticed your shoulder issue has it gotten better, worse, or stayed the same?
     - Understanding trajectory is key.
       If improving, may be reasonable to continue conservative management
   - Do you have pain, weakness, or both?
     - Clarifying patient's primary complaint can guide treatment and give some indication of the integrity of the rotator cuff. Weakness is often suggestive of more significant tendon injury including full-thickness tearing or involvement of multiple tendons.

N. Quinlan · R. Z. Tashjian (✉)
Department of Orthopaedics, University of Utah School of Medicine,
Salt Lake City, UT, USA
e-mail: noah.quinlan@hsc.utah.edu; Robert.tashjian@hsc.utah.edu

(b) Pain
  • Where does your shoulder hurt?
    – With one finger point to location of maximum pain.
       Rotator cuff derived pain is typically located over the lateral or
       posterolateral aspect of the arm in the region of the deltoid.
  • What exacerbates your symptoms?
    – Rotator cuff injuries are often exacerbated by overhead activities and
       heavy lifting.
  • What improves your symptoms?
    – Rest and activity below shoulder height is often associated with
       improved symptoms. Cervical spine-derived referred pain improves
       with arm elevation and therefore is a way to differ from rotator cuff-
       related pain.
  • Does your shoulder wake you up at night?
    – Rotator cuff pain commonly interferes with sleep although other dis-
       ease processes including glenohumeral arthritis and adhesive capsuli-
       tis do as well; therefore, they need to be ruled out.
  • Do you notice any crepitus with shoulder motion?
    – Subacromial crepitus correlates with cuff disease when the tuberosity
       contacts the acromial undersurface.
(c) Strength
  • Does your shoulder feel weak?
    – Is this due to pain, reduced stamina, or inherent weakness from struc-
       tural detachment of the tendon?
  • What are the activities where you notice weakness?
    – Do certain planes seem more affected than others? Elevation weak-
       ness suggests supraspinatus dysfunction, external rotation infraspina-
       tus dysfunction, and internal rotation subscapularis dysfunction.
  • Any other functional limitations?
    – Is range of motion affected?
       If so, may just be due to pain and weakness, but consider alternate
       diagnoses such as glenohumeral arthritis or adhesive capsulitis
(d) Prior injury/surgery
  • Did you have shoulder pain or weakness previously?
    – May indicate acute on chronic or a chronic injury
  • Have you had any prior shoulder injuries?
    – May indicate a chronic injury
  • Have you had any prior shoulder surgeries?
    – May have injured a previously repaired tendon that either healed or
       did not heal but was asymptomatic and now has become symptomatic
  • Do you have any known issues with your neck (cervical spine)?
    – Shoulder and cervical spine pathology can overlap so differentiating
       between these is crucial in guiding treatment.
    – Check for subjective pain radiating past elbow.

(e) Interventions
- Have you had any prior treatment such as:
  - Non-steroidal anti-inflammatory medication
  - Activity modification including rest
  - Physical therapy
  - Injections—corticosteroids or platelet-rich plasma
  - Modalities—ice, TENS, ultrasound
  - Acupuncture
  - Surgery

(f) Activity level/goals
- What activities do you enjoy participating in that require use of your shoulder?
- What activities do you hope to resume?
- Is your primary goal of treatment improvement in pain, weakness, or both?
- If surgery were an option, is this something you would want to proceed with knowing it will likely be a 6- to 12-month recovery?
- If it weren't for your shoulder, do you have any other conditions limiting your activity?

2. Physical exam
   (a) Inspection
   - Swelling
   - Ecchymosis
   - Intact skin/wounds
     - Assess for prior surgical scars
   - Bulk muscle mass
     - Evaluate for deltoid, supraspinatus, and infraspinatus atrophy

   (b) Palpation
   - Isolate points of tenderness
     - Clavicle
     - Acromioclavicular joint
     - Scapular spine
     - Posterolateral shoulder (rotator cuff insertion)
     - Biceps tendon
     - Superomedial angle of the scapula

   (c) Range of motion
   - General
     - Compare to contralateral side
     - Note if associated with pain
     - Crepitus that may indicate glenohumeral arthritis
   - Active
     - Flexion in the scapular plane (scaption)
     - Abduction
     - External rotation and internal rotation with elbow at side

- External rotation and internal rotation with shoulder abducted to 90°
- Reaching behind back (note most proximal spinous process level they are able to reach)
  - Passive
    - Flexion in the scapular plane (scaption)
    - Abduction
    - External rotation and internal rotation with elbow at side
    - External rotation and internal rotation with shoulder abducted to 90°
    - Check posterior capsule stiffness with a 90° abduction and internal rotation
      May cause secondary impingement
- (d) Strength testing
  - General
    - Graded muscle strength (0 through 5)
      5—full strength
      4—able to resist force though weak
      3—able to resist gravity, but no additional force
      2—unable to resist gravity, but able to move in anti-gravity plane
      1—muscle flicker only, without movement in any plane
      0—not muscle activity
    - Asses for weakness, pain, or both with each maneuver
    - Try to isolate which muscles are involved
      Tear may be isolated to single muscle or any combination
  - Supraspinatus
    - Empty can (Jobe's test)
      Bring patient's affected extremity to 90° abducted in scapular plane of motion
      Point thumb down to the ground
        "Drop arm" if unable to hold this position even without resistance
      Patient resists examiner downward direct pressure on the arm
  - Infraspinatus
    - External rotation strength at 0° shoulder abduction
      Elbow flexed to 90° and held against patient's side
        "External rotation lag" if unable to hold this position even without resistance suggests a large complete injury
      Patient resists examiner medial directed force on the arm (internal rotation)
  - Teres Minor
    - External rotation strength at 90° shoulder abduction
      Elbow flexed to 90°
      Shoulder abducted to 90° and externally rotated to 90°
        "Hornblower's sign" if unable to hold this position even without resistance
      Patient resists examiner anterior directed force on the arm (internal rotation)

- Subscapularis
  - Internal rotation strength at 0° shoulder abduction
    Elbow flex to 90° and held against patient's side
    Patient resists examiner laterally directed force on the arm (external rotation)
  - Belly press test
    Elbow flexed to 90°
    Arm internally rotated so hand rests on patient's belly with elbow anterior to the plane of the body
      "Internal rotation lag" if unable to hold this position without resistance
    Patient resists examiner attempt to pull arm anteriorly off belly and patient compensates by dropping elbow posterior to the plane of the body
  - Bear hug
    Reach across to contralateral shoulder and resist pull off
  - Lift off test
    Elbow flexed to 90°
    Patient position hand on small of their back
    Patient attempts to lift hand off their back as examiner resists
(e) Directed tests based on history or mechanism of injury
  - Assess for impingement
    - Hawkins
      Shoulder abducted to 90° and elbow maximally flexed
      Examiner applies internal rotation force by pushing up on elbow and down on hand distally
        Continue with progressive degrees of cross body adduction
      Recreates painful impingement in subacromial space if present
    - Neer
      Pain associated with passive forward flexion of the shoulder
        Hold scapula down while performing maneuver
        Reproduces subacromial impingement
  - General neurovascular exam
    - Focused axillary nerve evaluation
      Assess deltoid firing by directly palpating while having patient abduct or extend their shoulder
      Sensory over lateral deltoid
  - Consider cervical spine exam, including Spurling's test, if concern that spine pathology may be contributing to clinical picture
  - Assess for concomitant pathology particularly biceps tendonitis, glenohumeral arthritis or focal glenohumeral articular cartilage injuries, instability or labral tearing, adhesive capsulitis, calcific tendonitis, acromioclavicular joint arthritis, suprascapular nerve dysfunction, or quadrilateral space syndrome

3. Imaging
   (a) X-rays
      • Standard shoulder series to include:
         – AP
            Evaluate for glenohumeral arthritis and acromioclavicular joint arthritis; evaluate for fractures of the proximal humerus, scapula, or clavicle.
            Superior humeral head migration indicates some degree of chronicity of rotator cuff injury.
         – Grashey (True AP)
            Enhances evaluation of the glenohumeral joint; superior head migration with loss of contour between calcar of proximal humerus and axillary border of the scapula
         – Lateral (Scapular Y view)
            Evaluate anterior/posterior translation of the humeral head in the setting of dislocations or fracture morphology
         – Axillary
            Evaluate anterior/posterior translation of the humeral head suggestive of subluxation (anterior due to possible subscapularis injury; posterior often due to arthritis); evaluate glenohumeral joint for narrowing or glenoid wear morphology associated with arthritis
   (b) MRI
      • Gold standard for diagnosis of rotator cuff tears [2]
         – Arthrogram may be helpful especially in the setting of evaluating the healing of a repaired tendon [3]. Not necessary in the setting of a tear without prior surgery.
         – Understanding tear shape may assist in determining appropriate type of repair.
            Crescent
            U shape
            L shape
               Reverse L
            Massive and immobile
            Check if anterior cable is intact on sagittal obliques
      • Series
         – T2 series for inflammation, tendinopathy, and tears
         – T1 for evaluation of muscle quality (atrophy and fatty infiltration)
      • Coronal
         – Evaluate tendon tearing at the rotator cuff footprint (Fig. 4.1)
            May be partial- or full-thickness tear (complete from articular to bursal side)
               If full thickness, glenohumeral joint space communicates with subacromial space.
               Partial further subdivided into articular sided, intra-substance, bursal sided.

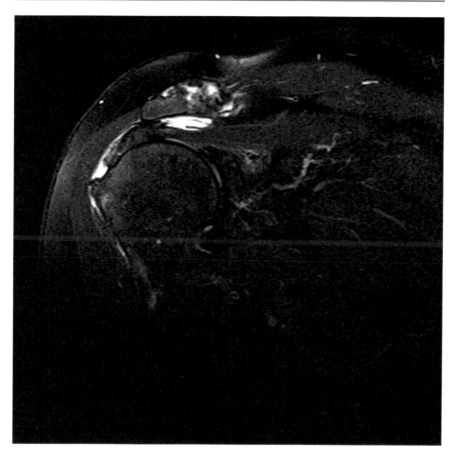

**Fig. 4.1** Coronal T2 image with fluid in tear site of a minimally retracted full-thickness rotator cuff tear

If no tear present, but increased signal within the tendon, then consider it tendinopathy.

Cystic bone changes may be present at rotator cuff insertion.
- If a tear is present, measure retraction of the lateral aspect of the rotator cuff stump to the greater tuberosity footprint.

The larger the retraction, the more concern it may be difficult to mobilize back to the footprint for repair [4].

Patte classification—stage 1, tendon edge close to insertion; stage 2, tendon edge at the level of the humeral head; stage 3, tendon edge at the level of the glenoid.
- Sagittal
  - Evaluate anterior to posterior tear length (Fig. 4.2).

Grade tear size

Small—0–1 cm

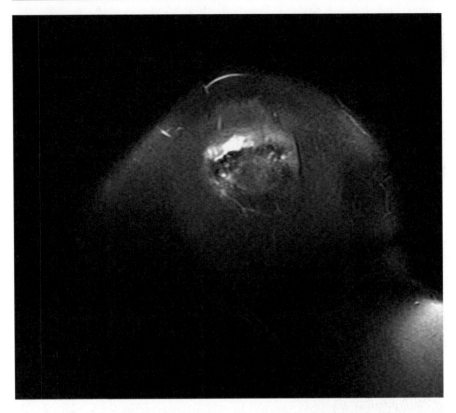

**Fig. 4.2** Sagittal view of the supraspinatus showing a medium-sized full-thickness rotator cuff tear

        Medium—1–3 cm

        Large—3–5 cm

        Massive—over 5 cm or involves more than 1 tendon

– Medially in the supraspinatus fossa on T1 sequence, assess muscle atrophy and fatty infiltration which takes months to years to develop after a tear (Fig. 4.3).

    More advanced fatty infiltration or muscle atrophy indicates degree of chronicity and worse outcomes/poor healing when repaired.

    Tangent sign—residual supraspinatus muscle lies below a line draw between the scapular spine and acromion.

        Indicates more severe atrophy, as muscle belly usually crosses this plane; indicator for poor healing after repair

    Goutallier classification

        0—no fat infiltration

        1—fatty streaks with muscle

        2—more muscle than fat

        3—equal muscle and fat

        4—less muscle than fat

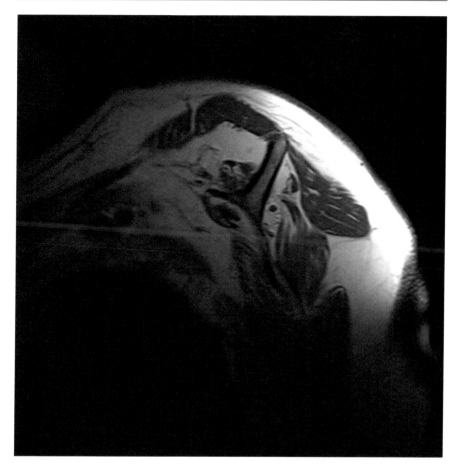

**Fig. 4.3** Sagittal T1 image showing cross sections of the supraspinatus, subscapularis, and infraspinatus with severe grade IV fatty infiltration of all three muscle bellies

  – Acromion morphology may be a source of impingement.
      Bigliani classification
          Type 1: flat
          Type 2: curved
          Type 3: hooked
 • Axial
  – Evaluate for subscapularis pathology; subluxation of the biceps tendon is an indicator of a subscapularis tear.
(c) CT scan
 • Commonly utilized to evaluate rotator cuff pathology in Europe with intraarticular contrast; more limited role in US
 • CT arthrogram useful if patient is contraindicated for MRI; easily able to evaluate tear size, retraction, and muscle quality
 • Useful when considering arthroplasty for rotator cuff arthropathy to assess bony morphology

   (d) Ultrasound
- Allows for dynamic evaluation of the rotator cuff which may improve the ability to determine the healing status of a repair
- Can be useful for immediate evaluation and monitor injury progression especially in patients contraindicated for an MRI
- Highly user dependent
  - Requires training and equipment
- Does not allow for evaluation of additional shoulder pathology

4. Treatment algorithm based on diagnosis
  (a) Nonoperative treatment
- A trial of conservative management is appropriate with the following diagnoses:
  - Tendinopathy
  - Partial tears
  - Chronic full-thickness tears in older patients (>65 years of age)
  - Acute on chronic tear with severe fatty infiltration and atrophy already preexisting
- Options
  - Non-steroidal anti-inflammatories
  - Activity modification including rest
    
    Avoid exacerbating activities, particularly those overhead
    
    Gradual return to activity once symptoms subside
  - Physical therapy for rotator cuff, deltoid, and periscapular strengthening and stretching in all planes of motion
  - Corticosteroid injection
    
    Beneficial to reduce pain, end cycle of inflammation, and allow patient to progress with therapy
    
        Recommended for patients significantly limited by pain to allow for participation in physical therapy
    
        Avoid in potential operative candidates due to increased infection risk or worse healing with injection performed within 3 months of surgery
    
    Locations
    
      Subacromial
    
        Indications: subacromial impingement, tendinopathy, bursal-sided partial tears, full-thickness tear
    
        Will not be beneficial for intra-articular pathology if the cuff remains intact as subacromial and glenohumeral space remain separate
    
      Intra-articular glenohumeral
    
        Indications: partial articular-sided tear, additional intra-articular pathology (biceps or labral injury)
    
        Most reliably performed under image guidance
  - Biologics are not currently supported by the literature [5]

(b) Operative treatment (options, approaches, and complications)
  • Rotator cuff repair
    – Indications:
        Acute full-thickness tear
        Acute on chronic tear with limited fat infiltration or atrophy
        Chronic full-thickness tears in young patients (<65 years of age)
        Chronic full-thickness tears in older patients (>65 years of age) refractory to conservative measures
        Partial tears refractory to conservative measures
            Articular-sided tears involving greater than 50% of the footprint
            Bursal-sided tears with evidence of subacromial impingement
    – Historically an open procedure, though vast majority is now performed arthroscopically; arthroscopic repairs significantly reduce the incidence of complications including infection [6], stiffness, and deltoid detachment.
    – Diagnostic arthroscopic evaluation of the glenohumeral and subacromial spaces.
    – Suture anchor repair:
        Tear is debrided back to healthy appearing tissue.
            If partial tear, tear completion may be performed to debride diseased edges and fully repair tendon back to bone; alternatively, an in situ repair without completion can be performed for bursal-sided tears using retrograde suture passing or a PASTA repair for articular-sided tears passing anchors through the cuff and then tying stitches in the subacromial space [2].
        Cuff footprint is debrided to allow area of tendon to bone healing.
            Bone stimulation techniques (microfracture) may be used at footprint to promote healing [5].
        Single vs. double row repair of tendon back to footprint.
            Double row biomechanically stronger; improved healing rates and functional outcome scores for large and massive tears with no difference for small- and medium-sized tears compared to single row [7].
            Double row often used for larger tears (Figs. 4.4 and 4.5).
        Risks and complications—Risks of arthroscopic rotator cuff repair include infection (<0.1%), failure of healing (<5% to >50% depending on patient age, tears size, tendon retraction, and muscle quality), stiffness and persistent pain.
    – Augments
        Indications: irreparable tear or reparable tears at severe risk for healing failure.
        Release cuff extensively (coracohumeral ligament, rotator cuff interval, posterior at scapular spine, at junction between cuff and labrum) in an effort to reduce cuff to footprint.

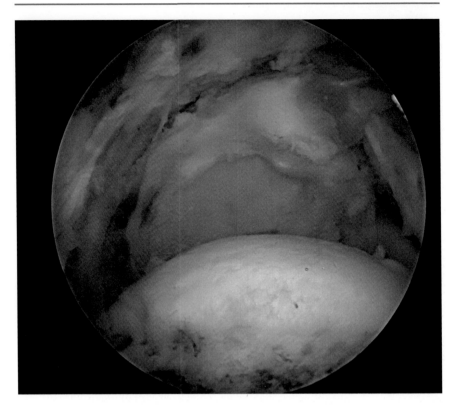

**Fig. 4.4** Massive retracted rotator cuff tear viewed from the lateral portal

If cuff tear under significant tension with high risk for re-tear, consider repair with augmentation utilizing acellular dermal matrix or synthetic patch graft.

If partially reparable or irreparable, options include:

   Leaving as a partial repair

   Structural autograft

      Long head of biceps tendon interposition between edge of tendon and footprint

   Synthetic patch interposition scaffold between tendon edge and rotator cuff footprint

   Acellular dermal matrix patch

      Superior capsular reconstruction—between glenoid and rotator cuff footprint (Fig. 4.6)

      Interposition—between edge of irreparable tendon and rotator cuff footprint

Healing failure after augmented repair vs. repair alone improves approximately 20–30%. Risks include increased operating room time and the addition of allograft tissue which may increase the risk for infection.

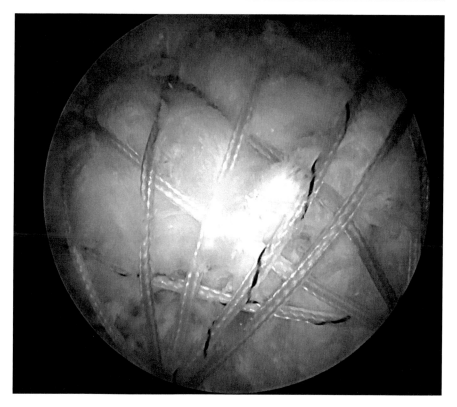

**Fig. 4.5** Arthroscopic suture bridge double row rotator cuff repair of massive retracted rotator cuff tear viewed from the lateral portal

- Additional procedures
  - Subacromial decompression
    - Reduce impingement that may be contributing to cuff pathology
  - Biceps tenotomy/tenodesis
    - If concomitant biceps pathology
- Tendon transfer
  - Indications: massive irreparable tear, significant fat atrophy; goals of improvement of both pain and strength; preferred in younger, higher demand patients.
  - Contraindications—significant glenohumeral arthritis; combined irreparable tears of the subscapularis, supraspinatus and infraspinatus.
  - Options:
    - Latissimus dorsi (± teres major) or lower trapezius tendon augmented with graft for deficient posterosuperior rotator cuff (supraspinatus and infraspinatus)
    - Pectoralis major or latissimus dorsi for deficient subscapularis

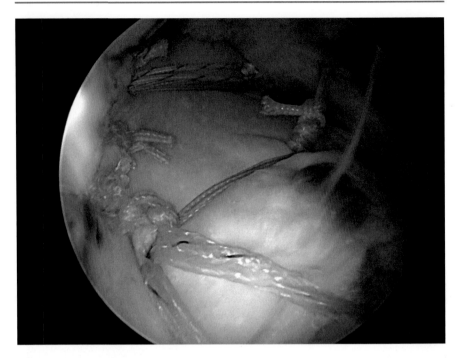

**Fig. 4.6** Superior capsule reconstruction of the previous massive retracted irreparable rotator cuff tear viewed from the lateral portal

  – Risks include failure of the tendon graft to heal and inability to restore function due to limited ability to recruit the transfer to improve function.
- Reverse total shoulder
  – Functioning deltoid is required for placement of reverse total shoulder arthroplasty along with no active infection. Bone loss on humerus or glenoid may be either reconstructed with allograft or autograft or replaced using metallic augments.
  – Indications:
      Rotator cuff arthropathy (Figs. 4.7 and 4.8)
      Massive irreparable rotator cuff tear without arthritis
  – Risks include dislocation (1–5%), scapular spine or acromion fracture (1–5%), infection (1–5%), scapular notching (10–60%), periprosthetic fracture (1%), baseplate loosening (<1%), and persistent shoulder pain.

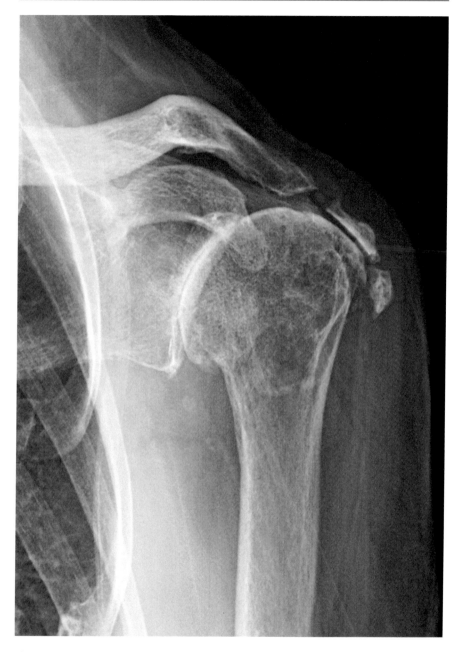

**Fig. 4.7** Rotator cuff arthropathy (shoulder arthritis with an irreparable rotator cuff tear)

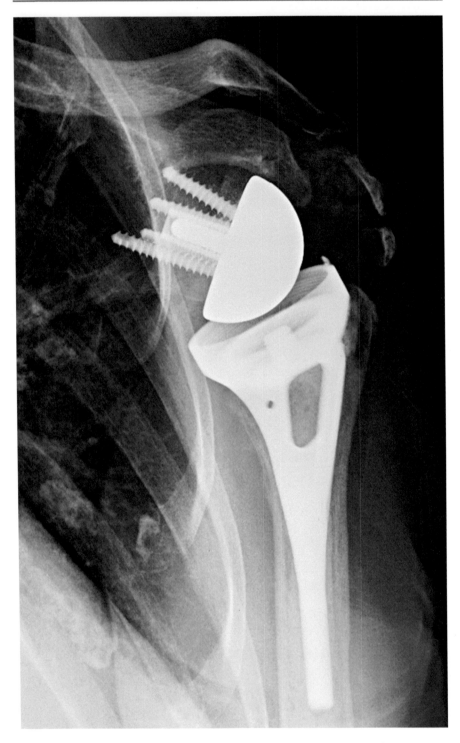

**Fig. 4.8** Reverse total shoulder arthroplasty for treatment of rotator cuff arthropathy

# References

1. Gutman MJ, Joyce CD, Patel MS, Kirsch JM, Gutman BS, Abboud JA, Namdari S, Ramsey ML. Early repair of traumatic rotator cuff tears improves functional outcomes. J Shoulder Elb Surg. 2021;30:2475. https://doi.org/10.1016/j.jse.2021.03.134. PMID: 33774173.
2. Plancher KD, Shanmugam J, Briggs K, Petterson SC. Diagnosis and management of partial thickness rotator cuff tears: a comprehensive review. J Am Acad Orthop Surg. 2021;29:1031. https://doi.org/10.5435/JAAOS-D-20-01092. PMID: 34520444.
3. Ball CM. Arthroscopic rotator cuff repair: magnetic resonance arthrogram assessment of tendon healing. J Shoulder Elb Surg. 2019;28(11):2161–70. https://doi.org/10.1016/j.jse.2019.02.024. PMID: 31078406.
4. Cvetanovich GL, Waterman BR, Verma NN, Romeo AA. Management of the irreparable rotator cuff tear. J Am Acad Orthop Surg. 2019;27(24):909–17. https://doi.org/10.5435/JAAOS-D-18-00199. PMID: 31206436.
5. Weber S, Chahal J. Management of rotator cuff injuries. J Am Acad Orthop Surg. 2020;28(5):e193–201. https://doi.org/10.5435/JAAOS-D-19-00463. PMID: 31599763.
6. Danilkowicz R, Levin J, Crook B, Long J, Vap A. Analysis of risk factors, complications, reoperations, and demographics associated with open and arthroscopic rotator cuff repair: an Analysis of a Large National Database. Arthroscopy. 2021;38:737. https://doi.org/10.1016/j.arthro.2021.09.001. PMID: 34508821.
7. Dines JS, Bedi A, ElAttrache NS, Dines DM. Single-row versus double-row rotator cuff repair: techniques and outcomes. J Am Acad Orthop Surg. 2010;18(2):83–93. https://doi.org/10.5435/00124635-201002000-00003. PMID: 20118325.

# Anterior Shoulder Instability

# 5

Caroline Vonck and Seth Gamradt

1. *Evaluation of Anterior Shoulder Instability*
   (a) Anatomy of the shoulder as a shallow ball and socket joint gives the shoulder the highest range of motion of any joint in the body.
   (b) Despite the constraint provided by capsule, labrum, and rotator cuff, the shoulder is inherently a non-constrained bony construct (as opposed to the hip, for example), and this joint is prone to instability.
   (c) Anterior shoulder instability is more common than posterior instability, affecting 1–2% of the population each year.
   (d) The first component of evaluating a patient with shoulder instability or dislocation is to take a thorough history (Box 5.1).

---

**Box 5.1 History Taking in Shoulder Instability**
- Patient age
- Handedness
- Unilateral or bilateral
- Family history
- Position of arm when instability occurs
  - Abduction/external rotation is typically anterior instability
  - Adduction/internal rotation is typically posterior instability

---

C. Vonck
Department of Orthopaedic Surgery, University of Southern California Keck School of Medicine, Los Angeles, CA, USA
e-mail: Caroline.Vonck@med.usc.edu

S. Gamradt (✉)
Orthopaedic Athletic Medicine, Clinical Orthopaedic Surgery, Keck Medicine of USC, University of Southern California, Los Angeles, CA, USA
e-mail: gamradt@usc.edu; https://www.gamradtortho.com/

© The Author(s), under exclusive license to Springer Nature Switzerland AG 2022
C. M. Chebli, A. M. Murthi (eds.), *The Resident's Guide to Shoulder and Elbow Surgery*, https://doi.org/10.1007/978-3-031-12255-2_5

- Number and frequency of dislocations or instability events
- Degree of trauma provoking the instability
  - Did the patient need an emergency room reduction?
  - Did the shoulder dislocate with minimal trauma? This often indicates multidirectional instability.
  - Does the shoulder dislocate during sleep?
  - Can the patient dislocate the shoulder voluntarily?
- Current pain level
- Sensory or motor complaints in the affected extremity
- Mechanical symptoms
- Sports participation
  - Contact/collision athletes
  - Throwing athletes
- Occupation
  - Military personnel
- Previous shoulder surgeries

2. Physical Examination
   (a) Cervical spine range of motion.
   (b) Palpation of the shoulder for any tenderness over the biceps tendon, AC joint, acromion, or coracoid.
   (c) Range of motion in forward elevation, abduction, external rotation, and internal rotation is measured actively and passively.
      - In the acutely injured or recently reduced shoulder, we are very careful with range of motion evaluation until the full extent of the clinical situation is evaluated with imaging.
   (d) Strength testing: Deltoid and rotator cuff are evaluated in standard fashion, but a complete strength testing is often not possible after an acute dislocation.
   (e) Provocative testing
      - Apprehension/relocation (Fig. 5.1), the patient is placed supine, which stabilizes the scapula against the examination table. The arm is abducted to 90°, and external rotation of the shoulder produces a feeling of instability/apprehension in the anterior shoulder instability patient. This feeling is typically eliminated by the relocation maneuver which is a posteriorly directed force from the examiner on the anterior aspect of the humeral head.
      - Supine load and shift test (Fig. 5.2) starts with the arm positioned in the plane of the scapula with 45–60° of abduction. In that position, an anterior followed by posterior translational forces are applied to the humerus, and the examiner assesses for translation, stability, pain, and/or a palpable click. The load and shift test are graded 1–3 based on the amount of humeral translation with respect to the glenoid (Fig. 5.3).

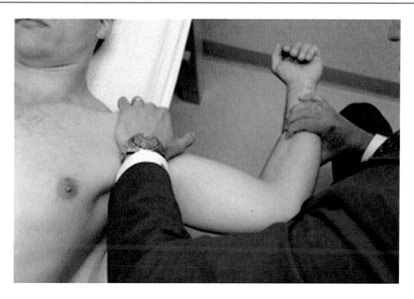

**Fig. 5.1** Apprehension/relocation. In a supine position, the scapula is stabilized. The arm is abducted and externally rotated. A positive test occurs if the patient experiences apprehension or instability in this position. In the same position, a posteriorly directed force is applied to the anterior aspect of the humeral head. A positive test occurs when the patient feels relief of the apprehension from this maneuver. (*Reproduced from Lizzio VA, Meta F, Fidai M, Makhni EC. Clinical Evaluation and Physical Exam Findings in Patients with Anterior Shoulder Instability. Curr Rev Musculoskelet Med. 2017;10(4):434–441*)

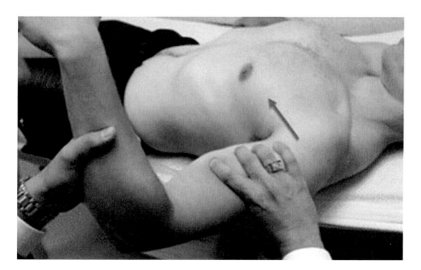

**Fig. 5.2** Load and shift. In a supine position, the scapula is stabilized. The arm is positioned in the plane of the scapula and stabilized distally. An axial force is applied to the arm, followed by anteriorly (depicted here) and posteriorly directed forces to the humeral head. (*Reproduced from Lizzio VA, Meta F, Fidai M, Makhni EC. Clinical Evaluation and Physical Exam Findings in Patients with Anterior Shoulder Instability. Curr Rev Musculoskelet Med. 2017;10(4):434–441*)

Glenohumeral Translation

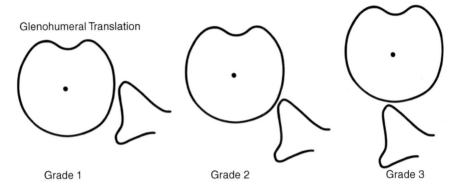

Grade 1                          Grade 2                          Grade 3

**Fig. 5.3** Grading glenohumeral translation. Progressive anterior translation of the humeral head relative to the glenoid results in subluxation and ultimately dislocation

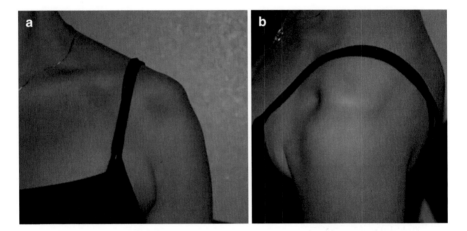

**Fig. 5.4** Sulcus sign. (**a**) Anterior and (**b**) lateral views of the shoulder with a positive sulcus sign. Not pictured is the inferiorly directed force applied to the arm while the scapula and shoulder are stabilized. (*Reproduced from Didinger T, Cooper JD, Gamradt SC. Multidirectional Shoulder Instability [Internet]. 2018. Available from:* https://musculoskeletalkey.com/multidirectional-shoulder instability/)

- The sulcus sign (Fig. 5.4) is assessed beginning with the shoulder in adduction and neutral rotation, and an inferiorly directed force is applied to the whole arm. Grading is as follows: 1+ = 1 cm, 2+ = 1–2 cm, 3+ = >3 cm. A more significant sulcus sign is commonly associated with multidirectional instability.
3. Imaging (Table 5.1)
4. Diagnoses/Abbreviations (Box 5.2)

**Table 5.1** Imaging evaluation in shoulder instability

| Standard radiographs | | Three-dimensional imaging | |
|---|---|---|---|
| AP | Evaluates for fracture and glenohumeral alignment | CT scan | Confirms reduction of dislocated shoulder, rules out humeral or glenoid fracture, and evaluates for humeral and glenoid bone loss in chronic instability |
| True AP (Grashey) | Evaluates for fracture and glenohumeral alignment | MRI scan | Evaluates rotator cuff which is critical in dislocated shoulders above 40 years old. Evaluates cartilage, labrum, effusion, bone bruising, and long head of biceps tendon |
| Scapular Y | Humeral head should be centered within Y formed by scapula | MRI arthrogram | Intraarticular contrast is more sensitive for labral injury |
| Axillary | An axillary view is critical to confirm reduction of dislocated shoulder. If the patient is unable to abduct arm or an axillary view cannot be obtained, a Velpeau view or CT scan can be acceptable alternatives | | |

---

**Box 5.2 Acronyms, Definitions, and Diagnoses in Anterior Shoulder Instability**

- *TUBS*: Traumatic, Unidirectional, Bankart lesion, usually requires Surgery. A classic acronym described by Thomas and Matsen that summarizes the typical characteristics of anterior shoulder instability (compared with AMBRI) [1].
- *AMBRI*: Atraumatic, Multidirectional, Bilateral, gets better with Rehabilitation, Infrequently requires surgery. A classic acronym describing MDI (multidirectional instability).
- *Bankart lesion*: Tear from 3 to 6 o'clock on the anterior rim of the glenoid which is the typical labrum injury resulting from an anterior shoulder dislocation.
- *Bony Bankart lesion*: Glenoid injury due to anterior dislocation which involves a fracture of the anterior rim of the glenoid.
- *GLAD lesion*: GlenoLabral Articular Disruption. A Bankart lesion that disrupts the articular cartilage in addition to the labrum.
- *ALPSA Lesion*: Anterior Labroligamentous Periosteal Sleeve Avulsion. In this Bankart lesion variant, the labrum pulls the glenoid with capsule and periosteum, typically ending up *medial and inferior* to its anatomic location. Failure to recognize this lesion and mobilize the labrum back to its anatomic location during Bankart repair is a risk factor for recurrent instability after surgery.

- *Hill-Sachs deformity*: Posterior-superior humeral bone injury resulting from contact with anterior glenoid rim during anterior shoulder dislocation. This can manifest as a minimal bone bruise or as severe as a large defect from chronic instability that engages with glenoid in external rotation.
- *AIGHL*: Anterior band of Inferior GlenoHumeral Ligament. Commonly tested static stabilizer of the shoulder in abduction external rotation.
- *PIGHL*: Posterior band of Inferior GlenoHumeral Ligament. Static stabilizer of the shoulder in abduction and posterior translation.
- *MGHL*: Middle GlenoHumeral Ligament. Static stabilizer of the shoulder in 45° of abduction.
- *SGHL*: Superior GlenoHumeral Ligament. Static stabilizer of the shoulder in adduction.
- *Inverted pear glenoid*: With repetitive dislocations, the antero-inferior glenoid bone begins to wear away and the glenoid takes on the shape of an upside-down pear due to loss of the antero-inferior glenoid bone.
- *HAGL lesion*: Humeral Avulsion of the Glenohumeral Ligament. An avulsion of the shoulder capsule after shoulder dislocation from the humeral side. Important to recognize this pathology on MRI because a standard Bankart repair will not stabilize the shoulder. This condition is usually treated by open or arthroscopic HAGL repair.

5. Classification of Shoulder Instability: There are many classification schemes for shoulder instability. No one classification strategy is all encompassing, but an excellent example is the FEDS classification by Jed Kuhn [2] (Table 5.2).
6. Initial Management of Acute Instability
    (a) A typical presentation of anterior shoulder instability is an athlete that has fallen and suffered immediate shoulder pain and an inability to move the shoulder.
    (b) The patient will present with a prominent acromion and a fullness in the anteromedial aspect of the shoulder.
    (c) An attempt at reduction is typically made at the athletic venue by qualified personnel (e.g., team physician, ski patrol, athletic trainer).
    (d) If the shoulder does not reduce easily, EMS can be activated.
    (e) The most common method of shoulder reduction is a traction countertraction method of reduction (Fig. 5.5). To perform this maneuver, the patient is supine on the examination table with a sheet wrapped around the torso and under the axilla. The dislocated shoulder is abducted to 45° with the elbow flexed to 90°. Traction is pulled on the affected arm in this position with countertraction performed using the sheet. This can be done with or without another sheet around the proximal arm to apply a lateral and cephalad force to the proximal humerus to aid in the reduction.

**Table 5.2**  FEDS classification of shoulder instability

| | |
|---|---|
| *Frequency* | Acute |
| | Recurrent |
| | Locked |
| *Etiology* | Traumatic |
| | Atraumatic |
| *Direction* | Unidirectional |
| | • Anterior |
| | • Posterior |
| | • Inferior |
| | Multidirectional |
| *Severity* | Dislocation |
| | Subluxation (an instability event where the shoulder does not entirely dislocate) |

*Adapted from Kuhn JE, Helmer TT, Dunn WR, Throckmorton V TW. Development and reliability testing of the frequency, etiology, direction, and severity (FEDS) system for classifying glenohumeral instability. J Shoulder Elbow Surg. 2011;20(4):548–556*

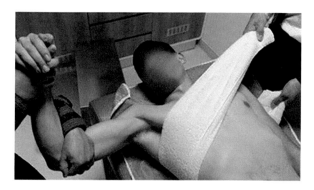

**Fig. 5.5**  Traction/countertraction reduction method. The most common method for reducing an anterior shoulder dislocation. (*Reproduced from Guler O, Ekinci S, Akyildiz F, et al. Comparison of four different reduction methods for anterior dislocation of the shoulder. J Orthop Surg Res. 2015;10:80*)

    (f) Radiographs of an anterior shoulder dislocation pre- and post-reduction are shown in Fig. 5.6. An axillary lateral radiograph and/or CT scan should always confirm reduction.

7. Nonoperative Treatment of Anterior Shoulder Instability
    (a) Treatment of an acutely dislocated shoulder involves an initial period of sling immobilization following successful reduction.
    (b) There was initially some interest in immobilization in external rotation as a means of decreasing recurrence [3], but further studies have shown that the position and duration of sling immobilization are not the key factors in reducing recurrent dislocation [4].
    (c) An MRI is not usually a necessity in treating shoulder instability, although it is commonplace in most orthopedic practices to obtain MRI after shoulder dislocation to assess the pathology at hand. Figure 5.7 demonstrates

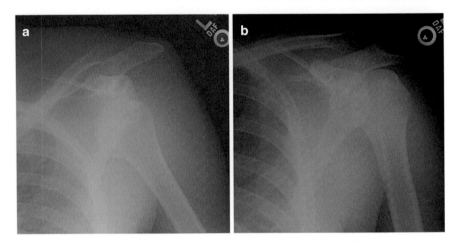

**Fig. 5.6** Anterior shoulder dislocation radiographs. (**a**) Pre-reduction and (**b**) post-reduction radiographs of a 22-year-old college student who dislocated his shoulder playing basketball. Pre-reduction, note the anterior-inferior position of the humerus with respect to the glenoid. Even with an obviously successful reduction on AP radiograph, this must be confirmed with axillary radiograph or CT scan

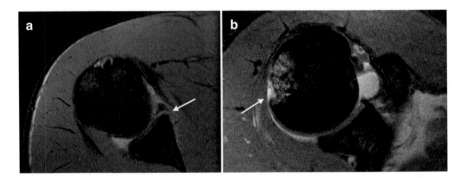

**Fig. 5.7** Anterior shoulder dislocation MRI. (**a**) Noncontrast image of axial MRI of a recent anterior shoulder dislocation showing Bankart lesion anteriorly. (**b**) Noncontrast image of axial MRI of a recent anterior shoulder dislocation showing acute Hill-Sachs deformity

typical MRI findings after anterior dislocation. MRI is considered critical in patients above the age of 40 to avoid missing a torn rotator cuff associated with dislocation, which is more common with increasing age.

(d) After an initial period of sling immobilization (about 2 weeks in our practice), physical therapy is initiated. When motion is full, rotator cuff strengthening is initiated. A return to physical activity is delayed until the shoulder is both objectively and subjectively close to normal.

(e) Typically, we tell our anterior instability patients to avoid forced abduction and external rotation (e.g., pullups, monkey bars, rings) for a period of 6 months.

(f) A second or third instability event or a persistent feeling of instability or apprehension warrants a surgical discussion.

8. In-Season Management of Shoulder Instability

   (a) The treatment of in-season athletes, competitive athletes (especially contact/collision athletes), and military personnel differs from this protocol. The following paragraphs address the interest in the treatment of in-season collision athletes and surgical stabilization in select cases of first-time dislocators.

   (b) Management of the athlete who has an in-season shoulder dislocation deserves special discussion, as players and coaches desire expeditious return to play.

   (c) Higher than the general population, the incidence of shoulder instability is 0.12 per 1000 athlete exposures; male football players, males wrestlers, and female ice hockey players are the most affected [5].

   (d) Buss et al. studied 30 athletes who sustained a first-time anterior shoulder dislocation during the season. Ninety percent returned to the same season play. Most were able to complete the season after missing an average of 10.2 days; however, 37% experienced additional instability [6].

   (e) In a prospective study of 45 collegiate contact sport athletes sustaining a first episode of anterior instability, Dickens and colleagues demonstrated 73% returned to the same season play at a median of 5 missed days; however, only 27% were able to finish the season without recurrent instability. Athletes who sustained a subluxation event as opposed to dislocation were 5.3 times more likely to return to the season [7].

   (f) In our practice, following an initial anterior instability event in collegiate football players—provided that the MRI pathology is not severe (e.g., bony Bankart or very high energy labrum injury)—we will allow return to play in the same season if they can regain full motion and strength without apprehension. A brace is sometimes helpful in football as it can strap to shoulder pads and limit abduction/external rotation.

   (g) A second instability event results in a recommendation of surgery. Regardless of the success or failure of return to play, we typically recommend off-season shoulder stabilization surgery in any athlete with a confirmed dislocation due to the very high chance of recurrent instability.

9. Surgical Treatment of Anterior Shoulder Instability in the First-Time Dislocator

   (a) Certain risk factors are associated with a higher risk of recurrent anterior shoulder instability and/or dislocation after index dislocation.

   (b) Demographics at risk include younger age, male sex, and activity level (i.e., participation in contact/collision sports).

   (c) Associated pathology about the shoulder—glenoid fractures, Hill-Sachs lesions, and capsuloligamentous injury—also contribute.

   (d) While reported early on in a randomized trial by Kirkley et al. in 1999 [8], prospective and randomized trials have continued to demonstrate that patients with these risk factors have reduced rates of recurrence if treated with surgery after their first dislocation [9–13].

(e) A recent meta-analysis of ten prospective studies consisting of 569 patients following first-time anterior shoulder instability reported an overall 67.4% rate of recurrent instability following nonoperative treatment compared with 9.7% following arthroscopic Bankart repair, a sevenfold decrease [14].

(f) Without surgical treatment, a recurrent instability event can result in more severe damage to the labrum, cartilage, capsule, humeral head, glenoid, and surrounding soft tissue, making future surgery more difficult.

(g) In our practice, contact/collision athletes and military personnel are offered surgery after a first-time dislocation, as they have a very high risk of re-dislocation without surgery.

(h) The surgical outcomes are also typically better when the shoulder has dislocated fewer times (ideally only once).

10. Principles of Arthroscopic Bankart Repair

(a) Typically, the first-line surgical treatment for anterior glenohumeral instability is to perform a Bankart repair. The goal of this surgery is to strengthen the damaged anterior capsular-labral complex.

(b) Robins et al. studied football players following anterior and/or posterior shoulder instability surgery from seven PAC-12 programs. They found 82.4% return to play in anterior stabilization surgeries. Overall, 15.6% sustained additional shoulder injury, and 10.3% necessitated reduction or revision surgery [15].

(c) Figure 5.8 shows the steps of an arthroscopic anterior stabilization surgery for a collision athlete with a first-time anterior shoulder dislocation.

(d) Pearls and Pitfalls of arthroscopic anterior shoulder stabilization are discussed in Table 5.3.

(e) Augmenting stability in arthroscopic shoulder stabilization:
- Remplissage: This involves placing suture anchors into the Hill-Sachs deformity and arthroscopically tenodesing the infraspinatus into the Hill-Sachs deformity [16]. This is particularly effective and indicated when there is a humeral Hill-Sachs deformity present but minimal glenoid bone loss.
- Rotator interval closure: This involves arthroscopically closing the rotator interval, which can limit external rotation and further tighten the shoulder capsule [17]. This is effective in shoulders where the anterior instability is caused in part by global laxity or MDI.
- Posterior plication or a "7 o'clock" anchor: Tightening the posterior shoulder capsule is also an option in higher risk arthroscopic stabilization or in shoulders with patulous inferior capsule [18].

11. Risk Factors for Failure of Arthroscopic Anterior Shoulder Stabilization

(a) Hyperlaxity of the shoulder, young age, bone loss of the glenoid or humeral head, and number of dislocation or instability events should be considered.

(b) The Instability Severity Index (ISIS) score, first published by Balg and Boileau in 2007 [19], was created to predict failure of arthroscopic anterior shoulder stabilization surgery based on preoperative patient factors/demographics, physical examination findings, and radiographic findings (Table 5.4).

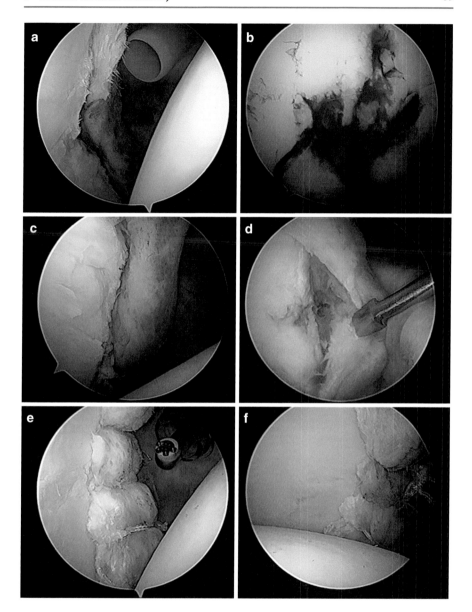

**Fig. 5.8** Arthroscopic Bankart repair. (**a**) Posterior portal view of acute Bankart tear. (**b**) Posterior portal view of acute Hill-Sachs deformity with hemorrhage and cartilage damage of the posterosuperior humeral head. (**c**) Bankart tear viewed from anterosuperior portal. (**d**) Bankart tear viewed from anterosuperior portal while labrum is mobilized via an elevator through the anterior portal. Mobilizing the labrum to an anatomic position is one of the most critical steps of arthroscopic Bankart repair. (**e**) Completed Arthroscopic Bankart repair viewed from posterior portal with reattachment of labrum and plication of capsule with a combination of traditional and knotless suture anchors. (**f**) Completed Arthroscopic Bankart repair viewed from anterosuperior portal

**Table 5.3** Pitfalls and technical pearls of arthroscopic anterior stabilization in the beach chair position

| Pearl | Pitfall |
|---|---|
| Accurate cannula placement for anterior and anterolateral working portals | Rapid placement of patient in beach chair position and inadequate maintenance of blood pressure for cerebral perfusion |
| Visualize from anteriorly while mobilizing labrum from neck of glenoid | Failure to identify associated pathology |
| A properly mobilized labrum will "float" into anatomic position | Performing arthroscopic stabilization in the setting of severe glenoid or humeral bone loss |
| Use three or more suture anchors, low on the glenoid ("3 below 3:00") and slightly on the glenoid face to avoid a medial repair | Inadequate mobilization of capsule and labrum resulting in inadequate reduction of tissue and poor restoration of labral anatomy |
| Trans-subscapularis access can allow placement of lowest (5:30) anchor; posterior traction can assist in placing this anchor | Inability to place inferior-most anchor at the 5:30 position |
| Grasp capsule and labral tissue lower than each anchor | Mechanical abrasion of knots on glenohumeral cartilage |
| Tie knots on the capsular side, restoring bumper effect and avoiding abrasion | |

*Used with permission from Chambers L, Kremen T, Snell C, et al. Arthroscopic Anterior Shoulder Stabilization in the Beach Chair Position Using Trans-Subscapularis Drilling of the 5: 30 Anchor. Techniques in Shoulder and Elbow Surgery 2011; 12: 60*

**Table 5.4** Instability Severity Index Score (ISIS)

| Prognostic factors | | Points |
|---|---|---|
| Age at surgery | ≤20 years | 2 |
| | >20 years | 0 |
| Sport participation | Competitive | 2 |
| | Recreational or none | 0 |
| Type of sport | Contact or overhead throwing | 1 |
| | Non-contact, non-throwing, or none | 0 |
| Hyperlaxity | Anterior or inferior shoulder hyperlaxity | 1 |
| | No hyperlaxity | 0 |
| Humeral head on AP radiographs | Hill-Sachs in external rotation | 2 |
| | No Hill-Sachs in external rotation | 0 |
| Glenoid on AP radiographs | Loss of contour of glenoid | 2 |
| | No loss of contour | 0 |
| Total | | X/10 |

*Adapted from Di Giacomo G, Peebles LA, Pugliese M, et al. Glenoid Track Instability Management Score: Radiographic Modification of the Instability Severity Index Score. Arthroscopy. 2020 Jan;36(1):56–67*

(c) A score of six or less was associated with recurrence risk of 10%, thus making arthroscopic repair a viable option. Seven or more points was associated with recurrence risk of 70%, in which case open stabilization was recommended [19].

(d) Patients with high risk for failure after arthroscopic repair should be considered for either primary open Bankart repair or primary Bristow/Latarjet procedure.

**Table 5.5** Risk factors for failure of arthroscopic anterior stabilization

| Patient-related factors | Surgeon-related factors |
| --- | --- |
| Generalized hyperlaxity | Failure to recognize contraindications to arthroscopic stabilization |
| Inferior hyperlaxity | Failure to place anchors low on the glenoid (e.g., 5:30 position) |
| Increased number of previous dislocations | Failure to adequately mobilize the Bankart lesion |
| Large Hill-Sachs deformity | Placement of suture anchors medially rather than on the face of glenoid |
| Anteroinferior glenoid bone loss | Use of fewer than 3 suture anchors |
| Previous attempt at stabilization | Inappropriate rehabilitation |
| Return to contact/collision athletics | |

*Used with permission from Chambers L, Kremen T, Snell C, et al. Arthroscopic Anterior Shoulder Stabilization in the Beach Chair Position Using Trans-Subscapularis Drilling of the 5: 30 Anchor. Techniques in Shoulder and Elbow Surgery 2011; 12: 60*

    (e) Patient and surgeon factors that contribute to failure following arthroscopic repair can be found in Table 5.5.

12. Arthroscopic Versus Open Stabilization Surgery

    (a) In patients with high risk of recurrent instability, open Bankart repair has historically had a lower failure rate than arthroscopic stabilization, as it confers increased stability. Arthroscopic repair may be associated with greater rates of recurrent instability.

    (b) Pagnani et al. studied 58 football players, all of whom had recurrent instability following arthroscopic Bankart repair and subsequently underwent open repair. Following open repair, only 3.4% had recurrent subluxation, none had recurrent dislocation, range of motion was nearly preserved, and 90% returned to play [20].

    (c) However, in the United States, arthroscopic Bankart repair remains the surgery of choice for anterior instability without bone loss due to training bias and patient preference [21], despite cited failure rates from 5% to 30% especially in contact/collision athletes [22–24].

    (d) In addition to patient and surgeon preference, an arthroscopic approach is associated in some studies with less soft tissue insult, shorter operative times, preserved shoulder range of motion, and even comparable clinical outcomes [25].

    (e) Given this and despite the failure rate, arthroscopic Bankart repair remains a viable treatment option, particularly in patients without bone loss and low number of instability events.

    (f) Revision arthroscopic stabilization surgery should only be used in the setting of a technical failure of the first operation or a traumatic failure of a well-functioning anterior stabilization surgery with high quality labrum *and without significant glenoid or humeral bone loss.*

13. Bristow/Latarjet Procedure for Bone Loss in Anterior Instability
    (a) Significant glenoid and/or humeral bone loss is a relative contraindication
        for arthroscopic stabilization. Thorough history taking will typically tip off
        the surgeon as to those patients with glenoid bone loss, large Hill-Sachs
        deformities, or both.
    (b) Typically, the patients will have the following characteristics, which are
        clues for bone loss associated with anterior shoulder instability:
        • Failed one or more shoulder instability operations
        • Numerous dislocations (more than five)
        • Increasingly easy dislocations and relocations without the need for the
          emergency room
        • Midrange instability: shoulder dislocates without abduction and exter-
          nal rotation
        • Mechanical symptoms
        • Seizure disorder
        • Dislocating during sleep
    (c) Surgeries used in anterior stabilization involving bone loss, both in the past
        and at present include:
        • Putti-Platt—Subscapularis shortening procedure to limit external rota-
          tion [26]. No longer frequently used, predictably causes arthritis in the
          shoulder.
        • Magnussen-Stack—Lesser tuberosity transfer from medial to biceps
          groove to lateral to biceps groove to limit external rotation [27]. No
          longer frequently used, predictably causes arthritis in the shoulder.
        • Latarjet—Two screw coracoid transfer with the conjoined tendon.
        • Bristow—One screw coracoid transfer (smaller amount of bone trans-
          ferred) with the conjoined tendon.
        • Eden-Hybbinette—Conjoined tendon transfer without bone [28].
        • Distal tibial allograft—The articular surface of the distal tibia happens
          to match up well with the congruity of the glenoid and therefore the
          distal tibia allograft is a useful salvage operation [29].
        • Distal clavicle autograft—The ipsilateral distal clavicle can be used for
          a graft source in glenoid bone loss [30].
        • Iliac crest bone graft—The ipsilateral anterior iliac crest is a good graft
          source in salvage glenoid bone loss surgery [31].
        • The Latarjet coracoid transfer is the most commonly utilized of these
          operations for primary bone loss surgery and revision of failed
          arthroscopic surgery. We consider Latarjet as a primary surgery in those
          athletes with more than 12.5% glenoid bone loss.
          – First introduced by Michel Latarjet in 1954 [32], it has since been
            refined and adapted to remain frequently used today. It involves
            transferring part of the coracoid and its muscular attachments to the
            anterior aspect of the glenoid to promote increased stability of the
            glenohumeral joint via both a bony block and musculotendi-
            nous sling.

- This operation is successful in restoring stability to shoulders with bone loss from 15% to 25% on the glenoid quite predictably, with a recurrent instability occurring in less than 5% of patients with high rates of patient satisfaction [33–35].
- The complication rate is much higher than in arthroscopic stabilization surgery (15–30%), including infection, recurrent instability, neurologic injury (musculocutaneous, radial, or axillary nerves), nonunion, resorption, graft malposition, screw fracture, and graft fracture [36, 37].
- The key steps of a Latarjet are critical to know. Figure 5.9 illustrates typical imaging of a patient before and after Latarjet coracoid transfer (Box 5.3).

---

**Box 5.3 Latarjet Coracoid Transfer Steps**
1. Expose coracoid through deltopectoral interval
2. Release coracoacromial ligament and pectoralis minor
3. Osteotomize coracoid process with a bent saw from medial to lateral
4. Flatten coracoid and prepare with two drill holes
5. Subscapularis split at junction of upper 2/3 and lower 1/3 of muscle belly at joint line
6. Expose capsule, capsulotomy, and insert humeral head retractor (e.g., Fukuda)
7. Resect labrum and freshen bone
8. Drill hole at 5 pm on glenoid 7 mm medial to articular surface as parallel as possible to joint
9. Fixate coracoid to bone inferiorly
10. Drill upper screw through coracoid and place second screw
11. Close capsule to CA ligament remnant

---

14. Return to Sport After Instability Surgery
    (a) Typically, immobilization after an instability operation is for 1 month, followed by 3 months of physical therapy and 2 months of weight lifting.
    (b) We prefer near full range of motion and near full strength prior to return to play.
15. Summary
    (a) Anterior shoulder instability is a common condition resulting from trauma typically in the abducted externally rotated position.
    (b) Closed reduction and immobilization followed by physical therapy can result in clinical success in the non-athlete.
    (c) A rotator cuff tear should be ruled out in any shoulder dislocation patient over the age of 40 with an MRI scan.

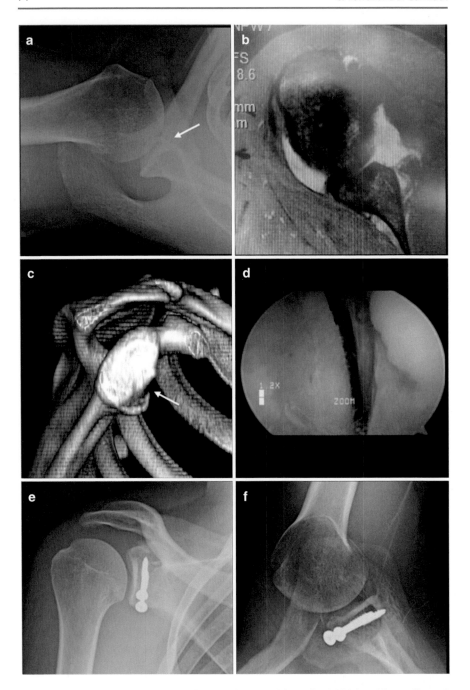

**Fig. 5.9** Imaging findings before and after Latarjet coracoid transfer. (**a**) Plain axillary radiograph of patient with anterior glenoid bone loss. (**b**) Axillary MRI arthrogram of patient with anterior glenoid bone loss. (**c**) Three-dimensional CT scan of patient with anteroinferior glenoid bone loss and inverted pear glenoid. (**d**) Arthroscopic image viewed from posterior portal of engaging Hill-Sachs deformity and antero-inferior glenoid bone loss. (**e**) Grashey view post-Latarjet coracoid transfer. (**f**) Axillary view post-Latarjet coracoid transfer

(d) A collision athlete who regains full range of motion with good strength and without apprehension can return to play the same season; however, a second instability event results in a surgical discussion, and surgery is typically recommended at the end of the season regardless.

(e) Based on data from randomized trials, collision and contact athletes, as well as military personnel, are probably better treated with initial stabilization surgery rather than nonoperative management.

(f) Open stabilization surgery historically has a slightly lower failure rate for cases of re-dislocation or recurrent instability when compared to arthroscopic stabilization, but it is much less common in the United States.

(g) Generalized laxity, young age, bone loss, collision athletics, and a high number of dislocations are the main risk factors for re-dislocation after stabilization surgery.

(h) Failed stabilization surgery and bone loss on the glenoid side are the main indications for Latarjet coracoid transfer surgery.

## References

1. Thomas SC, Matsen FA III. An approach to the repair of avulsion of the glenohumeral ligaments in the management of traumatic anterior glenohumeral instability. J Bone Joint Surg Am. 1989;71:506–13.
2. Kuhn JE. A new classification system for shoulder instability. Br J Sports Med. 2010;44:341–6. https://doi.org/10.1136/bjsm.2009.071183.
3. Itoi E, Hatakeyama Y, Kido T, et al. A new method of immobilization after traumatic anterior dislocation of the shoulder: a preliminary study. J Shoulder Elb Surg. 2003;12:413–5. https://doi.org/10.1016/s1058-2746(03)00171-x.
4. Finestone A, Milgrom C, Radeva-Petrova DR, et al. Bracing in external rotation for traumatic anterior dislocation of the shoulder. J Bone Joint Surg (Br). 2009;91:918–21. https://doi.org/10.1302/0301-620X.91B7.22263.
5. Owens BD, Agel J, Mountcastle SB, et al. Incidence of glenohumeral instability in collegiate athletics. Am J Sports Med. 2009;37:1750–4. https://doi.org/10.1177/0363546509334591.
6. Buss DD, Lynch GP, Meyer CP, et al. Nonoperative management for in-season athletes with anterior shoulder instability. Am J Sports Med. 2004;32:1430–3. https://doi.org/10.1177/0363546503262069.
7. Dickens JF, Owens BD, Cameron KL, et al. Return to play and recurrent instability after in-season anterior shoulder instability: a prospective multicenter study. Am J Sports Med. 2014;42:2842–50. https://doi.org/10.1177/0363546514553181.
8. Kirkley A, Griffin S, Richards C, et al. Prospective randomized clinical trial comparing the effectiveness of immediate arthroscopic stabilization versus immobilization and rehabilitation in first traumatic anterior dislocations of the shoulder. Arthroscopy. 1999;15:507–14. https://doi.org/10.1053/ar.1999.v15.015050.
9. Bottoni CR, Wilckens JH, DeBerardino TM, et al. A prospective, randomized evaluation of arthroscopic stabilization versus nonoperative treatment in patients with acute, traumatic, first-time shoulder dislocations. Am J Sports Med. 2002;30:576–80. https://doi.org/10.1177/03635465020300041801.
10. Jakobsen BW, Johannsen HV, Suder P, et al. Primary repair versus conservative treatment of first-time traumatic anterior dislocation of the shoulder: a randomized study with 10-year follow-up. Arthroscopy. 2007;23:118–23. https://doi.org/10.1016/j.arthro.2006.11.004.

11. Kirkley A, Werstine R, Ratjek A, et al. Prospective randomized clinical trial comparing the effectiveness of immediate arthroscopic stabilization versus immobilization and rehabilitation in first traumatic anterior dislocations of the shoulder: long-term evaluation. Arthroscopy. 2005;21:55–63. https://doi.org/10.1016/j.arthro.2004.09.018.

12. De Carli A, Vadala AP, Lanzetti R, et al. Early surgical treatment of first-time anterior glenohumeral dislocation in a young, active population is superior to conservative management at long-term follow-up. Int Orthop. 2019;43:2799–805. https://doi.org/10.1007/s00264-019-04382-2.

13. Gigis I, Heikenfeld R, Kapinas A, et al. Arthroscopic versus conservative treatment of first anterior dislocation of the shoulder in adolescents. J Pediatr Orthop. 2014;34:421–5. https://doi.org/10.1097/BPO.0000000000000108.

14. Hurley ET, Manjunath AK, Bloom DA, et al. Arthroscopic Bankart repair versus conservative management for first-time traumatic anterior shoulder instability: a systematic review and meta-analysis. Arthroscopy. 2020;36:2526–32. https://doi.org/10.1016/j.arthro.2020.04.046.

15. Robins RJ, Daruwalla JH, Gamradt SC, et al. Return to play after shoulder instability surgery in National Collegiate Athletic Association Division I Intercollegiate Football Athletes. Am J Sports Med. 2017;45:2329–35. https://doi.org/10.1177/0363546517705635.

16. Camp CL, Dahm DL, Krych AJ. Arthroscopic remplissage for engaging Hill-Sachs lesions in patients with anterior shoulder instability. Arthrosc Tech. 2015;4:e499–502. https://doi.org/10.1016/j.eats.2015.05.003.

17. Frank RM, Golijanan P, Gross DJ, et al. The arthroscopic rotator interval closure: why, when, and how? Oper Tech Sports Med. 2014;22:48–57. https://doi.org/10.1053/j.otsm.2014.02.005.

18. Wolf EM, Eakin CL. Arthroscopic capsular plication for posterior shoulder instability. Arthroscopy. 1998;14:153–63. https://doi.org/10.1016/s0749-8063(98)70034-9.

19. Balg F, Boileau P. The instability severity index score. A simple pre-operative score to select patients for arthroscopic or open shoulder stabilisation. J Bone Joint Surg (Br). 2007;89:1470–7. https://doi.org/10.1302/0301-620X.89B11.18962.

20. Pagnani MJ, Dome DC. Surgical treatment of traumatic anterior shoulder instability in American football players. J Bone Joint Surg Am. 2002;84:711–5. https://doi.org/10.2106/00004623-200205000-00002.

21. Zhang AL, Montgomery SR, Ngo SS, et al. Arthroscopic versus open shoulder stabilization: current practice patterns in the United States. Arthroscopy. 2014;30:436–43. https://doi.org/10.1016/j.arthro.2013.12.013.

22. Ee GW, Mohamed S, Tan AH. Long term results of arthroscopic Bankart repair for traumatic anterior shoulder instability. J Orthop Surg Res. 2011;6:28. https://doi.org/10.1186/1749-799X-6-28.

23. Panzram B, Kentar Y, Maier M, et al. Mid-term to long-term results of primary arthroscopic Bankart repair for traumatic anterior shoulder instability: a retrospective study. BMC Musculoskelet Disord. 2020;21:191. https://doi.org/10.1186/s12891-020-03223-3.

24. Tordjman D, Vidal C, Fontes D. Mid-term results of arthroscopic Bankart repair: a review of 31 cases. Orthop Traumatol Surg Res. 2016;102:541–8. https://doi.org/10.1016/j.otsr.2016.04.013.

25. Bottoni CR, Smith EL, Berkowitz MJ, et al. Arthroscopic versus open shoulder stabilization for recurrent anterior instability: a prospective randomized clinical trial. Am J Sports Med. 2006;34:1730–7. https://doi.org/10.1177/0363546506288239.

26. Truchly G, Thompson WA. Simplified Putti-Platt procedure. JAMA. 1962;179:859–62. https://doi.org/10.1001/jama.1962.03050110027005.

27. Miller LS, Donahue JR, Good RP, et al. The Magnuson-Stack procedure for treatment of recurrent glenohumeral dislocations. Am J Sports Med. 1984;12:133–7. https://doi.org/10.1177/036354658401200208.

28. Villatte G, Spurr S, Broden C, et al. The Eden-Hybbinette procedure is one hundred years old! A historical view of the concept and its evolutions. Int Orthop. 2018;42:2491–5. https://doi.org/10.1007/s00264-018-3970-3.

29. Provencher MT, Frank RM, Golijanin P, et al. Distal tibia allograft glenoid reconstruction in recurrent anterior shoulder instability: clinical and radiographic outcomes. Arthroscopy. 2017;33:891–7. https://doi.org/10.1016/j.arthro.2016.09.029.
30. Tokish JM, Fitzpatrick K, Cook JB, et al. Arthroscopic distal clavicular autograft for treating shoulder instability with glenoid bone loss. Arthrosc Tech. 2014;3:e475–81. https://doi.org/10.1016/j.eats.2014.05.006.
31. Malahias MA, Chytas D, Raoulis V, et al. Iliac Crest bone grafting for the management of anterior shoulder instability in patients with glenoid bone loss: a systematic review of contemporary literature. Sports Med Open. 2020;6:12. https://doi.org/10.1186/s40798-020-0240-x.
32. Latarjet M. A propos du traitement des luxations réecidivante de l'épaule. Lyon Chir. 1954;49:994–1003.
33. Walch G, Boileau P. Latarjet-Bristow procedure for recurrent anterior instability. Tech Should Elbow Surg. 2000;1:256–61. https://doi.org/10.1097/00132589-200001040-00008.
34. Hovelius L, Sandstrom B, Olofsson A, et al. The effect of capsular repair, bone block healing, and position on the results of the Bristow-Latarjet procedure (study III): long-term follow-up in 319 shoulders. J Shoulder Elb Surg. 2012;21:647–60. https://doi.org/10.1016/j.jse.2011.03.020.
35. Imam MA, Shehata MSA, Martin A, et al. Repair versus Latarjet Procedure for recurrent anterior shoulder instability: a systematic review and meta-analysis of 3275 shoulders. Am J Sports Med. 2020;49:1945. https://doi.org/10.1177/0363546520962082.
36. Shah AA, Butler RB, Romanowski J, et al. Short-term complications of the Latarjet procedure. J Bone Joint Surg Am. 2012;94:495–501. https://doi.org/10.2106/JBJS.J.01830.
37. Gupta A, Delaney R, Petkin K, et al. Complications of the Latarjet procedure. Curr Rev Musculoskelet Med. 2015;8:59–66. https://doi.org/10.1007/s12178-015-9258-y.

# Posterior Instability

Ryan Bicknell

## Introduction

- Posterior shoulder instability is often a challenging condition to diagnose and treat.
- Posterior instability makes up only 5% of cases of shoulder instability [1, 2].

1. **History**
   (a) Posterior shoulder instability usually presents with one of two presentations: acute traumatic dislocations and recurrent posterior instability.
   - **Acute Posterior Dislocations**
     – This usually presents following a traumatic episode with the shoulder in a flexed, adducted, and internally rotated position.
     – A classic example is a football player who sustains a posterior dislocation while blocking (i.e., lineman).
   (b) Other common presentations include electrocution and with seizure activity.
   - **Recurrent Posterior Instability**
     – This usually presents with deep pain within the posterior aspect of the shoulder [1, 3].
     – This is usually associated with worsening athletic performance and endurance [4, 5].
     – However, this can present with vague symptoms, so keep high index of clinical suspicion for posterior shoulder instability [6].

R. Bicknell (✉)
Shoulder and Elbow Surgery, Surgery and Mechanical and Materials Engineering, Kingston Health Sciences Centre, Kingston General Hospital Site - Watkins 3, Queen's University, Kingston, ON, Canada
e-mail: Ryan.Bicknell@kingstonhsc.ca

- This is often associated with repetitive microtrauma, including repetitive bench press, overhead weight lifting, rowing, swimming, and blocking linemen in football.
- Also, a predisposition in patients with generalized ligamentous laxity, with a gradual presentation of pain and sensation of instability.
- Finally, this can occasionally be a symptom of voluntary instability, including positional subluxation in a provocative position.

2. **Physical Examination**
   (a) **Inspection/Palpation**
   - With acute dislocation, shoulder often positioned in internal rotation with a prominent coracoid process and posterior fulness in the axilla [7].
   - Crepitus is sometimes noted with internal rotation [1].
   (b) **ROM**
   - With acute dislocation, there may be a block to external rotation and forward elevation.
   - With forward elevation, internal rotation patient may subjectively or objectively become unstable.
   (c) **Strength Testing**
   - Cuff strength testing is usually symmetric to contralateral shoulder.
   (d) **Directed Tests**
   - **Jerk Test** [8]
     - The patient is standing or seated.
     - The examiner stands next to the affected shoulder and grasps the elbow in one hand and the distal clavicle and scapular spine in the other.
     - The arm is placed in a flexed and internally rotated position and the flexed elbow is pushed posteriorly while the shoulder girdle is pushed anteriorly.
     - This causes the humeral head to subluxate posteriorly.
     - The arm is then slowing horizontally abducted, and the test result is positive when a sudden jerk associated with pain occurs as the subluxated humeral head relocates into the glenoid fossa.
   - **Kim Test** [9]
     - The patient is seated, with the arm in 90° of abduction.
     - With one hand, the examiner grasps the patient's elbow; with the other hand, the examiner grasps the lateral aspect of the patient's proximal arm, applying an axial loading force.
     - While elevating the patient's arm to 45°, the examiner applies a downward and posterior force to the upper arm.
     - A sudden onset of pain signifies a positive test result.
     - The combination of positive Kim and Jerk test results reportedly had 97% sensitivity for posterior instability [9].
   - **Posterior Stress Test** [10]
     - The patient is in a seated position.

- While stabilizing the medial border of the scapula, the examiner uses her or his free hand to apply a posterior force to the arm while it is held in a 90° forward flexed, adducted, and internally rotated position.
- A positive test result occurs with subluxation or dislocation, with reproduction of the patient's pain or apprehension.
- **Load and Shift Test** [11]
  - The patient is in a supine position with the symptomatic arm in approximately 20° of forward flexion and abduction.
  - The humeral head is then loaded while anterior and posterior stresses are applied.
  - The direction and amount of translation is then graded.
- **Sulcus Sign**
  - The patient is seated with the arm at the side in a neutral position.
  - The examiner grasps the patient's elbow or wrist and applies downward traction while observing the shoulder for a sulcus (depression) lateral or inferior to the acromion.
  - The sulcus sign suggests inferior glenohumeral instability; however, excessive inferior translation of the humerus on the glenoid is often associated with posterior subluxation and may indicate bidirectional or multidirectional instability when the inferior sulcus test reproduces the patient's symptoms.
  - Suggests rotator interval insufficiency.

3. **Imaging**
   (a) **X-rays**
      - AP (Grashey) view—A posterior dislocation is often missed on this view. Some indirect signs that can be seen include a light bulb sign and a trough line (Fig. 6.1a, b).
      - Scapular Y view—A posterior dislocation is often missed on this view (Fig. 6.1c).
      - Axillary view—This is essential for diagnosis as a posterior dislocation can often be missed on other views (Fig. 6.1d).
   (b) **MRI**
      - Important for assessment of soft tissue injuries.
      - In an irreducible dislocation, can aid in diagnosis of responsible structure, most commonly rotator cuff, capsule, or long head of biceps.
      - MR arthrography: essential for recurrent instability to assess posterior capsulolabral complex, SLAP tears, and rotator cuff tears [1, 4, 6, 12–14].
   (c) **CT Scan**
      - With 3D reconstructions and humeral head subtraction—Essential for assessment of associated fractures and quantification of glenoid bone loss or retroversion and reverse Hill-Sachs impaction (Fig. 6.2a, b).
      - Reverse Hill-Sachs lesions with posterior shoulder dislocation are common, seen in up to 89% in one series of 36 patients, while reverse Bankart lesion incidence is 60% in the same series [3].

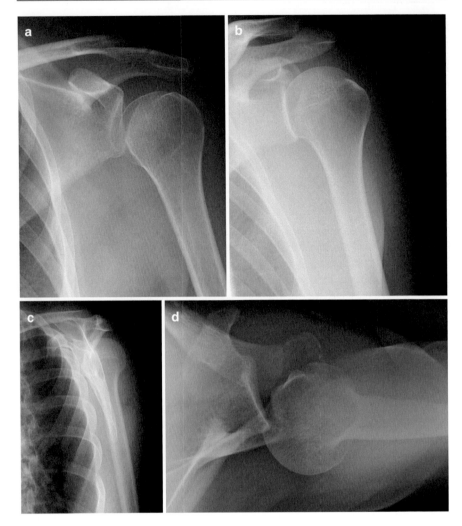

**Fig. 6.1** X-rays: (**a**) An AP X-ray shows a trough line, a dense vertical line in the medial humeral head due to impaction of the humeral head. (**b**) An AP X-ray shows a light bulb sign, due to fixed internal rotation of the humeral head which takes on a rounded appearance. (**c**) A posterior dislocation is often missed on a scapular Y X-ray. (**d**) An axillary X-ray shows a posterior dislocation with a reverse Hill-Sachs lesion

4. **Treatment**
    (a) The decision on the definitive management must be based on several factors:
        • Patient age
        • Duration of the dislocation event or instability symptoms
        • Patient's functional level
        • Risk of recurrence—based on clinical findings such as bone defects, presence of multiple ligamentous laxity (MDI), and comorbidities

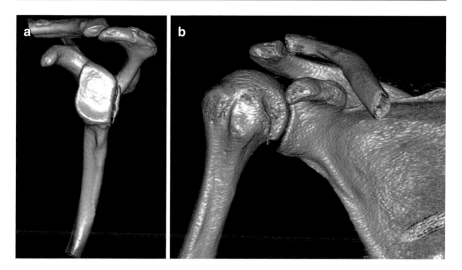

**Fig. 6.2** CT scan: (**a**) A CT scan with 3D reconstruction and humeral head subtraction shows posterior glenoid bone loss. (**b**) A CT scan with 3D reconstruction shows a reverse Hill-Sachs impaction fracture

(b) **Nonoperative Treatment**
  • **Patient Considerations**
    – Important to consider medical optimization of patient's seizures as part of nonoperative management or presurgical management [15].
    – Even with a locked dislocation, in older patients with impaired cognitive function and reasonable motion, nonoperative management can be considered [7, 15–17].
    – A patient with a single traumatic dislocation is at risk of recurrent dislocation especially with large bone defect or ligamentous laxity.
    – However, it is still unclear if immediate surgical intervention is indicated versus a trial of nonoperative management [6, 18].
    – In general, the presence of large bone defect, either reverse Hill-Sachs or reverse Bankart lesion, is suggestive for surgical intervention even if it is first time dislocation [18].
    – The aim of nonsurgical management is pain control, restoring shoulder stability and mobility, and maintaining the shoulder reduced in an anatomic position [6].
  • **Closed Reduction**
    – Careful imaging prior to closed reduction is crucial to prevent further shoulder injury (specifically humeral head or neck fractures).
    – Requires complete sedation and muscle relaxation to avoid any forceful movement [6, 7, 16].
    – Needs to be done in timely fashion, preferably less than 3 weeks [6, 7, 16].
    – Performed with gentle longitudinal traction.

- If the humeral head is locked behind the glenoid rim, shoulder adduction, anterior flexion, and internal rotation may help to stretch posterior shoulder capsule and disengaging the humeral head.
- Then progressive and gentle shoulder manipulation to external rotation and extension with anteriorly directed pressure on the humeral head to reduce the joint.
- Next, the shoulder joint stability is assessed through gentle range of motion.
- If the shoulder is stable in internal rotation, the shoulder can be kept immobilized in neutral rotation; otherwise, keeping the shoulder in 20° of external rotation is preferred [16].
- Immobilization for 6 weeks to prevent internal rotation.

- **Rehabilitation**
  - Passive ROM to full active ROM is the target between 6 and 12 weeks.
  - Strengthening exercises are concentrating on rotator cuff muscles, deltoid, and periscapular muscles which usually begin at 3 months.
  - The patient can return to sports once able to have full ROM, appropriate muscle strength, and coordination without signs of shoulder instability which usually take 9–12 months [6, 19].
  - Further rehabilitation focuses on proprioception exercises, strengthening the posterior deltoid and external rotators [6, 16], maintaining the scapula in neutral rotation by strengthening serratus and lower trapezius with pectoralis and latissimus stretching to prevent scapula anterior winging, as well as humeral head posterior translation which will keep the glenohumeral joint concentric in the joint [20].
  - Also, the patient should avoid any activity that causes worsening instability symptoms [6, 16].

(c) **Operative Treatment**

- **Open Reduction**
  - Can be performed by either an anterior or posterior approach based on patient findings and surgeon preference [1, 7, 16].
  - **Anterior approach**
    A standard deltopectoral approach.
    Conjoint tendon may be tight which can be eased by shoulder flexion, release, or tenotomy.
    The joint can often be exposed by opening the rotator interval.
    Then, the glenohumeral joint is reduced under direct vision either manually or by using a cobb or any appropriate instrument.
    If not reducible, a formal arthrotomy is necessary.
    The subscapularis tendon is managed either by a horizontal split or a formal release (i.e., tenotomy, peel, or lesser tuberosity osteotomy).
    After humeral head reduction, direct assessment of the humeral head can occur.
    The shoulder joint is tested for stability through a range of motion.

An isolated open reduction may lead to a stable shoulder, especially in reverse Hill-Sachs lesion less than 20% [7, 16].

– **Posterior approach**

Alternatively, a posterior shoulder approach can be performed with a vertical incision from mid posterior acromion to posterior axillary fold.

Careful inferior dissection in to avoid axillary nerve injury.

Then, the deltoid is elevated superiorly to expose infraspinatus tendon (IT).

A horizontal split or vertical tenotomy of IT can be performed or the interval between IT and teres minor can be used.

Then, a horizontal or vertical capsulotomy is used to expose the joint [21].

- **Arthroscopic Posterior Shoulder Stabilization**
  – Contraindicated in large glenoid defect more than 25%, or reverse Hill-Sachs more than 30% as those lesions may be better to be managed with an open technique.
  – Failure of previous arthroscopic stabilization is considered a relative contraindication.
  – Arthroscopic stabilization can be performed in either the beach chair or lateral decubitus position based on surgeon preference.
  – Examination under anesthesia (EUA) is useful to assess the degree and direction of instability and comparison with the contralateral shoulder.
  – Diagnostic arthroscopy is performed through a standard posterior portal.
  – After establishing the anterior portal and lateral portals, a posterolateral 7 o'clock portal is created with a spinal needle just posterior and inferior to posterior viewing portal to access posterior inferior aspect of glenoid.
  – Inferior labral repair is better to be addressed first due to small repair space and difficult access.
  – Then, the remaining area should be repaired anterior to posterior.
  – It is usually enough to have 3–4 suture anchor; however, the surgeon should assess the labrum as extensive repair may be required in some cases.
  – Capsular rasp, shaver, and burr are used to prepare the bone before an anchor insertion.
  – Capsular plication is an additional procedure that can be done in patients with excessive laxity.
  – It is critical to be careful in the 5–7 o'clock positions which is close to the axillary nerve.
  – The surgeon must be aware of postoperative stiffness secondary to excessive soft tissue tensioning during plication.

- Finally, rotator interval closure may be added when the shoulder is still unstable after labral stabilization and plication; however, the role of this procedure is still controversial [6, 19–21].

(d) **Open Posterior Shoulder Stabilization**
- Indicated in irreducible shoulder with minimal reverse Hill-Sachs or recurrent shoulder subluxation.
- Posterior shoulder approach is used to reduce the shoulder and access the reverse Bankart lesion.
- Similar labral repair is performed as explained in the previous section.
- The capsulotomy can be performed either T-capsulotomy or H-capsulotomy to allow for capsular shift as an additional procedure in patients with laxity [21].

(e) **Glenoid Bone Augmentation**
- Indicated in the setting of significant glenoid bone defect (>20%) [6].
- Iliac crest bone autograft (ICBG), distal clavicle autograft, or distal tibial allograft (DTA) are commonly used.
- DTA is an appealing alternative to ICBG as it shows better contact area, similar peak force, and normal glenoid contact pressure in a biomechanical study [22].
- Furthermore, DTA is an osteochondral bone graft and lack of donor site morbidity.
- Can be done arthroscopically or through an open posterior shoulder approach [23, 24].

(f) **Opening Wedge Glenoid Osteotomy**
- May be indicated in severe congenital glenoid retroversion >20°.
- The medial aspect of the glenoid is accessed through the posterior approach.
- The osteotomy is made based on the required retroversion correction.
- An ICBG is press-fit in the osteotomy site and can be fixed with an additional screw if necessary [1].
- Controversial, since Galvin et al. showed no difference in the outcome of arthroscopic stabilization in patients with glenoid dysplasia (14°) compared with normal glenoid version [25].

(g) **Reverse Hill-Sachs Remplissage**
- For smaller lesions, less than 20%.
- Similar to an infraspinatus remplissage in anterior instability, this involves filling the defect arthroscopically with subscapularis tendon using suture anchors.
- A 70° arthroscope can be helpful to better visualize the defect as well as subscapularis tendon.
- After diagnostic arthroscopy, the lesion is identified and prepared by using arthroscopic burr to reach subchondral bone to increase the chance of healing.
- Two suture anchors are placed from inferior to superior through the anterior superior portal.

- A suture-passing device is used to pass stitches through the tendon and tied in a mattress configuration [26].
- (h) **McLaughlin Procedure**
  - For lesions, 20–40%.
  - The subscapularis tendon is lifted off its origin and transposed into the humeral impression [7, 27].
  - Can also be performed with an osteotomy of lesser tuberosity (modified McLaughlin), which provides a better defect filling compared with tendon alone [28, 29].
- (i) **Rotational Humeral Osteotomy**
  - For lesions, 20–40%.
  - Rarely performed.
  - The humeral shaft is internally rotated and stabilized with a fixed angle device.
  - The rationale behind this osteotomy is to rotate the humeral defect anteriorly and facilitate shoulder ROM by moving the defect away from the glenoid.
  - The advantages of rotational osteotomy are sustaining the shoulder congruity with stable fixation, and immediate postoperative rehabilitation.
  - However, this procedure limits the shoulder external rotation [30].
- (j) **Humeral Head Bone Graft Reconstruction**
  - For defect size >40%.
  - Bone graft can be either ICBG autograft or allograft (humeral or femoral head) [31–33].
  - Fixed with headless screws or retrograde screw fixation.
- (k) **Shoulder Arthroplasty**
  - For defect size >40%.
  - Indicated in patients older than 55 years.
  - Hemiarthroplasty is a preferable option in patient with preserved glenoid cartilage [34].
  - Total shoulder arthroplasty (TSA) may be indicated in older patient with glenoid erosion [35].
  - Implant must be placed in adequate retroversion with anterior soft tissue release [7].
  - In severe cases with instability, labral repair may be useful to maintain the congruity of the shoulder joint in hemiarthroplasty [7].
  - Reverse shoulder arthroplasty (RSA) is another option in older patients with significant bone loss or failure of shoulder stabilization as a salvage procedure.
5. **Risks and Complications**
   - (a) **Bony Injury**
     - The incidence of associated injuries is 65% of which 34% are fractures of multiple sites of the humerus [36].
     - The most common areas are humeral neck fracture (55%), lesser tuberosity (42%), and greater tuberosity (23%) [36].

(b) **Rotator Cuff Injury**
   - Rotator cuff tear (RCT) is present in 13% of patient diagnosed with posterior shoulder dislocation, and the risk of RCT is fivefold higher in posterior shoulder dislocation [36].

(c) **Shoulder Stiffness**
   - Can occur secondary to posterior capsular tightness from prolonged immobilization or overtightening during capsular shift procedure.
   - It generally improves with postoperative stretching exercise [19].
   - Can occur due to delayed presentation, which can result in posttraumatic degenerative changes and bone deformities [37].

(d) **Recurrent Instability (<10%)**
   - Can be minimized with proper clinical evaluation and proper surgical intervention and rehabilitation postoperatively [19].

(e) **Glenoid Chondral Damage and Osteoarthritis**
   - Can occur at the time of dislocation or repetitive subluxation.
   - Iatrogenic glenoid chondral damage is avoided by proper anchor placement [19].

(f) **Neurovascular Injury**
   - The risk of nerve injury is very rare (<1%) [7].
   - Axillary nerve injury may occur during inferior capsular plication or using thermal device at the inferior aspect of glenoid.
   - The average distance between inferior glenoid rim and axially nerve is 12.4 mm in a cadaveric study [19].
   - Suprascapular nerve (SSN) injury and posterior circumflex artery (PCA) injury can occur with use of a posterolateral (7 o'clock) portal.
   - The mean distance between SSN and PCA with 7 o'clock portal in different arm position is $29 \pm 3$ mm and $39 \pm 4$ mm, respectively [29].
   - Proper instrument use during portal establishment can help avoid this complication, which includes using a blunted instrument, keeping the shoulder in one position, and direct visualization during portal placement [38].

(g) **Avascular Necrosis (AVN)**
   - Posterior shoulder fracture dislocation may increase the risk of AVN which depends on the degree of fracture displacement and the interval between dislocation and fixation.
   - Immediate reduction with fixation may decrease the risk of AVN [37].

## References

1. Millett PJ, Clavert P, Hatch GF III, Warner JJ. Recurrent posterior shoulder instability. J Am Acad Orthop Surg. 2006;14(8):464–76.
2. Robinson CM, Aderinto J. Recurrent posterior shoulder instability – current concepts review. J Bone Joint Surg Am. 2005;87:883–92.
3. Provencher MT, Bell SJ, Menzel KA, Mologne TS. Arthroscopic treatment of posterior shoulder instability: results in 33 patients. Am J Sports Med. 2005;33(10):1463–71.

4. Bradley JP, Baker CL III, Kline AJ, Armfield DR, Chhabra A. Arthroscopic capsulolabral reconstruction for posterior instability of the shoulder: a prospective study of 100 shoulders. Am J Sports Med. 2006;34(7):1061–71.

5. Kim SH, Ha KI, Park JH, et al. Arthroscopic posterior labral repair and capsular shift for traumatic unidirectional recurrent posterior subluxation of the shoulder. J Bone Joint Surg Am. 2003;85(8):1479–87.

6. Frank RM, Romeo AA, Provencher MT. Posterior glenohumeral instability: evidence-based treatment. J Am Acad Orthop Surg. 2017;25(9):610–23.

7. Rouleau DM, Hebert-Davies J, Robinson CM. Acute traumatic posterior shoulder dislocation. J Am Acad Orthop Surg. 2014;22(3):145–52.

8. Blasier RB, Soslowsky LJ, Malicky DM, Palmer ML. Posterior glenohumeral subluxation: active and passive stabilization in a biomechanical model. J Bone Joint Surg Am. 1997;79(3):433–40.

9. Kim SH, Park JS, Jeong WK, Shin SK. The Kim test: a novel test for posteroinferior labral lesion of the shoulder. A comparison to the jerk test. Am J Sports Med. 2005;33(8):1188–92.

10. Pollock RG, Bigliani LU. Recurrent posterior shoulder instability: diagnosis and treatment. Clin Orthop Relat Res. 1993;291:85–96.

11. Gerber C, Ganz R. Clinical assessment of instability of the shoulder: with special reference to anterior and posterior drawer tests. J Bone Joint Surg (Br). 1984;66(4):551–6.

12. Bey MJ, Hunter SA, Kilambi N, Butler DL, Lindenfeld TN. Structural and mechanical properties of the glenohumeral joint posterior capsule. J Shoulder Elb Surg. 2005;14(2):201–6.

13. Dewing CB, McCormick F, Bell SJ, et al. An analysis of capsular area in patients with anterior, posterior, and multidirectional shoulder instability. Am J Sports Med. 2008;36(3):515–22.

14. Smark CT, Barlow BT, Vachon TA, Provencher MT. Arthroscopic and magnetic resonance arthrogram features of Kim's lesion in posterior shoulder instability. Arthroscopy. 2014;30(7):781–4.

15. Goudie EB, Murray IR, Robinson CM. Instability of the shoulder following seizures. J Bone Joint Surg (Br). 2012;94(6):721–8.

16. Cicak N. Posterior dislocation of the shoulder. J Bone Joint Surg (Br). 2004;86(3):324–32.

17. Loebenberg MI, Cuomo F. The treatment of chronic anterior and posterior dislocations of the glenohumeral joint and associated articular surface defects. Orthop Clin North Am. 2000;31(1):23–34.

18. Moroder P, Danzinger V, Minkus M, Scheibel M. [The ABC guide for the treatment of posterior shoulder instability]. Orthopade 2018;47(2):139–47.

19. Thompson MMS. Posterior shoulder instability DeLee, Drez and Miller's orthopaedic sports medicine, vol. 2. 5th ed. Philadelphia, PA: Elsevier; 2019. p. 463–75.

20. Chalmers PN, Hammond J, Juhan T, Romeo AA. Revision posterior shoulder stabilization. J Shoulder Elb Surg. 2013;22(9):1209–20.

21. Donald Lee RN. Operative techniques: shoulder and elbow surgery. 2nd ed. Philadelphia, PA: Elsevier; 2018. p. 167–79.

22. Frank RM, Shin JJ, Saccomanno MF, Bhatia S, Shewman E, Wang V, et al. Comparison of glenohumeral contact pressures and contact areas after posterior glenoid reconstruction with iliac crest or distal tibia osteochondral allograft. Orthop J Sports Med. 2014;2(2 Suppl):2325967114S00101.

23. Parada SA, Shaw KA. Graft transfer technique in arthroscopic posterior glenoid reconstruction with distal tibia allograft. Arthrosc Techn. 2017;6(5):e1891–e5.

24. Gilat R, Haunschild ED, Tauro T, Evuarherhe A, Fu MC, Romeo A, et al. Distal tibial allograft augmentation for posterior shoulder instability associated with glenoid bony deficiency: a case series. Arthrosc Sports Med Rehabil. 2020;2(6):e743–e52.

25. Galvin JW, Morte DR, Grassbaugh JA, Parada SA, Burns SH, Eichinger JK. Arthroscopic treatment of posterior shoulder instability in patients with and without glenoid dysplasia: a comparative outcomes analysis. J Shoulder Elb Surg. 2017;26(12):2103–9.

26. Lavender CD, Hanzlik SR, Pearson SE, Caldwell PE III. Arthroscopic reverse remplissage for posterior instability. Arthrosc Techn. 2016;5(1):e43–e7.

27. McLaughlin LH. Posterior dislocation of the shoulder. J Bone Joint Surg Am. 1952;24A(3):584–90.

28. Castagna A, Delle Rose G, Borroni M, Markopoulos N, Conti M, Maradei L, et al. Modified MacLaughlin procedure in the treatment of neglected posterior dislocation of the shoulder. Musculoskelet Surg. 2009;93(1):1–5.

29. Hawkins RJ, Neer CS, Pianta RM, Mendoza FX. Locked posterior dislocation of the shoulder. J Bone Joint Surg Am. 1987;69(1):9–18.

30. Keppler P, Holz U, Thielemann FW, Meinig R. Locked posterior dislocation of the shoulder: treatment using rotational osteotomy of the humerus. J Orthop Trauma. 1994;8(4):286–92.

31. Begin M, Gagey O, Soubeyrand M. Acute bilateral posterior dislocation of the shoulder: one-stage reconstruction of both humeral heads with cancellous autograft and cartilage preservation. Chir Main. 2012;31(1):34–7. 22.

32. Barbier O, Ollat D, Marchaland JP, Versier G. Iliac bone-block autograft for posterior shoulder instability. Orthop Traumatol Surg Res. 2009;95(2):100–7. 23.

33. Gerber C, Lambert SM. Allograft reconstruction of segmental defects of the humeral head for the treatment of chronic locked posterior dislocation of the shoulder. J Bone Joint Surg Am. 1996;78(3):376–82.

34. Page AE, Meinhard BP, Schulz E, Toledano B. Bilateral posterior fracture-dislocation of the shoulders: management by bilateral shoulder hemiarthroplasties. J Orthop Trauma. 1995;9(6):526–9.

35. Cheng SL, Mackay MB, Richards RR. Treatment of locked posterior fracture-dislocations of the shoulder by total shoulder arthroplasty. J Shoulder Elb Surg. 1997;6(1):11–7.

36. Rouleau DM, Hebert-Davies J. Incidence of associated injury in posterior shoulder dislocation: systematic review of the literature. J Orthop Trauma. 2012;26(4):246–51.

37. Alepuz ES, Pérez-Barquero JA, Jorge NJ, García FL, Baixauli VC. Treatment of the posterior unstable shoulder. Open Orthop J. 2017;11:826–47.

38. Davidson PA, Rivenburgh DW. The 7-o'clock posteroinferior portal for shoulder arthroscopy. Am J Sports Med. 2002;30(5):693–6.

# Multidirectional Instability

**7**

Akshar H. Patel, Felix H. Savoie III, and Michael J. O'Brien

## Introduction

*Multidirectional instability* (MDI) is a term first coined in 1980 by Charles Neer and Craig Foster to describe a large redundant inferior capsule with rotator interval laxity as seen by bulging of the rotator interval on arthrogram [1]. Since that time, the definition has been refined with the advent of new research to currently describe a pathologic condition in which there is abnormal movement of the humeral head on the glenoid which produces *symptomatic instability in two or more directions*; instability encompasses subluxation or dislocation in multiple directions, with one direction including requisite inferior instability [2, 3].

1. History
   (a) Classification
   - Thomas and Matsen originally classified shoulder instability into two categories [4].
   - "TUBS" describes *T*raumatic *U*nilateral dislocations with a *B*ankart lesion requiring *S*urgery.
   - "AMBRI" describes *A*traumatic injuries occurring in patients prone to *M*ultidirectional instability who have *B*ilateral excessive laxity, which typically responds to *R*ehabilitation, but may require surgical intervention via an *I*nferior capsular shift [5].
   - Over the years, the classification of glenohumeral joint instability has been modified to incorporate different disease etiologies such as static instabilities, dynamic instabilities, and voluntary dislocation. Now there is a spectrum to describe shoulder instability.

A. H. Patel · F. H. Savoie III · M. J. O'Brien (✉)
Department of Orthopaedic Surgery, Tulane University School of Medicine, New Orleans, LA, USA
e-mail: apatel30@tulane.edu; fsavoie@tulane.edu; mobrien@tulane.edu

© The Author(s), under exclusive license to Springer Nature Switzerland AG 2022
C. M. Chebli, A. M. Murthi (eds.), *The Resident's Guide to Shoulder and Elbow Surgery*, https://doi.org/10.1007/978-3-031-12255-2_7

(b) Epidemiology
- The precise incidence of MDI is unknown due to the challenge of diagnosing this condition, but Blomquist et al. reported 7% of the operations for shoulder instability in Norway during 2008 were attributed to MDI [6].
- It typically presents during the second or third decade of life [7].
- It is less common after the age of 40 due to the natural stiffening of tissues around the shoulder [8].
- Current literature supports that MDI occurs equally among male and females [9, 10].
- MDI from repetitive stress is frequently seen in overhead athletes such as swimmers, gymnasts, and volleyball players [5].
- MDI from overt trauma may be seen in rugby players, collision and contact sports, and people who have been involved in motor vehicle accidents and explosions.

(c) Etiology
- MDI is multifactorial. It may be due to traumatic or atraumatic origins, with or without preexisting laxity [11].
- Many authors believe MDI is due to repetitive microtrauma imposed on a congenitally lax and redundant joint capsule [2, 3, 12–15].
- Can develop secondary to collagen tissue disorders.
- Patients with congenital conditions such as Ehlers-Danlos syndrome, Marfan syndrome, osteogenesis imperfecta, and benign joint hypermobility syndrome may be predisposed to developing MDI [16–19]. These connective tissue disorders affect the rate of collagen formation, number of collagen fibrils and crosslinks, and the type of collagen in tissues, which may contribute to glenohumeral joint instability [12, 20–22].
- MDI secondary to trauma may be due to a single or multiple traumatic dislocations. It is important to note that patients with significant trauma are more likely to have structural lesions to the glenoid labrum or joint capsule. Traumatic MDI will have one predominant direction of instability and may have better outcomes with early surgical stabilization [7, 23].
- In contrast, patients with an atraumatic or repetitive microtraumatic MDI, especially from overhead activities, are more likely to have an intact but attenuated capsule associated with globally increased capsular volume, signs of poor motor control, scapular dyskinesis, and instability in multiple directions. They generally respond well to nonoperative management and rehabilitation [23, 24].

(d) Pathogenesis
- MDI is due to alterations between the static (glenoid concavity and version, labral height, and glenohumeral ligaments and capsule) and dynamic stabilizers (rotator cuff, scapulothoracic muscles, proprioceptive and neuromuscular control) causing symptoms in two or more directions [25].
- Patients become symptomatic due to pain from rotator cuff tendonitis.
  - Laxity in the glenohumeral ligaments and joint capsule leads to shoulder instability, and the rotator cuff becomes overworked trying to

provide dynamic stability to the shoulder, which causes rotator cuff swelling, tendonitis, and pain.
- This pain leads to the development of scapular protraction with dyskinesia, as the patient tries to splint the arm in a position of comfort, which produces trapezial pain, weakness, and spasms.
- Poor posture and scapular protraction places an increased strain on the rotator cuff, producing more pain.
- The resulting rotator cuff weakness thereby increases shoulder subluxation, which creates a worsening cycle of instability, dyskinesia, tendonitis, and pain (Fig. 7.1).
- This ultimately manifests as pain at rest and with any activities as the inflamed rotator cuff struggles to provide stability to the dyskinetic and unbalanced shoulder.
• Athletes may exhibit symptoms if they have shoulder inferior subluxation at rest, especially in circumstances of poor core and hip strength. These patients are typically asymptomatic once a balance among shoulder muscle stabilizers is achieved.
• The progression of MDI can be thought of as a cyclical exacerbation of the disease process with initial rotator cuff tendonitis leading to shoulder pain and protraction, which causes further rotator cuff weakness, which increases shoulder subluxation, and thereby worsens the initial rotator cuff tendonitis.

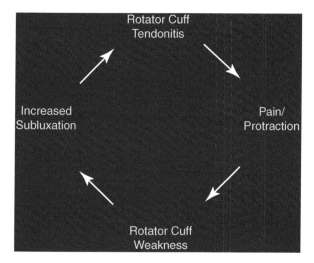

**Fig. 7.1** The cycle of multidirectional instability. Ligamentous laxity in two or more directions causes the rotator cuff to become overworked in an attempt to increase dynamic stability, causing rotator cuff tendonitis and pain. This leads to scapular protraction, dyskinesis, and poor posture, placing more stress on the rotator cuff resulting in swelling, weakness, and pain. Rotator cuff weakness further compromises stability of the glenohumeral joint worsening the cycle of MDI

- The final pathway results in shoulder pain and dysfunction. The glenohumeral joint remains subluxated inferiorly at rest, with the inflamed rotator cuff unable to provide dynamic stability to the joint, and severe pain that impairs all function.

(e) Eliciting a thorough history
- Patients may present with confounding symptoms, ranging from vague shoulder pain to outright instability.
- Patients will complain of feelings of instability with shoulder shifting or clunking. This may occur while lying in bed or in their sleep.
- Pain and instability can occur with simple activities such as walking, as is worsened with lifting, overhead function, and any athletic activities. Pain may occur at rest when rotator cuff inflammation is severe.
- Pain is more pronounced during the midrange of glenohumeral motion due to rotator cuff activation.
- Patients may report their shoulder "falls out the bottom."
- Symptoms that present when carrying heavy objects at one's side are indicative of inferior instability.
- Patients may experience transient neurologic symptoms from shoulder subluxation and neuropraxia.
- The shoulder pain described with MDI is consistent with pain exhibited secondary to rotator cuff tendonitis as there is an imbalance between shoulder muscles, scapular dyskinesia, and loss of proprioception.

2. Physical exam
(a) Inspection/palpation
- On examination, patients will exhibit poor posture and scapular protraction with shoulders rolled forward.
- Scapular dyskinesia is distinctly apparent in all cases by viewing scapular mechanics from posterior during active arm elevation.
- When palpating the shoulder, tenderness is present on the distal supraspinatus tendon as well as the coracoid with typical tightness over the pectoralis minor tendon.
- It is important to note that "instability" differs from "laxity." The term "laxity" describes the physiological looseness or tightness of the shoulder with variation between individuals. It is measured on exam under anesthesia and should be equal bilaterally. In contrast, the term "instability" is used to describe a pathologic condition in which there is abnormal movement of the humeral head on the glenoid producing *symptoms*. It represents a change from normal with multiple causes including but not limited to traumatic injury, overuse, tissue attenuation, and posture.

(b) ROM
- Range of motion may be limited secondary to pain. Pay particular attention to hyper-external rotation and hyper-abduction.

(c) Strength testing
- Shoulder stability and strength can be assessed with the patient sitting or supine, but may be easier to perform supine for patient comfort.

- Patients may have diminished rotator cuff (supraspinatus) and periscapular muscle strength due to inflammation and rotator cuff tendonitis.

(d)  Directed tests based on history or mechanism of injury

- It is paramount to observe scapula motion and mechanics from a posterior view during active arm elevation and abduction. As scapular position can influence physical exam findings, it is important to consider the position of the scapula and compensation from the rotator cuff when testing for instability.
- When assessing anterior and posterior instability, the load and shift test can provide critical information about instability in multiple directions. Perform the load and shift test with the patient supine for patient comfort. The shoulder usually can be subluxated over the rim of the glenoid (Grade 3 Laxity) anteriorly, posteriorly, and inferiorly, or dislocated outright [5]. Generalized laxity may be present in all three directions; however, it is important to determine the primary direction of instability that elicits pain and symptoms.
- When assessing inferior instability, it is important to assess for a positive sulcus sign (Fig. 7.2). While applying a downward traction force to the elbow of the patient with the arm resting at the side in a neutral position, greater than a fingerbreadth of depression under the lateral acromion is created. It is important to note that the positive sulcus does not diminish with external rotation and is increased in comparison to the contralateral shoulder when the shoulder is in adduction.
- When suspecting MDI, assess for a positive Whipple test with and without scapula stabilization (Fig. 7.3). The arm is placed in 90° of forward

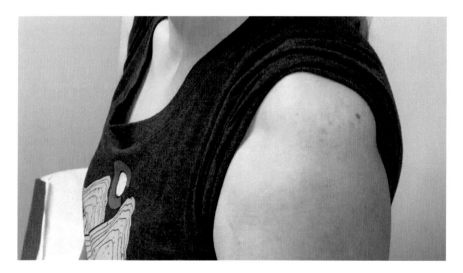

**Fig. 7.2**  A positive sulcus sign. With the arm resting at the side in a neutral position, a downward pull at the elbow creates greater than a fingerbreadth of depression under the lateral acromion. This does not correct with the arm in external rotation in MDI patients

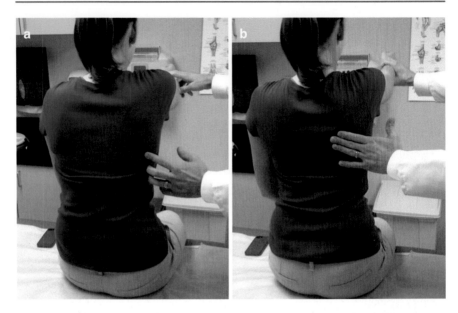

**Fig. 7.3** A positive Whipple test. The arm is brought into 90° of forward flexion. With poor posture and a protracted scapula (**a**), downward pressure on the arm creates pain and weakness, indicating scapular dyskinesis. The scapula is down and out. When posture is corrected and the scapula is pulled into retraction (**b**), the pain resolves, and strength improves

flexion with neutral forearm rotation, and the patient resists a downward force. A positive test recreates pain and weakness, indicating scapular dyskinesis.

- Pain with inferior subluxation of the arm in adduction is indicated with a positive Gagey test. To perform the Gagey test, the patient sits in an upright position in front of the examiner. Stabilize the patient's shoulder girdle by placing one hand on the clavicle and scapula to prevent the shoulder from elevating. Use the other hand to passively move the patient's arm into end-range abduction. A normal shoulder will abduct to 90°, while a positive Gagey test will abduct greater than 105° indicating inferior glenohumeral instability.
- Lafosse Hyperextension-Internal Rotation (HERI) test is a method that can evaluate the integrity of the inferior glenohumeral ligament (IGHL) by measuring the glenohumeral extension angle [26] (Fig. 7.4). The patient stands in front of the examiner facing away. To perform the HERI test and to measure the glenohumeral extension angle of the right shoulder, the examiner places the left elbow against the patient's left scapula and maximally elevates the patient's left arm to lock the thoracic spine and prevent the patient from bending forwards while also locking both scapulothoracic joints. The examiner then grasps the patient's right forearm, pulling it backwards and in pronation with the elbow extended, thereby inducing hyperextension and internal rotation of the patient's right

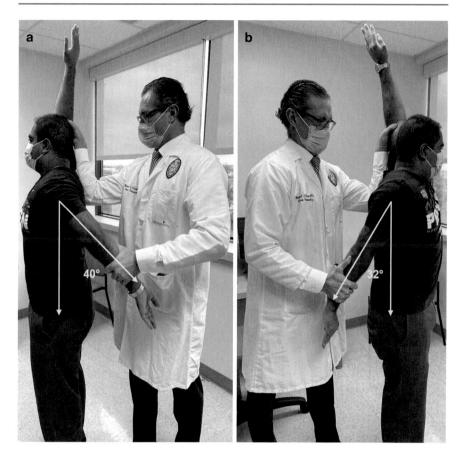

**Fig. 7.4** The HERI test. With the contralateral arm in full elevation, the arm under examination is pulled backwards in pronation with the elbow extended (**a**), thereby inducing hyperextension and internal rotation of the patient's glenohumeral joint. The HERI test should be performed on both sides for comparison (**b**). A side-to-side difference greater than 14.5° in the glenohumeral angle during maximal extension indicates IGHL laxity in the affected extremity. In this figure, a normal examination is seen when the HERI test was performed

glenohumeral joint. Internal rotation of the glenohumeral joint prevents anterior subluxation and apprehension. The examiner increases the degree of hyperextension until a hard resistance is felt, indicating maximal glenohumeral extension. When the right glenohumeral joint is maximally extended, the extension angle is measured, and any pain or apprehension reported by the patient is recorded. The HERI test should be performed on both sides and the results of the two tests compared. A side-to-side difference greater than 14.5° increase in the glenohumeral angle during maximal extension indicates IGHL injury in the affected extremity.

- Generalized ligamentous laxity should be suspected if there is a high Beighton score [24, 27] (Table 7.1).

**Table 7.1** The Beighton scoring system for measuring generalized joint hypermobility (the maximum possible score is 9)

| Assessment site | Right | Left |
|---|---|---|
| Hyperextension of elbow >10° | 1 | 1 |
| Ability of thumb to touch ipsilateral forearm | 1 | 1 |
| Hyperextension of 5th MCP joint | 1 | 1 |
| Hyperextension of the knee >10° | 1 | 1 |
| Ability to touch the floor with both hands with full palms and knees extended | 1 | |

- The presence of impingement syndrome and rotator cuff tendonitis on Neer and Hawkins impingement maneuvers in patients under the age of 20 should raise suspicion of possible MDI.
- Examine for scapular dyskinesis to gain additional information about alterations to muscle activation via the scapular assistance test and scapular retraction test.
  - The scapular assistance test is performed by stabilizing the patient's shoulder girdle by placing a hand on the clavicle and scapular spine. The other hand is used to grasp the inferior angle of the scapula on the same side. Ask the patient to abduct their arm and assist the movement of the scapula. A positive scapular assistance test is seen when a patient experiences less pain during the assisted movement in comparison to non-assisted movement due to weakness of scapular stabilizers.
  - The scapular retraction test can also be utilized to evaluate scapular dyskinesis by stabilizing the retracted scapula to test the rotator cuff. This is done by placing your hand over the patient's clavicle and scapular spine with your forearm supporting the medial border of the scapula. Ask the patient to perform an empty can test while providing resistance and a downward force with your other hand. A positive test is seen when a patient's rotator cuff strength is restored during the scapular retraction test.

3. Imaging
   (a) Radiographs
   - Plain radiographs should be obtained for initial workup in suspected MDI patients.
   - Obtain an anterior-posterior (AP) shoulder X-ray with both internal and external rotation, true AP or Grashey view, scapular-Y, and axillary and Bernageau radiographs. These will help assess for glenoid dysplasia, hypoplasia, humeral head subluxation or anomalies, and traumatic injuries such as a Hill-Sachs deformity or a bony Bankart lesion.
   - It should be noted that plain radiographs are usually normal in MDI patients.
   (b) MRI
   - Neer originally diagnosed MDI on traction roentgenograms [1].

- Magnetic resonance imaging (MRI) with arthrogram (MRA) is the imaging modality of choice in MDI patients.
  - It provides the most information about the shoulder, including normal anatomy and areas of structural damage.
  - It identifies excessive capsular volume, the presence of a patulous anterior or posterior capsule, rotator interval bulging, Bankart lesions, Kim lesions, glenoid erosions, and paralabral cysts.
  - Typical MDI findings on MRI arthrogram include capsular laxity, which can be seen with the presence of a patulous inferior capsule [28].
4. Treatment
   (a) Nonoperative treatment
   - Due to altered proprioception and neuromuscular control of the glenohumeral joint and scapulothoracic articulation, treatment always begins with nonoperative management of symptomatic MDI with shoulder rehabilitation in all patients.
   - The initial goal of nonoperative treatment is focused on reducing inflammation and correcting scapular position through proprioceptive training.
     - Inflammation is controlled with non-steroidal anti-inflammatory medications and selective corticosteroid injections.
     - Static bracing, dynamic bracing, and McConnell taping may be employed to correct dyskinesis and place the shoulder back into the correct position.
   - Pain-free rotator cuff exercises are initiated only after the correct scapular position has been reestablished.
   - Physical therapy is aimed at not only improving the strength of the rotator cuff and dynamic stabilizers but also improving neuromuscular control by retraining the pattern of shoulder muscle activation through exercise in order to compensate for static deficiencies.
     - The scapula in MDI patients is typically protracted; therefore, the rehabilitation protocol is directed towards restoring correct motor control of the scapulothoracic stabilizers.
     - Coordination and strength of both the rotator cuff muscles and the periscapular musculature should be achieved to provide stability [9].
     - Moreover, during the early rehabilitation course, closed chain kinetic exercises will provide patients with safe co-contraction of the scapular and rotator cuff muscles during muscle activation training.
     - Core and hip abduction strengthening exercises should be added to provide additional core stability.
     - Patients typically follow this regiment for 3–6 months.
     - Devices such as scapular posture shirts, bracing, taping, and electrical stimulation may provide additional support during rehabilitation [29, 30].
   (b) Operative treatment
   - Surgery for MDI is indicated when there is a failure of appropriate nonoperative treatment with persistent pain, instability, and functional

impairment that interferes with activities of daily living or prevents a return to sports.

- Rehabilitation is typically performed for 6 months before any surgical intervention is offered and must include appropriate scapular stabilization exercises and support in the form of scapular bracing and taping.
- Surgery is contraindicated in patients who are voluntary dislocators.
- Surgical options
  - Surgical options include an open capsular shift or arthroscopic shift with capsulorrhaphy and capsular plication.
  - In the setting of Ehlers-Danlos syndrome and other collagen tissue disorders, an allograft capsular reconstruction may be performed.
  - Arthroscopic surgery with true rotator interval plication is currently the preferred surgical treatment option at our institution based on 5-year outcomes with greater than 85% success. Therefore, the next section will focus on arthroscopic repair techniques.

5. Surgical approach
   (a) The primary goal of arthroscopic MDI surgery is to directly address the pathology.
   (b) Arthroscopic instability surgery is performed in the lateral decubitus position for the benefit of improved visibility and access of the axillary pouch.
   (c) On diagnostic arthroscopy, it is imperative to critically assess for a widened rotator interval, a loose patulous capsule, and possible associated labral tears, capsular tears, or humeral avulsion of the glenohumeral ligaments (HAGL lesions).
   - Initially, the shoulder may appear reduced in a native position. After the application of 5–10 pounds of balanced suspension, the shoulder will subluxate or dislocate in an inferior direction into the axillary pouch due to the attenuated rotator interval, coracohumeral ligament (CHL), and superior glenohumeral ligament (SGHL).
   - An arthroscopic "drive-through sign" of the glenohumeral joint is easily performed due to capsular laxity and attenuation.
   - The arthroscope can be placed in the anterior-superior portal to view the entire glenohumeral joint and evaluate for anterior or posterior capsular redundancy.
   (d) When performing a capsulorrhaphy for MDI, capsular abrasion is performed prior to the capsular shift.
   - This can be completed with an arthroscopic shaver or rasp.
   - Subsequently, a suture plication with a superior shift is performed, beginning in the inferior capsule and working superiorly with multiple plication sutures.
   - The first plication suture is placed at the 6 o'clock position. A pigtail suture passer is used to secure a portion of the capsule, and pass an absorbable suture through the capsule and glenoid labrum (Fig. 7.5). As the plication suture is tied, redundant capsular tissue is diminished and the IGHL is tightened.

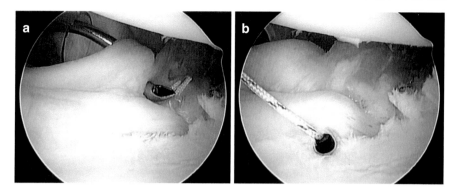

**Fig. 7.5** Arthroscopic suture plication with a superior shift. The first plication suture is placed at the 6 o'clock position. A pigtail suture passer is used to secure a portion of the capsule by passing a suture through the capsule as seen on the left (**a**) and then through the glenoid labrum as seen on the right (**b**). The suture is tried reducing the capsular volume. Additional sutures are placed until the capsular plication is complete

- Subsequent plication sutures are placed more superiorly to decrease capsular volume in the anterior and posterior capsule. We favor using absorbable sutures for most shoulder pathology related to MDI except at the rotator interval.
- If there is evidence of an absent, hypotrophic, or dysfunctional labrum, then a suture anchor must be placed for the capsulorrhaphy. The suture anchor is placed into the glenoid between the glenoid and the labrum, taking care not to place the suture anchor through the labrum.
- In patients with a thin or atrophic posterior capsule, additional stability may be provided to the posterior capsule by performing posterior plication through the capsule and infraspinatus tendon. A spinal needle is passed through infraspinatus and the lateral capsule on the humeral side, after which a retrograde retriever is utilized to pass the suture at a very low point above the axillary nerve with the starting point near the upper portion of teres minor. The resulting repair reinforces the posterior capsule repair without contributing to muscle weakness.
- (e) After completion of the capsulorrhaphy, an open or a true arthroscopic rotator interval closure may be performed.
  - Rotator interval closure is a necessary step in capsular shift surgery for MDI in order to tighten the SGHL and CHL to correct inferior joint subluxation.
  - The rotator interval closure is performed by placing 2–3 permanent plication sutures in oblique medial-to-lateral fashion between the supraspinatus and subscapularis, taking care not to incarcerate the long head of the biceps tendon.
  - The rotator interval is closed arthroscopically by tying the knots blindly in the subacromial and subdeltoid space, resulting in plication of the CHL and SGHL.

(f) Capsular reconstruction with an allograft is reserved for patients with collagen disorders who are refractory to previous treatment.
- During this procedure, it is necessary to address glenoid as well as capsule and labrum pathology.

(g) Postoperatively, rehabilitation protocols should be tailored to patients based on the individual's primary direction of instability and robustness of repair and progressed based on activity level and sport.
- Typically, patients are immobilized in an abduction brace for 4–6 weeks with scapular rehabilitation beginning in the first week.
- Active arm elevation is permitted at 6 weeks postoperatively.
- Although early bracing and taping is done, there is never any stretching allowed in therapy.
- Rotator cuff and periscapular strengthening are initiated at 8–10 weeks postoperatively and progressed as tolerated.

6. Risks and complications
(a) Recurrence of MDI has been reported to range between 8% and 30% following surgical repairs and plication [9, 13, 15, 31].
(b) The high rate of recurrence is thought to be due to inability to change the structural integrity of collagen, which contributes to future laxity. It is unknown if chondrolysis may be associated with MDI.
(c) A foreseen complication is postsurgical arthritis and capsulorrhaphy arthropathy.
(d) Due to the close proximity of the axillary nerve to the inferior glenohumeral pouch, axillary nerve injury may occur after open, thermal, and arthroscopic procedures.
(e) Although rare, stiffness and loss of motion may also be seen. Additionally, subscapularis insufficiency may result when an open procedure is performed.
(f) In cases of failure, a modified Gallie allograft reconstruction procedure may be performed, especially in Ehlers-Danlos patients. In the authors' experience, this has maintained stability in the setting of collagen tissue disorders for 7–8 years.
(g) In 1980, Neer and Foster first reported satisfactory results in 16 of 17 shoulders (94%) following an open inferior capsular shift technique with a follow-up of at least 2 years. Since Neer's original paper, treatment of MDI has progressed with the advent of arthroscopic techniques [1]. Functional outcomes for MDI are typically measured using a variety of shoulder scoring systems including but not limited to the Rowe scale, Constant score, Neer score, UCLA score, American Shoulder and Elbow Society (ASES) score, and the Western Ontario Shoulder Instability (WOSI) Index.
- Using laser-assisted capsulorrhaphy for MDI, Lyons reported 96% of patients remained stable and asymptomatic at a minimum of 2 years postoperatively [32].
- Thermal capsulorrhaphy has been largely abandoned due to capsular thermal necrosis and high failure rates.

- Gartsman demonstrated that 91% of patients had successful outcomes according to the Rowe score with arthroscopic plication surgery during a 2–5-year follow-up [33].
- In a 5-year follow-up study of MDI treated with arthroscopic shift, Treacy reported that 88% of patients had a satisfactory Neer score with maintained shoulder stability [34].
- In 4–10-year follow-up, Marquardt reported that 89% of patients treated with an open inferior capsular shift procedure had successful results according to the Rowe scale [35].
- Pollock reported a favorable outcomes in 94% of patients and 96% stability of MDI shoulders after an open inferior capsular shift at a mean 61-month follow-up [36].
- At a mean follow-up of 56 months, Alpert demonstrated an 85% satisfaction rate in MDI patients who underwent arthroscopic stabilization with labral repair and a median ASES score of 96.7 at the final follow-up.
- Wichman and Snyder demonstrated satisfactory results in 79% of patients the Neer criteria at a minimum follow-up of 2 years with the use of arthroscopic capsular plications for MDI [37].

## References

1. Neer CS, Foster CR. Inferior capsular shift for involuntary inferior and multidirectional instability of the shoulder. A preliminary report. J Bone Joint Surg Am. 1980;62:897–908.
2. Bahu MJ, Trentacosta N, Vorys GC, Covey AS, Ahmad CS. Multidirectional instability: evaluation and treatment options. Clin Sports Med. 2008;27:671–89.
3. An YH, Friedman RJ. Multidirectional instability of the glenohumeral joint. Orthop Clin North Am. 2000;31:275–83.
4. Thomas SC, Matsen FA. An approach to the repair of avulsion of the glenohumeral ligaments in the management of traumatic anterior glenohumeral instability. J Bone Jt Surg Ser A. 1989;71:506–13.
5. Schenk TJ, Brems JJ. Multidirectional instability of the shoulder: pathophysiology, diagnosis, and management. J Am Acad Orthop Surg. 1998;6:65–72.
6. Blomquist J, Solheim E, Liavaag S, Schroder CP, Espehaug B, Havelin LI. Shoulder instability surgery in Norway: the first report from a multicenter register, with 1-year follow-up. Acta Orthop. 2012;83:165–70.
7. VandenBerghe G, Hoenecke HR, Fronek J. Glenohumeral joint instability: the orthopedic approach. Semin Musculoskelet Radiol. 2005;9:34–43.
8. Longo UG, Rizzello G, Loppini M, Locher J, Buchmann S, Maffulli N, Denaro V. Multidirectional instability of the shoulder: a systematic review. Arthrosc J Arthrosc Relat Surg. 2015;31:2431–43.
9. Kiss J, Damrel D, Mackie A, Neumann L, Wallace WA. Non-operative treatment of multidirectional shoulder instability. Int Orthop. 2001;24:354–7.
10. Cameron KL, Duffey ML, Deberardino TM, Stoneman PD, Jones CJ, Owens BD. Association of generalized joint hypermobility with a history of glenohumeral joint instability. J Athl Train. 2010;45:253–8.
11. Gerber C, Nyffeler RW. Classification of glenohumeral joint instability. Clin Orthop Relat Res. 2002;400:65–76.

12. Mallon WJ, Speer KP. Multidirectional instability: current concepts. J Shoulder Elb Surg. 1995;4:54–64.
13. Misamore GW, Sallay PI, Didelot W. A longitudinal study of patients with multidirectional instability of the shoulder with seven- to ten-year follow-up. J Shoulder Elb Surg. 2005;14:466–70.
14. Beasley L, Faryniarz DA, Hannafin JA. Multidirectional instability of the shoulder in the female athlete. Clin Sports Med. 2000;19:331–49.
15. Ide J, Maeda S, Yamaga M, Morisawa K, Takagi K. Shoulder-strengthening exercise with an orthosis for multidirectional shoulder instability: quantitative evaluation of rotational shoulder strength before and after the exercise program. J Shoulder Elb Surg. 2003;12:342–5.
16. Maltz SB, Fantus RJ, Mellett MM, Kirby JP. Surgical complications of Ehlers-Danlos syndrome type IV: case report and review of the literature. J Trauma. 2001;51:387–90.
17. Malfait F, Hakim AJ, De Paepe A, Grahame R. The genetic basis of the joint hypermobility syndromes. Rheumatology. 2006;45:502–7.
18. Zweers MC, Hakim AJ, Grahame R, Schalkwijk J. Joint hypermobility syndromes: the pathophysiologic role of tenascin-X gene defects. Arthritis Rheum. 2004;50:2742–9.
19. Kitagawa T, Matsui N, Nakaizumi D. Structured rehabilitation program for multidirectional shoulder instability in a patient with Ehlers-Danlos syndrome. Case Rep Orthop. 2020;2020:1–4.
20. Shirley ED, DeMaio M, Bodurtha J. Ehlers-Danlos syndrome in orthopaedics: etiology, diagnosis, and treatment implications. Sports Health. 2012;4:394–403.
21. Hirakawa M. On the etiology of the loose shoulder–biochemical studies on collagen from joint capsules. Nihon Seikeigeka Gakkai Zasshi. 1991;65:550–60.
22. Guerrero P, Busconi B, Deangelis N, Powers G. Congenital instability of the shoulder joint: assessment and treatment options. J Orthop Sports Phys Ther. 2009;39:124–34.
23. Lewis A, Kitamura T, Bayley JIL. The classification of shoulder instability: new light through old windows! Curr Orthop. 2004;18:97–108.
24. Warby SA, Pizzari T, Ford JJ, Hahne AJ, Watson L. The effect of exercise-based management for multidirectional instability of the glenohumeral joint: a systematic review. J Shoulder Elb Surg. 2014;23:128–42.
25. Navlet MG, Asenjo-Gismero CV. Multidirectional instability: natural history and evaluation. Open Orthop J. 2017;11:861–74.
26. Lafosse T, Fogerty S, Idoine J, Gobezie R, Lafosse L. Hyper extension-internal rotation (HERI): a new test for anterior gleno-humeral instability. Orthop Traumatol Surg Res. 2016;102:3–12.
27. Smits-Engelsman B, Klerks M, Kirby A. Beighton score: a valid measure for generalized hypermobility in children. J Pediatr. 2011;158:119–23.
28. Dewing CB, McCormick F, Bell SJ, Solomon DJ, Stanley M, Rooney TB, Provencher MT. An analysis of capsular area in patients with anterior, posterior, and multidirectional shoulder instability. Am J Sports Med. 2008;36:515–22.
29. Paine RM, Voight M. The role of the scapula. J Orthop Sports Phys Ther. 1993;18:386–91.
30. Walker DL, Hickey CJ, Tregoning MB. The effect of electrical stimulation versus sham cueing on scapular position during exercise in patients with scapular dyskinesis. Int J Sports Phys Ther. 2017;12:425–36.
31. Alpert JM, Verma N, Wysocki R, Yanke AB, Romeo AA. Arthroscopic treatment of multidirectional shoulder instability with minimum 270° labral repair: minimum 2-year follow-up. Arthrosc J Arthrosc Relat Surg. 2008;24:704–11.
32. Lyons TR, Griffith PL, Savoie FH, Field LD. Laser-assisted capsulorrhaphy for multidirectional instability of the shoulder. Arthroscopy. 2001;17:25–30.
33. Gartsman GM, Roddey TS, Hammerman SM. Arthroscopic treatment of multidirectional glenohumeral instability: 2- to 5-year follow-up. Arthroscopy. 2001;17:236–43.
34. Treacy SH, Savoie FH, Field LD. Arthroscopic treatment of multidirectional instability. J Shoulder Elb Surg. 1999;8:345–50.

35. Marquardt B, Pötzl W, Witt KA, Steinbeck J. A modified capsular shift for atraumatic anterior-inferior shoulder instability. Am J Sports Med. 2005;33:1011–5.
36. Pollock RG, Owens JM, Flatow EL, Bigliani LU. Operative results of the inferior capsular shift procedure for multidirectional instability of the shoulder. J Bone Jt Surg Ser A. 2000;82:919–28.
37. Wichman MT, Snyder SJ. Arthroscopic capsular plication for multidirectional instability of the shoulder. Oper Tech Sports Med. 1997;5:238–43.

# SLAP Tears and Biceps Tendinopathy

**8**

Matthew J. Deasey and Stephen F. Brockmeier

Introduction: Injuries to the superior labrum and long head of biceps tendon complex are common in both the industrial and competitive athlete. These injuries can occur in isolation or coexist with other shoulder pathology, such as rotator cuff injuries. SLAP tears (*S*uperior *L*abrum *A*nterior to *P*osterior) are most often treated successfully without operative intervention [1]. Conservative treatment consists of physical therapy focused on peri-scapular retraining and strengthening along with stretching to promote rotational balance at the glenohumeral joint. Should the injury prove recalcitrant to conservative management, arthroscopic debridement of the superior labrum with biceps tenodesis is the standard of care for most patients [2, 3]. High level overhead athletes may warrant treatment with labral repair [4, 5].

1. History
   (a) Classic patients: overheard/throwing athlete, laborer ("industrial athlete") [6–8]
       - Acute injury
       - Acute-on-chronic injury
       - Chronic injury
   (b) Level of play (recreational, collegiate, professional, etc.)/jobsite requirements
       - Necessity of throwing/overhead motion to successful return to play—(i.e., pitcher versus position player, javelin thrower versus decathlete)
       - Percentage of work that requires shoulder abduction and forward flexion or that must be done overhead—(i.e., hanging sheetrock and painting versus project management)
   (c) Hand dominance
   (d) Instability events

M. J. Deasey (✉) · S. F. Brockmeier
Department of Orthopaedic Surgery, University of Virginia Health System,
Charlottesville, VA, USA
e-mail: Mjd7c@hscmail.mcc.virginia.edu; sfb2e@hscmail.mcc.virginia.edu

(e) Aggravating and relieving factors

(f) Prior treatment course

2. Physical exam

(a) Inspection

- Muscle bulk of injured versus contralateral extremity
- Morphology of biceps musculature
  - "Popeye sign" pathognomonic for proximal biceps tendon rupture
- Previous surgical incisions—remote arthroscopic incisions require careful exam

(b) Palpation

- Long head of biceps tendon in bicipital groove
- Assess clavicle for crepitus or bony step-off
- Fullness or wasting at posterior shoulder concerning for para-labral cyst

(c) Range of motion—compare to contralateral shoulder

- Forward elevation
- Abduction
- External rotation
  - Perform with arm at side as well as with arm abducted to 90 degrees
- Internal rotation
  - Patient is supine, elbow flexed to 90 degrees, arm abducted to 90 degrees
    Forearm neutral
  - Examiner passively externally and internally rotates shoulder with goniometer
  - Difference of >20° internal rotation relative to contralateral side is diagnostic for glenohumeral internal rotation deficit (GIRD) [9]

(d) Provocative maneuvers

- Speed's resisted forward elevation test (Fig. 8.1):
  - Patient seated or standing, extended elbow, arm forward flexed to 90°
  - Patient actively forward flexes against resistance from examiner
  - Pain elicited with attempted forward flexion is a positive test
- O'Brien's active compression test (Fig. 8.2):
  - Patient seated or standing, extended elbow, arm forward flexed to 90°
  - Arm adducted 10–15°; patient actively forward flexes against resistance from examiner first with fully pronated forearm, then with supinated forearm
  - Pain that is present with pronation and relieved with supination is a positive test
- Yergason's resisted supination test (Fig. 8.3):
  - Patient seated or standing, elbow flexed to 90°, arm at side.
  - Forearm fully pronated.
  - Patient actively supinates against resistance from examiner.
    Examiner palpates bicipital groove.
  - Pain with resisted supination is a positive test.
    Palpable tendon subluxation indicates torn transverse humeral ligament.

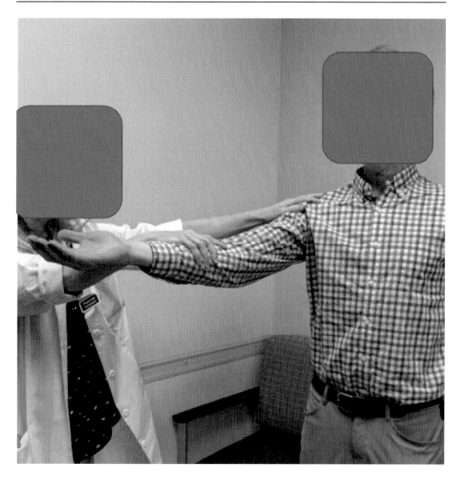

**Fig. 8.1** Speed's test: patient actively forward flexes against resistance from examiner. Pain elicited with attempted forward flexion is a positive test

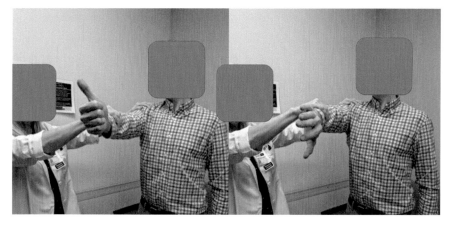

**Fig. 8.2** O'Brien's active compression test: patient actively forward flexes against resistance from examiner. Pain that is absent with a supinated arm, but present with a pronated arm is a positive test

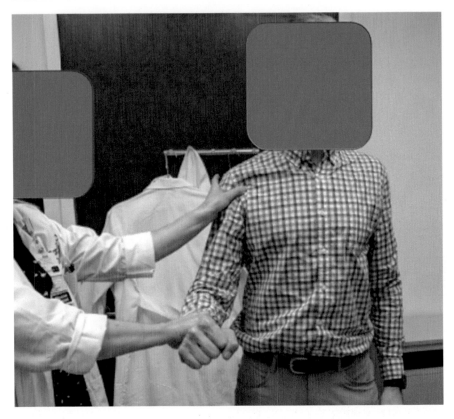

**Fig. 8.3** Yergason's resisted supination test: patient actively supinates against resistance from examiner. Examiner palpates bicipital groove. Pain at the groove with resisted supination is a positive test

- Dynamic labral shear test (Fig. 8.4):
  - Patient standing or supine, elbow flexed to 90°, arm abducted to 120°.
  - Arm passively externally rotated to tightness; examiner stabilizes scapula.
  - Examiner maintains external rotatory force while horizontally abducting the arm and simultaneously lowering arm from 120 to 60° of vertical abduction.
  - Painful click or catch during descent is a positive test [10].
- (e) Neurovascular exam:
  - Axillary nerve
    - Sensation over lateral shoulder
    - Active abduction
  - Musculocutaneous never
    - Lateral forearm sensation
    - Elbow flexion

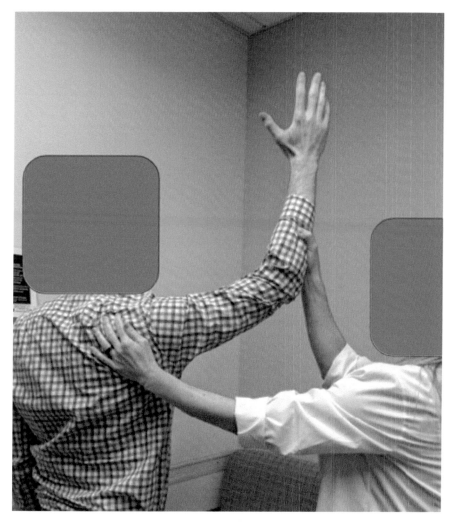

**Fig. 8.4** Dynamic labral shear: Examiner maintains external rotatory force while horizontally abducting the arm and simultaneously lowering arm from 120 to 60 degrees of vertical abduction. A painful click during this arc of motion is a positive test

- Hoffman's test—evaluate for cervical myelopathy
- Radial and ulnar arteries
  - Pulses at wrist
  - Capillary refill in fingertips
3. Imaging
   (a) X-rays—axillary, scapular Y, and AP in the plane of the joint (Grashey)
   - Useful to assess for bony lesions to the glenoid or humeral head
   - Osteophytes, joint space narrowing concerning for arthritis
   (b) MRI—gold standard diagnostic modality

- Arthrogram with gadolinium increases sensitivity/specificity [11–13]
- Mimics of superior labral lesions: the sublabral foramen and the Buford complex, which have incidences of 11% and 1.5%, respectively [14, 15].

4. Classification
   (a) Snyder classification (Fig. 8.5, Table 8.1) [6]
   - Type I: superior labrum frayed, biceps anchor intact
   - Type II: superior labrum intact, biceps anchor detached
   - Type III: bucket handle superior labral tear, biceps anchor intact
   - Type IV: bucket handle superior labral tear, biceps anchor detached

5. Treatment
   (a) First-line treatment for SLAP lesions with or without biceps tendinopathy is nonoperative in both the high level athlete and general populations.
   - Oral anti-inflammatory medications
   - Physical therapy and stretching exercises
     - Directed toward correction of both glenohumeral and scapular dyskinesia
     - Sleeper stretch for GIRD (Fig. 8.6) [9, 16]:
       Patient lying on affected side, elbow flexed to 90°, shoulder forward flexed to 90°
       Contralateral arm used to steadily and maximally internally rotate the affected shoulder
   (b) Operative treatment
   - Indicated in patients who have failed nonoperative treatment
   - Patients stratified in two domains: age and throwing motion dependence
     - Age <35 considered "young," <40 considered "older" [17, 18]
     - Pitchers, swimmers, volleyball attackers "dependent" versus baseball position players, basketball players "non-dependent" on overhead motion
   - Positioning
     - Beach chair or lateral decubitus with shoulder suspension
       SCDs/foot pumps to decrease VTE risk and increase cerebral perfusion [19]
       Drape out field to include sternal notch for potential extensile needs
   - Biceps tenodesis/tenotomy and labral debridement
     - Arthroscopic procedure done after standard diagnostic shoulder scope
       Indicated in patients >40 years of age
       Most non-dependent athletes, even high level
       Return to play still possible for high level athletes with biceps tenodesis [3, 20, 21]
       Tag the LHB tendon if tenodesis planned
         Spinal needle can be used to pass tag suture, clamp outside skin
       Transect LHB tendon at biceps anchor
       Debride stump and frayed labrum
     - Tenodesis of LHB tendon—prevents "Popeye" deformity and aids in forearm supination strength and endurance vs. tenotomy [22, 23]

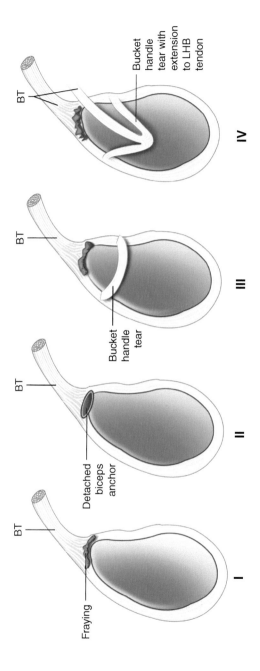

**Fig. 8.5** Schematic representing the Snyder classification of SLAP tears

**Table 8.1** The Snyder classification of SLAP tears

| Classification | Superior labrum | Biceps anchor | Surgical treatment |
|---|---|---|---|
| Type I | Frayed | Intact | Labral debridement |
| Type II | Frayed | Detached | Biceps tenodesis with labral repair vs. debridement |
| Type III | Bucket handle tear | Intact | Labral debridement |
| Type IV | Bucket handle tear | Detached | Biceps tenodesis with labral debridement |

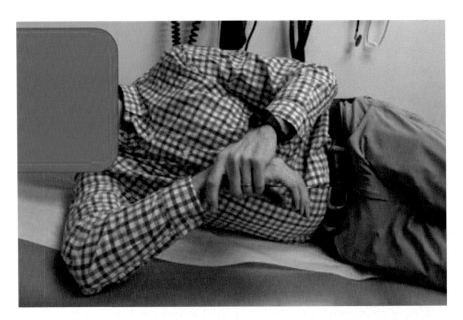

**Fig. 8.6** The sleeper stretch is performed with the patient lying on their affected side with the elbow flexed to 90° and the shoulder forward flexed to 90°. The contralateral arm is used to internally rotate the affected shoulder

Mini-open (subpectoral) [24, 25]

    1.5 cm incision, medial humerus, at the level of the inferior aspect of the pectoralis major tendon

        Tendon can be hooked from with a finger, medial to lateral to avoid neurovascular structures.

        Can be secured with unicortical biotenodesis or suspensory ("button") fixation.

Arthroscopic (suprapectoral)

    Anterior aspect of humerus just lateral to bicipital groove [26, 27]

        Accessed through careful subdeltoid dissection

    Biotenodesis screw fixation

- Superior labral repair ± tenodesis

  Restores bumper effect of superior labrum.

  Suture anchor fixation with traditional or knotless anchors – if using traditional anchor.

  Keep stack away from glenoid articular surface (Fig. 8.7)

  Biomechanical studies promote mattress configuration posterior to biceps anchor for great pull-out strength and decreased tendency for impingement on LHB [28, 29].

- Surgical risks/complications
  - Musculocutaneous neurapraxia

    Uncommon but devastating if too far medial with biceps tendon dissection or tenodesis.

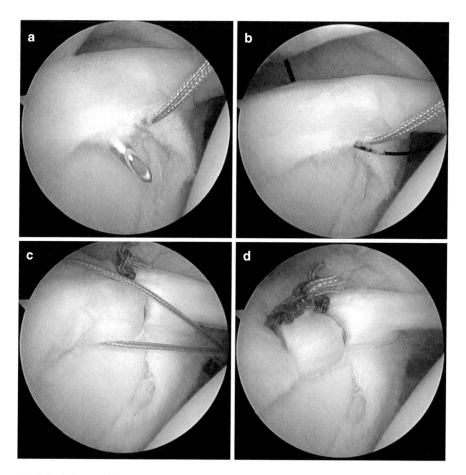

**Fig. 8.7** Arthroscopic images showing the process of labral repair: (**a, b**) suture passing; (**c**) step-wise repair; (**d**) knotted suture anchors place posterior to the biceps anchor with stacks directed away from the articular surface

Visualization of tag stitch motion proximally can decrease risk.
Elbow flexion/supination weakness, lateral forearm paresthesias.
– Stiffness
Clear PT protocol for early ROM
– Superficial wound infection

## References

1. Wilk KE, Macrina LC. Nonoperative and postoperative rehabilitation for injuries of the throwing shoulder. Sports Med Arthrosc. 2014;22(2):137–50.
2. Virk MS, Cole BJ. Proximal biceps tendon and rotator cuff tears. Clin Sports Med. 2016;35(1):153–61.
3. Griffin JW, Cvetanovich GL, Kim J, Leroux TS, Riboh J, Bach BR, et al. Biceps tenodesis is a viable option for management of proximal biceps injuries in patients less than 25 years of age. Arthrosc J Arthrosc Relat Surg. 2019;35:1036–41.
4. Gilliam BD, Douglas L, Fleisig GS, Aune KT, Mason KA, Dugas JR, et al. Return to play and outcomes in baseball players after superior labral anterior-posterior repairs. Am J Sports Med. 2018;46(1):109–15.
5. Calcei JG, Boddapati V, Altchek DW, Camp CL, Dines JS. Diagnosis and treatment of injuries to the biceps and superior labral complex in overhead athletes. In: Current reviews in musculoskeletal medicine. New York: Humana Press; 2018. p. 63–71.
6. Snyder SJ, Karzel RP, Del PW, Ferkel RD, Friedman MJ. SLAP lesions of the shoulder. Arthrosc J Arthrosc Relat Surg. 1990;6(4):274–9.
7. Andrews JR, Carson WG, Mcleod WD. Glenoid labrum tears related to the long head of the biceps. Am J Sports Med. 1985;13(5):337–41.
8. Provencher MT, McCormick F, Dewing C, McIntire S, Solomon D. A prospective analysis of 179 type 2 superior labrum anterior and posterior repairs. Am J Sports Med. 2013;41(4):880–6.
9. Rose MB, Noonan T. Glenohumeral internal rotation deficit in throwing athletes: current perspectives. Open Access J Sports Med. 2018;9:69–78.
10. Ben Kibler W, Sciascia AD, Hester P, Dome D, Jacobs C. Clinical utility of traditional and new tests in the diagnosis of biceps tendon injuries and superior labrum anterior and posterior lesions in the shoulder. Am J Sports Med. 2009;37(9):1840–7.
11. Schwartzberg R, Reuss BL, Burkhart BG, Butterfield M, Wu JY, McLean KW. High prevalence of superior labral tears diagnosed by MRI in middle-aged patients with asymptomatic shoulders. Orthop J Sports Med. 2016;4(1):232596711562321.
12. Hacken B, Onks C, Flemming D, Mosher T, Silvis M, Black K, et al. Prevalence of MRI shoulder abnormalities in asymptomatic professional and collegiate ice hockey athletes. Orthop J Sports Med. 2019;7(10):232596711987686.
13. Lansdown DA, Bendich I, Motamedi D, Feeley BT. Imaging-based prevalence of superior labral anterior-posterior tears significantly increases in the aging shoulder. Orthop J Sports Med. 2018;6(9):232596711879706.
14. Williams MM, Snyder SJ, Buford D. The buford complex—the "cord-like" middle glenohumeral ligament and absent anterosuperior labrum complex: a normal anatomic capsulolabral variant. Arthroscopy. 1994;10(3):241–7.
15. Ellman H, Gartsman G. Miscellaneous intra-articular conditions. In: Arthroscopic shoulder surgery and related procedures. Philadelphia: Lea & Febiger; 1993. p. 277–362.
16. Fedoriw WW, Ramkumar P, McCulloch PC, Lintner DM. Return to play after treatment of superior labral tears in professional baseball players. Am J Sports Med. 2014;42(5):1155–60.

17. Cvetanovich GL, Gowd AK, Agarwalla A, Forsythe B, Romeo AA, Verma NN. Trends in the management of isolated SLAP tears in the United States. Orthop J Sports Med. 2019;7(3):232596711983399.
18. Werner BC, Brockmeier SF, Gwathmey FW. Trends in long head biceps tenodesis. Am J Sports Med. 2015;43(3):570–8.
19. Kwak HJ, Lee JS, Lee DC, Kim HS, Kim JY. The effect of a sequential compression device on hemodynamics in arthroscopic shoulder surgery using beach-chair position. Arthrosc J Arthrosc Relat Surg. 2010;26(6):729–33.
20. Gupta AK, Chalmers PN, Klosterman EL, Harris JD, Bach BR, Verma NN, et al. Subpectoral biceps tenodesis for bicipital tendonitis with slap tear. Orthopedics. 2015;38(1):48–53.
21. Douglas L, Whitaker J, Nyland J, Smith P, Chillemi F, Ostrander R, et al. Return to play and performance perceptions of baseball players after isolated SLAP tear repair. Orthop J Sports Med. 2019;7(3):232596711982948.
22. Patel KV, Bravman J, Vidal A, Chrisman A, McCarty E. Biceps tenotomy versus tenodesis. Clin Sports Med. 2016;35:93–111.
23. Slenker NR, Lawson K, Ciccotti MG, Dodson CC, Cohen SB. Biceps tenotomy versus tenodesis: clinical outcomes. Arthrosc J Arthrosc Relat Surg. 2012;28(4):576–82.
24. Johannsen AM, Macalena JA, Carson EW, Tompkins M. Anatomic and radiographic comparison of arthroscopic suprapectoral and open subpectoral biceps tenodesis sites. Am J Sports Med. 2013;41(12):2919–24.
25. Green JM, Getelman MH, Snyder SJ, Burns JP. All-arthroscopic suprapectoral versus open subpectoral tenodesis of the long head of the biceps brachii without the use of interference screws. Arthrosc J Arthrosc Relat Surg. 2017;33(1):19–25.
26. Duchman KR, DeMik DE, Uribe B, Wolf BR, Bollier M. Open versus arthroscopic biceps tenodesis: a comparison of functional outcomes. Iowa Orthop J. 2016;36:79–87.
27. Hurley DJ, Hurley ET, Pauzenberger L, Lim Fat D, Mullett H. Open compared with arthroscopic biceps tenodesis. JBJS Rev. 2019;7(5):4.
28. Domb BG, Ehteshami JR, Shindle MK, Gulotta L, Zoghi-Moghadam M, Macgillivray JD, et al. Biomechanical comparison of 3 suture anchor configurations for repair of type II SLAP lesions. Arthroscopy. 2007;23(2):135–40.
29. Yang HJ, Yoon K, Jin H, Song HS. Clinical outcome of arthroscopic SLAP repair: conventional vertical knot versus knotless horizontal mattress sutures. Knee Surgery Sport Traumatol Arthrosc. 2016;24(2):464–9.

# Adhesive Capsulitis

**9**

Marc S. Kowalsky

1. History
   (a) Epidemiology
      - The incidence of this condition in the general population has been estimated between 2% and 5%.
      - Women are more often affected by this condition than men, most frequently between the ages of 40 and 60.
   (b) Phases [1, 2]
      - Freezing
         - Can last 10–36 weeks and is characterized by insidious onset of diffuse shoulder pain and gradual loss in range of motion over time.
         - The pain can be quite severe, and the patient may have difficulty identifying a precise location of maximum pain.
         - While the patient may not recognize the loss of motion themselves or may attribute this loss of motion to pain rather than stiffness, he or she will often describe difficulty performing certain activities of daily living that require certain motions, including movement behind the back, across the body, or overhead.
         - This loss of motion can be quite subtle initially, which perhaps is a reason early adhesive capsulitis can be misconstrued for other painful shoulder conditions.
      - Frozen
         - Can last between 4 and 12 months and is characterized fundamentally by persistent limitation in motion.
         - Oftentimes, the pain decreases substantially during this phase.
         - In some cases, the patient may not describe any pain at all and may instead notice isolated stiffness.

M. S. Kowalsky (✉)
Orthopaedic and Neurosurgery Specialists, ONS Foundation for Clinical Research and Education, Greenwich, CT, USA

- This loss of motion can be quite severe and therefore can significantly limit the patient's daily function.
- Due in part to the duration of this phase, patients often express profound frustration over their limitations.
  - Thawing
    - Can last 12 months or longer.
    - As this is typically described as a self-limited condition, the symptoms of pain and stiffness typically resolve on their own, but this process can take a significant amount of time.
  (c) Components of a Detailed History
    - Causes
      - Most patients who develop this condition have no clear associated medical history; however, a higher incidence of this condition in patients with thyroid disease or diabetes has been identified [3–5].
      - There is often no specific traumatic injury or antecedent event, though some patients may recall a minor injury or recent associated increase in activity.
    - Age, sex, hand dominance, and occupation of the patient
      - The physician can have a high index of suspicion for adhesive capsulitis in a woman between ages 40 and 60 with a history of diabetes or thyroid disease [4, 5].
      - Information such as hand dominance, occupation, and preferred recreational activities help the physician to better understand the impact of the patient's symptoms on everyday life and what the patient's expectations might be for recovery.
    - Parameters of pain, including duration, intensity, location, and nature or type of pain
      - Pain and stiffness associated with adhesive capsulitis are often insidious in onset and therefore may be associated with a prolonged duration of symptoms.
      - The intensity and nature of pain vary tremendously in these patients, dependent in large part on the phase of disease. Symptoms of pain are far more intense during the freezing phase and improve gradually as the condition evolves.
      - Location of pain often varies as well. As the condition is characterized by profound, global inflammation of the glenohumeral joint capsule and rotator interval tissues, patients often describe pain as diffuse. This contrasts with the more focal pain associated with other conditions such as biceps tendonitis, bursitis, or acromioclavicular joint arthritis.
2. Physical examination
  (a) General concepts
    - A focused musculoskeletal examination should always move through the same progression of components: inspection, palpation, range of motion, strength testing, special tests, and neurovascular assessment.

- A cervical spine examination should always be included, as there are certainly cervical spine conditions that can cause shoulder pain.
- When examining a patient with shoulder pain, it is imperative to expose the shoulder for inspection.
  - Men should be asked to remove their shirts to expose the extremity, and women should be asked to dress down to a shirt that exposes the shoulder or instead to wear a gown for the examination.

(b) Inspection
- The shoulder should be inspected from various perspectives, and any evidence of swelling, deformity, ecchymosis, asymmetry, healed incisions, or scars should be documented.
- The subcutaneous osseous anatomy can also be assessed, including the sternoclavicular and acromioclavicular joints, clavicle, as well as the acromion and scapular spine.
- Static winging of the scapula can be appreciated when viewing the exposed extremity from the posterior perspective.
- The examiner should also evaluate the appearance of certain soft tissue structures about the shoulder.
  - Namely, careful attention should be paid to inspection of the supraspinatus and infraspinatus fossae of the scapula.
  - In the case of chronic rotator cuff tearing, or denervation injury, atrophy of these rotator cuff muscles can be appreciated.
  - If the long head of biceps brachii tendon has ruptured, the patient will present with an obvious cosmetic "Popeye" deformity due to the distal retraction of the muscle, which can only be appreciated on the exposed arm.
- In the case of adhesive capsulitis, however, inspection may not reveal any significant abnormality about the shoulder visible to the examiner.

(c) Palpation
- The examiner should spend time palpating the accessible structures that may contribute to shoulder pain.
  - Sternoclavicular and acromioclavicular joints.
  - The biceps tendon as it passes anteriorly along the bicipital groove.
  - Palpation along the trapezius may elicit pain in the case of spasm or strain, which can often accompany adhesive capsulitis.
  - Palpation lateral to the lateral edge of the acromion, deep to the deltoid origin, may create tenderness in the case of subacromial bursitis, rotator cuff tendonitis, or tearing.
  - Palpation along the periphery of the scapula can often elicit tenderness from periscapular strain and can allow for the identification of crepitus or popping consistent with snapping scapula.
- The challenge with adhesive capsulitis rests with the fact that the entire shoulder can be painful, and the patient may present with more diffuse tenderness rather than focal findings.

(d) Range of Motion
  • As with any patient presenting with shoulder pain, it is important to assess both active and passive motion.
  • Simple motion in forward elevation, abduction, and external rotation at the side is evaluated (Fig. 9.1a, b).
  • Composite motion such as internal rotation and extension measured by the most cephalad achievable spinous process, and external rotation in abduction are also quantified.
  • The defining physical examination finding in patients with adhesive capsulitis is a limitation in both active and passive range motion [4, 5].
  • Early in the natural history of adhesive capsulitis, the limitation in motion can be quite subtle, but during the frozen phase, the difference in motion compared to the contralateral side can be significant.
  • Limitation of active motion with preserved passive motion might instead suggest rotator cuff dysfunction, including tearing or denervation. Injury to the deltoid muscle or axillary neuropathy can also present in this way.
(e) Strength
  • At minimum, strength is assessed in abduction, external rotation at the side, external rotation in abduction, and internal rotation at the side. Including these four parameters allows for evaluation of the four components of the rotator cuff: supraspinatus, infraspinatus, teres minor, and subscapularis, respectively.
  • Manual muscle testing is done by asking the patient to resist the examiner in the mid-arc of motion, and strength is qualitatively graded as follows: grade 5, full strength; grade 4, less than full strength; grade 3, able to move the extremity against gravity; grade 2, able to move the extremity with gravity eliminated; and grade 1, fasciculations of muscle present.

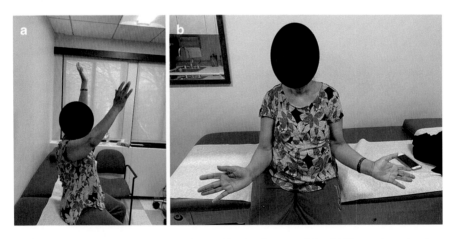

**Fig. 9.1** (a) Forward elevation in a patient with adhesive capsulitis. (b) External rotation in a patient with adhesive capsulitis

- Typically, patients with adhesive capsulitis will present with full strength; however, pain-mediated weakness may be present depending on the stage of the condition at the time of presentation.
- If true weakness exists in a patient with suspected adhesive capsulitis, then either an alternative or concomitant diagnosis should be considered.

(f) Directed Tests

- Special tests have limited utility in the evaluation of a patient with adhesive capsulitis.
- As this condition is characterized fundamentally by the combination of significant pain and limited range of motion, most sensitive though nonspecific tests for other painful conditions of the shoulder may be positive and therefore may mislead the examining physician.
    - These include special tests for the rotator cuff (Neer, Hawkins, Jobe signs), for the biceps tendon (Speed, Yergason signs), and for the labrum (active compression, biceps load, and crank tests), among others.
    - Moreover, many of these tests, including lag signs for rotator cuff tears, simply may not be possible in the setting of limited range of motion.
- The role of directed tests in the evaluation of these patients is significantly limited; therefore, physicians should rely instead on the components of the examination described previously for the identification of adhesive capsulitis among their patients.

3. Imaging

(a) X-rays

- General concepts
    - The single most important imaging modality in the assessment of a patient who might have adhesive capsulitis is plain radiographs.
    - The primary distinction that must be made when evaluating these patients is whether they have adhesive capsulitis, or instead osteoarthritis, since these are the two common conditions that can cause both pain and limited passive range of motion.
    - Plain radiographs will easily reveal which patients have osteoarthritis, with a constellation of findings including joint space narrowing, osteophyte and loose body formation, subchondral sclerosis, cyst formation, and posterior migration of the humeral head.
    - Plain radiographs can also reveal findings consistent with calcific tendonitis, with radio-opaque calcific deposits within the rotator cuff insertion.
    - While plain radiographs are mostly used to rule out alternative pathology, relative osteopenia has been described as a subtle radiographic finding in patients with adhesive capsulitis.

- Views
    - Anteroposterior

        An internally rotated view will provide visualization of the lesser tuberosity.

        An externally rotated view will provide visualization of the greater tuberosity.

        A true Grashey view is obtained by angling the patient 30–45° toward the affected side, with the shoulder slightly internally rotated. This technique provides a perpendicular view of the glenohumeral joint, without overlap between the humeral head and glenoid.
    - Scapular lateral view
    - Axillary view
- (b) MRI
    - Advanced imaging has a limited role in the evaluation of a patient with adhesive capsulitis. It is uncommon for a patient with adhesive capsulitis to have concomitant structural injury such as a rotator cuff tear.
    - In fact, MRI can be misleading in revealing minor structural findings including partial rotator cuff tearing or incidental labrum tearing. The treating physician should exercise extreme caution in interpreting an MRI in a patient with adhesive capsulitis and must place incidental findings in context.
        - A partial tear of the rotator cuff or a labrum tear is rarely the primary source of pain and stiffness in these patients; therefore, formal treatment of this pathology should be deferred.
    - Only in occasional cases should a physician consider obtaining an MRI for patients with adhesive capsulitis.
        - First, if risk factors are found to be consistent with a possible concomitant rotator cuff tear, such as recent trauma or rotator cuff weakness on examination.
        - Second, if a patient does not progress as expected with appropriate treatment for adhesive capsulitis, then an MRI can be obtained.
        - Except for these rare cases, MRI and other advanced imaging modalities should be avoided in the evaluation of patients with adhesive capsulitis.
        - When obtained, positive findings include contracture and thickening of the glenohumeral joint capsule, particularly in the axillary recess.
4. Treatment
    - (a) Nonoperative management
        - General concepts
            - Adhesive capsulitis has been described as a self-limited condition, because for most patients it will typically resolve on its own if given enough time.
            - The vast majority of patients will improve without operative intervention.

- Formal conservative management can perhaps expedite recovery somewhat and possibly help some patients recover without the need for surgery [6].
- Establishing appropriate expectations for the patient with adhesive capsulitis is critical. He or she should be informed that even with structured conservative management, recovery may require 6 months or longer [3, 7–9].

• Components of nonoperative management
    - Nonsteroidal anti-inflammatory medication
    - Rest from strenuous activities
    - Periodic icing for symptomatic relief
    - Physical therapy

    Early in the condition, particularly during the freezing phase, therapy will focus on anti-inflammatory modalities.

    As pain improves, rehabilitation will begin to focus on therapeutic exercises to improve range of motion.

    - Corticosteroid

    Corticosteroid, administered orally or via injection, may play an important role in the management of adhesive capsulitis, depending on the stage of the condition when a patient presents for treatment.

    These medications are particularly useful during the freezing phase; however, they may also provide benefit even later in the disease, primarily with respect to pain.

    Oral corticosteroid

    Typically prescribed as a scheduled tapering dose of methylprednisolone, can be prescribed for patients who present with evidence of significant inflammation or for those who choose to defer an injection [10]

    Corticosteroid injection

    Allows for direct delivery of the medication in the glenohumeral joint and its capsule, the structure primarily affected by the condition.

    Can be administered with the physician's corticosteroid of choice, combined with local anesthetic, with or without ultrasound guidance.

    The patient is typically advised to rest and ice the shoulder for several days, to use non-steroidal anti-inflammatory medication, and to begin physical therapy 1 week after the injection.

    A single injection is typically sufficient; repeat injections are rarely required and risk damage to the soft tissue structures in close proximity to the glenohumeral joint [2, 11, 12].

    Hydrodilation

    Hydrodilation has been described as an alternative to steroid injection alone.

With this procedure, also referred to as capsular distension, normal saline is injected into the intra-articular space, often with ultrasound guidance, in order to distend the contracted glenohumeral joint capsule.

Local anesthetic and corticosteroid are often included in the injection. The amount of fluid injected varies in the literature.

There is data to support the effectiveness of this treatment modality in the nonoperative management of adhesive capsulitis [13, 14].

Other modalities

Hyaluronic acid injection

Platelet-rich plasma injection

Extracorporeal shock wave therapy

TNF alpha inhibitors

Others

(b) Operative management
- General concepts
  - Operative intervention only becomes necessary when symptoms persist despite appropriate nonsurgical management and after a prolonged period of time.
  - While specific recommendations for a mandatory minimum amount of time for conservative management before surgery is considered are perhaps lacking, it has been recommended to wait 6 months before considering operative intervention [3, 14–16].
  - Operating earlier on these patients risks subjecting certain individuals to surgery unnecessarily, as they may have otherwise improved with additional time and conservative treatment.
- Positioning and anesthesia
  - This procedure is typically performed under general anesthesia together with a peripheral nerve block.
    Historically, indwelling catheters were often used to provide durable anesthesia to assist in immediate range of motion exercises.
    Currently, similar pain relief can be achieved with a long-acting nerve block using liposomal bupivacaine.
  - The patient is placed in the beach chair position with the cervical spine in a neutral position.
- Principles
  - When operative intervention is required, it typically consists of arthroscopic capsular release and manipulation under anesthesia.
  - An examination under anesthesia is performed to document preoperative range of motion.
  - Some surgeons will begin the procedure with a manipulation of the shoulder. However, others will instead begin with arthroscopy and reserve manipulation for later in the procedure.

- A diagnostic arthroscopy is then performed through a standard posterior viewing portal and anterior rotator interval portal.

  The surgeon should move through his or her typical progression of assessment of all visible structures within the glenohumeral joint, including the humeral head and glenoid articular surfaces, glenoid labrum, biceps tendon including its anchor on the superior labrum and its extra-articular groove portion, rotator cuff tendons, and the axillary recess.

  It is extremely important always to remember to insert the arthroscope through the anterior portal to allow for comprehensive evaluation of the posterior structures.

  The most remarkable finding in patients with adhesive capsulitis will be extensive synovitis throughout the glenohumeral joint space (Fig. 9.2).

  It is rare to encounter significant concomitant structural tearing of the rotator cuff. Less significant degenerative changes can be seen, but rarely require formal treatment.
- Technique

  Capsular release

  This portion of the procedure is typically performed while viewing from the posterior portal and working through the anterior portal (Fig. 9.3).

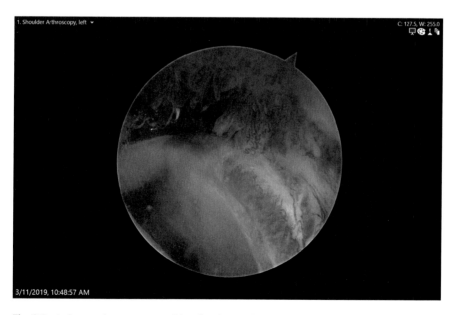

**Fig. 9.2** Arthroscopic appearance of the glenohumeral space in a patient with adhesive capsulitis, with extensive synovitis throughout the joint

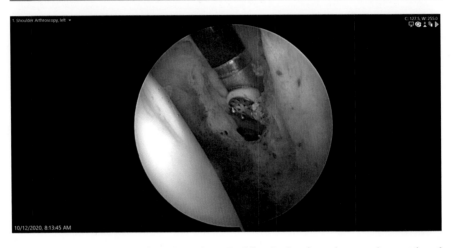

**Fig. 9.3** Anterior capsular release is performed while viewing from the posterior portal, and working through the anterior rotator interval portal. The anterior capsule is released using a radiofrequency ablation instrument as seen here, or with a capsular biting instrument, to the level of the muscular subscapularis, while taking care to avoid the axillary nerve

The rotator interval tissue is first debrided, primarily using the radiofrequency ablation instrument.

Care is taken to avoid the anterior leading edge of the supraspinatus, the biceps tendon, and subscapularis.

After thorough debridement of the interval tissue, the coracoid process and origin of the conjoined tendon can be visualized.

The release is the continued toward the anterior capsule along the articular aspect of the subscapularis tendon.

This aspect of the procedure can be performed either with the radiofrequency ablation instrument or a capsular biter, an instrument with one blunt tip that can be inserted in the interval between capsular and subscapularis tissue.

Regardless of approach, care should be taken to avoid the axillary nerve as the release progressed toward the inferior capsule.

Manipulation

Once the initial anterior capsular release is performed, some surgeons will then perform the manipulation.

A brief reevaluation of motion will reveal a significant improvement in external rotation at the side at this point in the procedure. The manipulation is then performed, primarily in forward elevation.

It is important to maintain a short lever arm on the humerus during manipulation to avoid risk of iatrogenic fracture.

Manipulation in rotation should not be performed for this same reason.

The arthroscope can then be reinserted into the glenohumeral joint to assess the release.

The surgeon will notice that the manipulation propagated the release from the point of instrumented release toward the inferior capsule and axillary recess.

The muscular subscapularis can be visualized superficial to the released capsular tissue (Fig. 9.4).

Oftentimes, the axillary nerve can be visualized as it travels from anterior to posterior inferior to the glenohumeral joint (Fig. 9.5).

Controversies

There is debate in the literature regarding the importance of posterior capsular release.

There is evidence that patients can ultimately regain motion in all directions following isolated anterior capsular release with manipulation [14].

However, some surgeons continue to prefer to include posterior capsular release as well.

This step in the procedure is often performed while viewing from the anterior portal and working posteriorly.

Using the radiofrequency ablation instrument with a hook tip can increase precision of the procedure, which is helpful to avoid the supraspinatus and infraspinatus, which are immediately adjacent to the rather thin posterior capsule.

The release can be continued from the anterior rotator interval release, along the superior capsule, toward the posterior capsule, culminating at the site of the posterior portal.

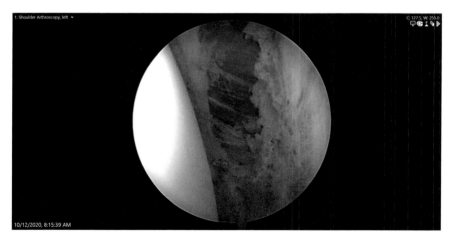

**Fig. 9.4** The initial anterior capsular release has been completed, and the subscapularis muscle fibers can be visualized deep to the released capsular tissue

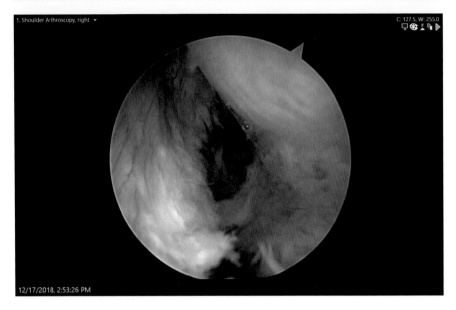

**Fig. 9.5** Following initial instrumented capsular release, followed by manipulation, the capsulotomy has been propagated through the inferior capsule as well in a safe, controlled manner

After this portion of the procedure, the motion can be reassessed, and the surgeon will notice improvement in internal rotation in abduction.

There is debate regarding the need to address concomitant pathology at the time of operative intervention for adhesive capsulitis.

It is very unlikely that the surgeon will encounter significant and symptomatic pathology that will require formal treatment.

A rare patient may present with a combination of a full-thickness rotator cuff tear and shoulder stiffness.

When required, patients can be effectively treated with concomitant capsular release with manipulation and repair of the rotator cuff.

However, there may still be a preference for staged treatment in this case, with initial management of stiffness, and treatment of the rotator cuff with a second procedure once a patient has regained adequate range of motion.

Debate also exists regarding appropriate treatment of the long head of biceps tendon.

As with the rotator cuff, it is very rare to encounter significant pathology of the biceps tendon that require formal treatment.

Unless the surgeon encounters significant tearing, disruption of the biceps anchor on the superior labrum, or disruption of the bicipital sling with instability, formal treatment of the biceps tendon should be deferred.

Finally, there is a question regarding the need for subacromial decompression when treating adhesive capsulitis.

If a surgeon inserts the arthroscope into the subacromial space, he or she should consider formal bursectomy and/or acromioplasty only if significantly pathology is encountered.

- Risks and complications
  - Operative intervention for adhesive capsulitis is a technically simple procedure with less risk compared to other procedures for the treatment of shoulder conditions. However, certain risks should be kept in mind.
  - Iatrogenic fracture

    When performing the manipulation, the surgeons should maintain a short lever arm by controlling the humerus as close to the glenohumeral joint as possible to mitigate risk of iatrogenic fracture, particularly in osteoporotic patients.
  - Axillary nerve injury

    As with any shoulder procedure, the axillary nerve must also be protected and may be at risk during the capsular release.

    Using the capsular biter with one blunt tip allows the surgeon to develop a plane between capsule and subscapularis before biting the capsule, thereby assuring that only capsular tissue is captured by the instrument.

    The surgeon can also protect the axillary nerve by continuing the capsular release only to the level of the muscular subscapularis.

    The manipulation can then be performed in order to propagate the release indirectly toward the axillary recess. Occasionally, once the arthroscope is reinserted, the surgeon can visualize the axillary nerve passing inferior to the joint immediately deep to the released capsule, underscoring the proximity of this structure.
  - Incorrect diagnosis or treatment

    As mentioned previously, it is rare to encounter concurrent pathology that is clinically important and requires operative intervention. Instead, this pathology is often incidental.

    If the surgeon fails to diagnose, and therefore appropriately treat, adhesive capsulitis, or if the surgeon diagnoses and inappropriately treats incidental pathology, this can have a detrimental impact on the patient's ultimate outcome.

    With a careful evaluation including a detailed physical examination, and with sufficient skepticism regarding associated conditions, this issue can be avoided.

# References

1. Kitridis D, Tsikopoulos K, Bisbinas I, Papaioannidou P, Givissis P. Efficacy of pharmacological therapies for adhesive capsulitis of the shoulder: a systematic review and network meta-analysis. Am J Sports Med. 2019;47(14):3552–60.
2. Sun Y, Zhang P, Liu S, et al. Intra-articular steroid injection for frozen shoulder: a systematic review and meta-analysis of randomized controlled trials with trial sequential analysis. Am J Sports Med. 2017;45(9):2171–9.
3. Le HV, Lee SJ, Nazarian A, Rodriguez EK. Adhesive capsulitis of the shoulder: review of pathophysiology and current clinical treatments. Should Elb. 2017;9(2):75–84.
4. Hsu JE, Anakwenze OA, Warrender WJ, Abboud JA. Current review of adhesive capsulitis. J Shoulder Elb Surg. 2011;20(3):502–14.
5. Dias R, Cutts S, Massoud S. Frozen shoulder. BMJ. 2005;331(7530):1453–6.
6. Hand C, Clipsham K, Rees JL, Carr AJ. Long-term outcome of frozen shoulder. J Shoulder Elb Surg. 2008;17(2):231–6.
7. Zhang J, Zhong S, Tan T, et al. Comparative efficacy and patient-specific moderating factors of nonsurgical treatment strategies for frozen shoulder: an updated systematic review and network meta-analysis. Am J Sports Med. 2020;2020:363546520956293.
8. Griggs SM, Ahn A, Green A. Idiopathic adhesive capsulitis. A prospective functional outcome study of nonoperative treatment. J Bone Joint Surg Am. 2000;82(10):1398–407.
9. Levine WN, Kashyap CP, Bak SF, Ahmad CS, Blaine TA, Bigliani LU. Nonoperative management of idiopathic adhesive capsulitis. J Shoulder Elb Surg. 2007;16(5):569–73.
10. Buchbinder R, Hoving JL, Green S, Hall S, Forbes A, Nash P. Short course prednisolone for adhesive capsulitis (frozen shoulder or stiff painful shoulder): a randomised, double blind, placebo controlled trial. Ann Rheum Dis. 2004;63(11):1460–9.
11. Lorbach O, Anagnostakos K, Scherf C, Seil R, Kohn D, Pape D. Nonoperative management of adhesive capsulitis of the shoulder: oral cortisone application versus intra-articular cortisone injections. J Shoulder Elb Surg. 2010;19(2):172–9.
12. Oh JH, Oh CH, Choi JA, Kim SH, Kim JH, Yoon JP. Comparison of glenohumeral and subacromial steroid injection in primary frozen shoulder: a prospective, randomized short-term comparison study. J Shoulder Elb Surg. 2011;20(7):1034–40.
13. Yoon JP, Chung SW, Kim JE, et al. Intra-articular injection, subacromial injection, and hydrodilatation for primary frozen shoulder: a randomized clinical trial. J Shoulder Elb Surg. 2016;25(3):376–83.
14. Yip M, Francis AM, Roberts T, Rokito A, Zuckerman JD, Virk MS. Treatment of adhesive capsulitis of the shoulder: a critical analysis review. JBJS Rev. 2018;6(6):e5.
15. Rangan A, Brealey SD, Keding A, et al. Management of adults with primary frozen shoulder in secondary care (UK FROST): a multicentre, pragmatic, three-arm, superiority randomised clinical trial. Lancet. 2020;396(10256):977–89.
16. Favejee MM, Huisstede BM, Koes BW. Frozen shoulder: the effectiveness of conservative and surgical interventions–systematic review. Br J Sports Med. 2011;45(1):49–56.

# Impingement and Acromioclavicular Arthritis

# 10

Lauren Zurek and Bradford Parsons

## Introduction

Subacromial impingement syndrome is a spectrum of pathology involving the structures of the subacromial space, ranging from subacromial bursitis to rotator cuff tendinopathy and ultimately, can lead to degenerative partial and full-thickness tears of the rotator cuff [1]. Subacromial impingement syndrome and acromioclavicular arthritis are common sources of shoulder pain for which nonoperative management is typically successful. Surgery is reserved for those who do not respond to nonoperative modalities.

1. Background
   (a) Subacromial space is defined by the undersurface of the acromion superiorly, the humeral head inferiorly, and the margin of the subacromial bursa laterally.
       • The subacromial space contains the subacromial bursa, the bursal aspect of the rotator cuff tendons, and the coracoacromial ligament [2].
           – The subacromial bursa reduces friction and thus facilitates movement, between the overlying coracoacromial arch and the rotator cuff below [3].
           – The coracoacromial ligament is a stout triangular band that spans between the undersurface of the acromion and the coracoid process.
       • The coracoacromial ligament, acromion, and coracoid process form an osseoligamentous structure referred to as the coracoacromial arch [4].
       • Acromion

L. Zurek (✉) · B. Parsons
Mount Sinai Hospital, New York, NY, USA
e-mail: Bradford.Parsons@mountsinai.org

- Forms from the union of four ossification centers.

  Basi-acromion, meta-acromion, meso-acromion, and pre-acromion.

  Failure of the ossification centers to unite results in an os acromiale, which can be a rare source of pain.

  Reported prevalence in the population is 8% [5].

  Occurs most frequently at the junction between the meso- and meta-acromion [5].

  Frequently found incidentally on radiographs or advanced imaging.

- Bigliani classification of acromial morphology [6]

  Type I, flat

  Type II, curved

  Type III, hooked

  Associated with rotator cuff degeneration [6]

- Etiology
  - Intrinsic tendon degeneration, either from diminished vascular supply, aging, trauma, or tensile forces, leads to rotator cuff weakness and, ultimately, humeral ascent against the overlying structures creating subacromial impingement [7].
  - Extrinsic compression from extratendinous structures leads to tendon inflammation and, ultimately, degeneration [7].

    Main source of compression is felt to be the anterior acromion and coracoacromial ligament.

    Other potential causes of compression include degeneration of the acromioclavicular (AC) joint, glenohumeral instability, tuberosity fracture nonunion or malunion, mobile os acriomale, calcific tendinitis, and iatrogenic factors.

  - Despite ongoing debate on the etiology, subacromial impingement syndrome is likely multifactorial, involving both extrinsic compression and intrinsic degeneration.

(b) The AC joint is a diarthrodial articulation between the acromion process of the scapula and the distal end of the clavicle.

- Fibrocartilaginous disk, analogous to the meniscus of the knee, provides cushion to the joint [8].
- Fibrous capsule inserts around the articular margin of the joint.
- The AC ligaments are confluent with the fibrous capsule and resist anterior and posterior translation of the joint [8].
  - The posterior and superior AC ligaments are the most important for stability [8].
- The coracoclavicular ligament is composed of the conoid and trapezoid ligaments [8].
  - Resists superior and axial translation of the joint, primarily.
  - In the absence of AC ligaments, resists anterior and posterior translation.
  - Conoid ligament is the strongest of the components.

- Despite the small surface area, the AC joint withstands significant axial and rotational forces [8].
- Degeneration of the AC joint can occur due to a multitude of factors including age-related degeneration of the intra-articular meniscus, post-traumatic arthropathy, distal clavicle osteolysis, inflammatory arthropathy, septic arthritis, joint instability, and impingement [9].
  - Distal clavicle osteolysis is a distinct entity felt to be caused by hyper-vascularization, and ultimately, bone resorption after repetitive micro-trauma causes small subchondral fractures [10].

2. History
   (a) Subacromial impingement
   - Anterolateral shoulder pain which radiates into the lateral deltoid region [11].
   - Typically, insidious with a gradual increase in symptoms, although can follow a specific inciting event which led to an acute traumatic bursitis [11].
   - Aggravation of pain with certain arm positions, such as overhead shoulder elevation, lifting objects away from the body, or terminal internal rotation [11].
     - Reaching for an object on a high shelf
     - Putting on a coat
   - Night pain or disturbance is often present [11].
   (b) AC arthritis and distal clavicle osteolysis
   - Anterior or superior shoulder pain.
   - Young adult and middle-aged patients.
   - Pain is aggravated by overhead and crossbody movements [12].
   - Commonly, patients have a history of weightlifting or other repetitive overhead activities [12].
   - Mechanical symptoms such as popping, catching, or grinding are frequently reported [12].

3. Physical exam
   (a) Inspect or palpate for any muscle atrophy, swelling, deformity, or prominence of the distal clavicle as compared to the contralateral side.
   - Direct palpation of the AC joint frequently yields tenderness in the patient with symptomatic arthritis or osteolysis [13].
   (b) Passive and active shoulder range of motion should be performed to differentiate impingement from adhesive capsulitis.
   (c) Rotator cuff strength should be assessed, as weakness would suggest a possible rotator cuff tear as opposed to isolated impingement.
   (d) If patient has a known os acromiale, palpation of the nonunion site as a potential site of tenderness or an unstable fragment should be performed [14].
   (e) Provocative maneuvers
   - Subacromial impingement
     - Neer impingement sign is performed by standing behind the patient and passively elevating the arm in the scapular plane while stabilizing the scapula and is considered positive if elevation beyond 90° produces pain [15].

- Hawkins test is performed by forcibly internally rotating the arm after passively elevating the shoulder to 90° and is considered positive if pain is elicited [16].
- These maneuvers decrease the subacromial space while also increasing contact between the rotator cuff and the bony and ligamentous borders of the subacromial space [17].
- AC arthritis and distal clavicle osteolysis
  - Crossbody adduction test is considered positive if pain is elicited when the shoulder is brought into 90° of forward flexion and maximal adduction [18].
  - The AC resisted extension test involves bringing the shoulder into 90° of forward flexion and the patient actively extends against resistance. This is considered positive if it elicits pain [18].
  - O'Brien active compression test involves bringing the shoulder to 90° of forward flexion and 10° of adduction. The patient performs resisted shoulder flexion with the arm in maximal internal rotation and then again with maximal supination. Pain when the arm is in maximal supination is consistent with AC pathology [18].
  - The Bell-van Riet test is a combination of the crossbody adduction and O'Brien tests. The affected shoulder is flexed to 90°, the arm is maximally adducted across the body, and the patient actively elevates against resistant with the shoulder in internal rotation. The test is considered positive if pain is elicited [18].
4. Imaging
   (a) X-rays
   - The anteroposterior (AP) view in the normal plane is used to evaluate the AC joint, specifically for any osteophyte formation or osteolysis.
     - Common radiographic findings with AC arthritis include joint space narrowing, subchondral cysts, osteophytes, and subchondral sclerosis [19].
       Radiographic degeneration of the AC joint is common and can be seen as early as the second decade of life, but is not necessarily symptomatic [20].
     - This view may reveal ossification of the coracoacromial ligament or the presence of a subacromial spur which is common with subacromial impingement.
   - The AP view in the scapular plane, also known as a Grashey view, is used to evaluate the glenohumeral joint and may show sclerotic or cystic changes in the greater tuberosity in later stages of impingement.
   - The Zanca view obtains the best visualization of the AC joint by eliminating the overlay of the scapular spine. It is an AP view obtained with 10–15° of cephalad tilt to the beam.
   - The axillary view should be assessed for the presence of an os acromiale and any displacement of the AC joint.
   - The scapular Y view is best used for determining acromial morphology.

(b) MRI
- Can be useful for obtaining additional detail about concomitant pathology and potential sites of subacromial impingement, although not always necessary as this can typically be seen on plain radiographs.
- Should be obtained if there is a suspicion for rotator cuff tear based on either patient history or exam.
- Capsular hypertrophy, effusion, and subchondral edema are commonly seen with AC pathology [21].

(c) Ultrasound
- Can be used as an alternative to MRI for evaluation of rotator cuff integrity, but results are highly technician dependent.

5. Treatment algorithm based on diagnosis
   (a) Nonoperative treatment
   - Mainstay of initial management for subacromial impingement syndrome, symptomatic os acromiale, acromioclavicular arthritis, and distal clavicle osteolysis.
   - Activity modification with avoidance of pain aggravating activities.
   - Non-steroidal anti-inflammatory drugs (NSAIDs) can be clinically effective in treating the inflammation of the subacromial bursa seen with impingement syndrome [22] and the inflammation associated with AC pathology.
   - Physical therapy with a specific rehabilitation protocol is a modality commonly used and that is effective in lowering the percentage of patients who need surgical intervention [23].
     - A specific rehabilitation protocol for subacromial impingement includes stretching, eccentric rotator cuff strengthening, and scapular stabilization exercises [23].
   - Subacromial corticosteroid injections are an adjunct treatment for impingement which can be used to help facilitate participation with physical therapy [22].
   - AC intra-articular corticosteroid injections can serve both a diagnostic and therapeutic role in patients with findings consistent with AC arthritis or distal clavicle osteolysis [24].
     - Despite the subcutaneous location of the AC joint, intra-articular injections can be difficult and accuracy can be improved with use of ultrasound guidance [25].
   - Platelet-rich plasma (PRP) contains specific growth factors believed to promote healing, such as platelet-derived growth factor, vascular endothelial growth factor, and insulin-like growth factor [26].
     - Although there is some evidence demonstrating a positive effect of PRP in the treatment of tendinopathies, there is inconclusive data evaluating its specific effectiveness for the treatment of subacromial impingement or rotator cuff tendinopathy [26].
   - The American Academy of Orthopaedic Surgeons practice guidelines recommend management of impingement syndrome with physical

therapy and NSAIDs, but neither support nor refute the use of corticosteroid injections or other modalities such as pulsed electromagnetic fields, iontophoresis, phonophoresis, transcutaneous electrical nerve stimulation, ice, heat, massage, or activity modification [27].

(b) Operative treatment
- Surgical intervention is reserved for patients with persistent pain after a trial of nonoperative treatment.
- In the absence of a full-thickness rotator cuff tear or a partial-thickness tear of more than 50% thickness, subacromial decompression alone can be an effective treatment for subacromial impingement.
  - Prior to the advent of arthroscopy, a decompression was an open anterior acromioplasty, but this required detachment of the deltoid from the acromion to access the subacromial space and failure of the deltoid to heal can lead to dysfunction [28].
  - Arthroscopic decompression consists of removing the subacromial bursa, an anterior acromioplasty, and excision of the coracoacromial ligament with an arthroscope through standard arthroscopic portals [28].
     There is some ongoing debate whether a bursectomy without acromioplasty is adequate treatment for subacromial impingement syndrome [29].
  - To adequately eliminate extrinsic compression of the rotator cuff with an acromioplasty, the anterior third of the acromion should be flattened with an arthroscopic bur to resemble a type I acromion [2].
  - If an os acromiale is present, but not felt to be symptomatic, during a subacromial decompression, care must be taken to not violate the deltoid attachment, or the fibrous membrane that spans the unfused area of the os, as this could destabilize the fragment.
- Open reduction and internal fixation of a symptomatic os acromiale has more favorable outcomes than excision of the fragment, but nonunion rates and need for hardware removal remains high [30].
- Distal clavicle resection has proven good to excellent results for both AC arthritis and distal clavicle osteolysis, but has less predictable results for post-traumatic arthropathy [31].
  - With an open procedure, an incision is made overlying the AC joint and the distal clavicle is resected with an oscillating saw or osteotome. The approach does require disruption of the deltotrapezial fascia and the superior AC capsule and ligaments, which if not adequately repaired, can lead to destabilization and persistent pain [8].
  - Arthroscopic technique includes two approaches: direct and bursal. Direct approach is considered more technically demanding and typically reserved for patients with isolated AC joint disease as it does not violate the bursal space.

Bursal approach with standard arthroscopic portals is recommended in patients with other concurrent pathology, as it allows the surgeon to address all of the pathology.

Resection is performed with the use of an arthroscopic bur under direct visualization, regardless of arthroscopic approach.

While the surgeon wants an even and adequate resection so that there is no residual contact between the clavicle and acromion, excess resection can lead to instability from compromise of the bony insertions of the stabilizing ligaments.

There is no exact resection length that has been definitively recommended, but most surgeons would agree that a resection of 8 to 10 mm is adequate while avoiding iatrogenic instability [10].

- Most common complication after distal clavicle resection is persistent pain, which can result from either over- or under-resection [10].

The most common site for insufficient resection with an arthroscopic approach is posterior and superior, but moving the arthroscope to a direct anterior portal for better visualization can aid in avoiding this complication [10].

Less frequently, instability of the AC joint can occur, either from excessive bony resection which disrupts the coracoclavicular ligaments or from violation of the superior AC capsule, and is more common with an open approach.

# References

1. Neer CS II. Anterior acromioplasty for the chronic impingement syndrome in the shoulder: a preliminary report. J Bone Joint Surg Am. 1972;54(1):41–50.
2. Flatow EL, Soslowsky LJ, Ticker JB, Pawluk RJ, Helper M, Ark J, Mow VC, Bigliani LU. Excursion of the rotator cuff under the acromion. Patterns of subacromial contact. Am J Sports Med. 1994;22:779–88.
3. Bigliani LU, Ticker JB, Flatow EL, Soslowsky LJ, Mow VC. The relationship of acromial architecture to rotator cuff disease. Clin Sports Med. 1991;10:823–38.
4. Soslowsky LJ, An CH, Johnston SP, Carpenter JE. Geometric and mechanical properties of the coracoacromial ligament and their relationship to rotator cuff disease. Clin Orthop Relat Res. 1994;304:10–7.
5. Kurtz C, Humble B, Rodosky M, Sekiya J. Symptomatic os acromiale. J Am Acad Orthoped Surg. 2006;14:12–9.
6. Bigliani BU, Morrison ES, April EW. The morphology of the acromion and its relationship to rotator cuff tears. Orthop Trans. 1986;10:216.
7. Chansky HA, Iannotti JP. The vascularity of the rotator cuff. Clin Sports Med. 1991;10(4):807–22.
8. Corteen DP, Teitge RA. Stabilization of the clavicle after distal resection: a biomechanical study. Am J Sports Med. 2005;33(1):61–7.
9. DePalma AF. The role of the discs of the sternoclavicular and acromioclavicular joints. Clin Orthop Relat Res. 1959;13:7–12.

10. Aaron D, Parsons B, Cagle P, Flatow E. Arthroscopic treatment of subacromial and acromio-clavicular pathology. In: Nicholson G, editor. Orthopaedic knowledge update: shoulder and elbow 5. Alphen aan den Rijn: Wolters Kluwer; 2020. p. 223–38.
11. Bigliani LU, Levine WN. Subacromial impingement syndrome. J Bone Joint Surg Am. 1997;79(12):1854–68.
12. Shu B, Johnston T, Lindsey DP, McAdams TR. Biomechanical evaluation of a novel reverse coracoacromial ligament reconstruction for acromioclavicular joint separation. Am J Sports Med. 2012;40(2):440–6.
13. Hegedus EJ, Goode A, Campbell S, et al. Physical examination tests of the shoulder: a system-atic review with meta-analysis of individual tests. Br J Sports Med. 2008;42(2):80–92.
14. Ortiguera CJ, Buss DD. Surgical management of the symptomatic os acromiale. J Shoulder Elb Surg. 2002;11(5):521–8.
15. Neer CS II. Impingement lesions. Clin Orthop Relat Res. 1983;173:70–7.
16. Hawkins RJ, Kennedy J. C: Impingement syndrome in athletes. Am J Sports Med. 1980;8:151–8.
17. Codman EA. The shoulder. New York: G. Miller & Co. Medical Publishers; 1934.
18. Chronopoulos E, Kim TK, Park HB, Ashenbrenner D, McFarland EG. Diagnostic value of phys-ical tests for isolated chronic acromioclavicular lesions. Am J Sports Med. 2004;32(3):655–61.
19. Ernberg LA, Potter HG. Radiographic evaluation of the acromioclavicular and sternoclavicu-lar joints. Clin Sports Med. 2003;22(2):255–75.
20. Meyer AW. The minute anatomy of attritional lesions. J Bone Joint Surg Am. 1931;13:341–60.
21. Strobel K, Pfirrmann CW, Zanetti M, Nagy L, Hodler J. MRI features of the acromiocla-vicular joint that predict pain relief from intraarticular injection. AJR Am J Roentgenol. 2003;181(3):755–60.
22. Kim YS, Bigliani LU, Fujisawa M, et al. Stromal cell-derived factor 1 (SDF-1, CXCL12) is increased in subacromial bursitis and downregulated by steroid and nonsteroidal anti-inflammatory agents. J Orthop Res. 2006;24(8):1756–64.
23. Holmgren T, Bjornsson Hallgren H, Oberg B, Adolfsson L, Johansson K. Effect of specific exercise strategy on need for surgery in patients with subacromial impingement syndrome: randomized controlled study. BMJ. 2012;344:787.
24. Docimo S Jr, Kornitsky D, Futterman B, Elkowitz DE. Surgical treatment for acromioclavicu-lar joint osteoarthritis: patient selection, surgical options, complications, and outcome. Curr Rev Musculoskelet Med. 2008;1(2):154–60.
25. Borbas P, Kraus T, Clement H, et al. The influence of ultrasound guidance in the rate of success of acromioclavicular joint injection: an experimental study on human cadavers. J Shoulder Elb Surg. 2012;21(12):1694–7.
26. Nejati P, Ghahremaninia A, Naderi F, Garibzadeh S, Mazaherinezhad A. Treatment of sub-acromial impingement syndrome: platelet-rich-plasma or exercise therapy? A randomized controlled trial. Orthop J Sports Med. 2017;5:5.
27. Pedowitz RA, Yamaguchi K, Ahmad CS, et al. American Academy of Orthopaedic Surgeons clinical practice guideline on: optimizing the management of rotator cuff problems. J Bone Joint Surg Am. 2012;94(2):163–7.
28. Davis AD, Kakar S, Moros C, Kaye EK, Schepsis AA, Voloshin I. Arthroscopic versus open acromioplasty: a meta- analysis. Am J Sports Med. 2010;38(3):613–8.
29. Kolk A, Thomassen BJW, Hund H, et al. Does acromioplasty result in favorable clini-cal and radiologic outcomes in the management of chronic subacromial pain syndrome? A double-blind randomized clinical trial with 9 to 14 years' follow-up. J Shoulder Elb Surg. 2017;26(8):1407–15.
30. Harris JD, Griesser MJ, Jones GL. Systematic review of the surgical treatment for symptom-atic os acromiale. Int J Shoulder Surg. 2011;5(1):9–16.
31. Zawadsky M, Marra G, Wiater JM, et al. Osteolysis of the distal clavicle: Long-term results of arthroscopic resection. Arthroscopy. 2000;16(6):600–5.

# Proximal Humerus Fractures

# 11

Jack E. Kazanjian

## Introduction

Proximal humerus fractures are common injuries in general orthopedic practice and are increasing in frequency. They typically occur in the geriatric population and are true fragility fractures. Younger patients that sustain proximal humerus fractures are usually secondary to high energy trauma. Treatment and intervention ranges from nonsurgical management to osteosynthesis and in some cases arthroplasty. Understanding the fracture type, patient age, health status, and "personality" of the injury can guide the surgeon in treatment of these common injuries.

1. **History**
   (a) Bimodal distribution
   (b) Elderly population—most common
      - Low level fall
      - Reason for fall? Underlying medical issues and medications
      - Pre-injury activity level and living situation
      - Handedness
      - Expectations
      - Abuse??
   (c) Younger population
      - High energy trauma
2. **Physical examination**
   (a) Soft tissue swelling and ecchymosis common
   (b) Skin tenting and necrosis, deformity of shoulder
   (c) Concomitant shoulder girdle/extremity injuries

J. E. Kazanjian (✉)
Department of Orthopaedic Surgery, Philadelphia College of Osteopathic Medicine, Premier Orthopaedics and Sports Medicine Associates, Havertown, PA, USA

- (d) Neurologic exam
  - Axillary nerve injury most common—difficult to assess motor but sensory exam important
  - Brachial plexus—rare
  - 67–82% of all fractures have subclinical nerve injury—affects recovery
- (e) Vascular exam—high suspicion due to collateral circulation
  - High suspicion with significant acute swelling of limb, marked fracture displacement/dislocation
- (f) Range of motion—difficult, do not assess

3. **Imaging**
   - (a) Neer trauma series
     - True AP (Grashey), scapular Y, axillary
     - Upright when possible
     - Discomfort may impede quality
     - Axillary difficult but **necessary (r/o dislocation)**
       - Trauma axillary
       - Velpeau axillary
   - (b) CT scan—indications not clear
     - Assess dislocation and direction
     - Articular fractures
     - Tuberosity fractures and displacement
     - Poor initial films
     - **3D recons** aid in evaluation
   - (c) MRI—not widely used, rarely indicated
     - Rotator cuff tear—could influence outcome
       - Fracture dislocation
     - Preexisting cuff disease—influence ORIF versus arthroplasty and potential outcome
       - Up to 8% of all fractures

4. **Classifications**
   - (a) Fractures initially described by Codman, based upon epiphyseal lines
   - (b) **Neer classification**—anatomic relationship of four "parts"
     - Parts—greater tuberosity, lesser tuberosity, anatomic head, shaft
     - Separate part—displacement between parts
       - >1 cm; angulation >45°
       - Also includes head split and dislocation
     - Poor intra- and interobserver reliability
     - There are variants that also fall out of classification
     - Four-part valgus impacted—not part of classification, less chance of AVN despite four parts
   - (c) **OTA**—3 groups and subgroups
     - Fracture location, status of surgical neck, dislocation

5. **Anatomy**
   - (a) Muscle forces
     - Pectoralis major—shaft anterior and medial

- Supraspinatus, infraspinatus, teres minor—posterosuperior and rotational displacement of greater tuberosity
- Subscapularis—internal rotation of articular segment and/or lesser tuberosity

(b) Blood supply
  - Anterior humeral circumflex artery—large anastomosis
    - Anterolateral ascending branch—up through bicipital groove, terminates as Arcuate artery in the head
  - Posterior humeral circumflex artery
    - Recent studies show its main supply to the head
  - Pathoanatomy
    - Hertel criteria—**predictor of humeral head ischemia**
      <8mm of calcar attached to articular segment
      Disrupted medial hinge >2 mm
      Increased complexity of fracture
      Displacement >1 cm, angulation >45°
      Does not predict AVN; AVN also does not portend poor prognosis

6. **Surgical treatment protocol**
  (a) Two-part fractures
    - Surgical neck
      - Indications—increased varus, shaft translation, calcar/shaft comminution
      - Techniques—suture osteosynthesis (Fig. 11.1a, b), IM nail, ORIF with locked plating (Fig. 11.2a, b), CRPP
      - Increased of nonunion with nonoperative treatment in elderly, varus >30 degrees, osteoporosis

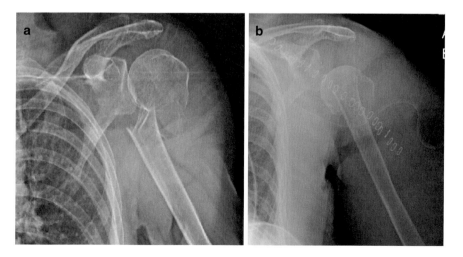

**Fig. 11.1** (a, b) 2 Part surgical neck fracture—suture technique

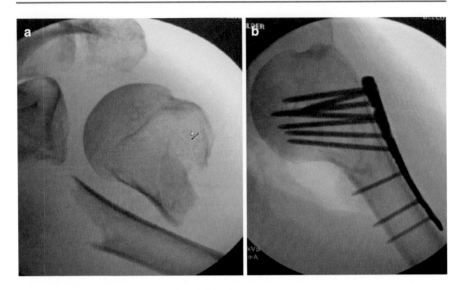

**Fig. 11.2** (**a**, **b**) 2 Part surgical neck—ORIF w/plate

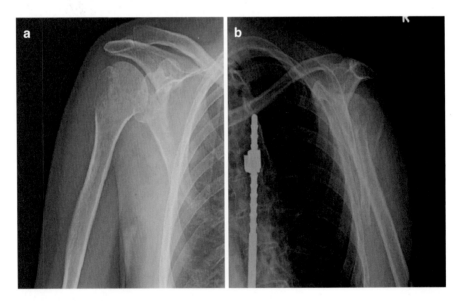

**Fig. 11.3** (**a**, **b**) 2 Part greater tuberosity fracture

- Greater tuberosity
  - Indications—>5–10 mm displacement (Fig. 11.3a, b), \*\*can consider 3–5 mm in young active patient\*\*
  - Techniques—suture osteosynthesis, ORIF with screws, ORIF with plate (Fig. 11.4a, b), ARIF with screws, ARIF with cuff repair constructs, tension band wiring
  - Can be missed, associated with anterior glenohumeral dislocation

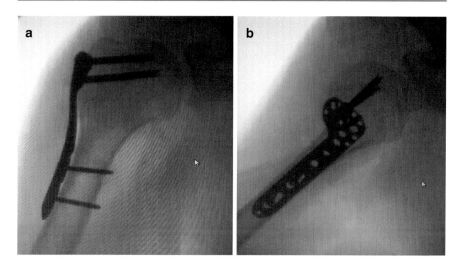

**Fig. 11.4** (**a**, **b**) 2 Part greater tuberosity—ORIF

**Fig. 11.5** 3 Part variant anatomic neck

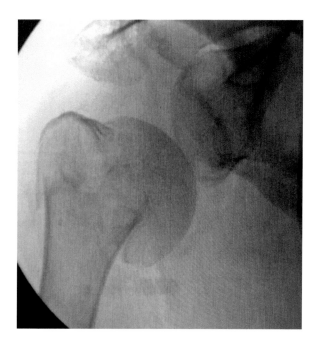

- Lesser tuberosity
  - Indications—3–5 mm of displacement, block to internal rotation
  - Techniques—ORIF with suture/suture anchors, ORIF with screws, excise with subscapularis repair
  - Rare, posterior dislocation until proven otherwise
- Anatomic neck—Fig. 11.5
  - Indications—displacement

- Techniques—ORIF in young (Fig. 11.6a, b), hemiarthroplasty/RSA in elderly
- Rare, increased risk of nonunion

(b) Three-part fractures
- Greater tuberosity and surgical neck—Fig. 11.7a, b
  - Indication—displaced fracture in young patient or physiologically young/active. Elderly amenable to surgical intervention
  - Techniques—ORIF with locked plating (Fig. 11.8a, b), IM nail, CRPP (young, good bone), RSA in select elderly patients
- Lesser tuberosity and surgical neck

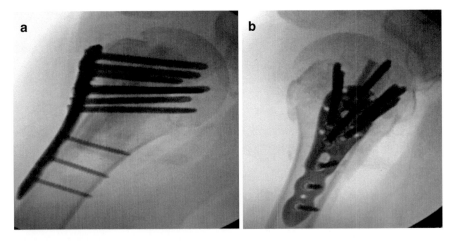

**Fig. 11.6** (**a, b**) 3 Part variant anatomic neck—ORIF w/fibula strut

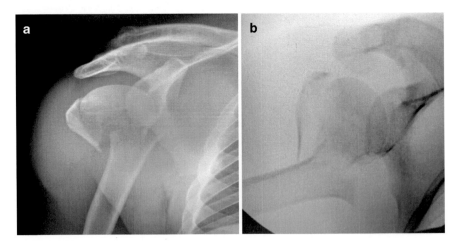

**Fig. 11.7** (**a, b**) 3 Part—surgical neck and greater tuberosity

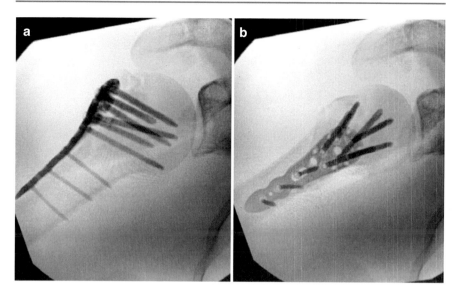

**Fig. 11.8** (**a, b**) 3 Part ORIF—GT and surgical neck

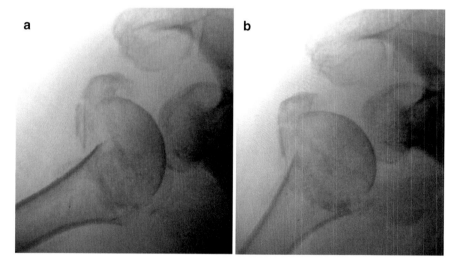

**Fig. 11.9** (**a, b**) 4 Part fracture

- Indication—displaced fracture in young patient or physiologically young/active, elderly amenable to surgical intervention
- Techniques—ORIF with locked plating, IM nail, CRPP (young, good bone), RSA in select elderly patients

(c) Four-part fractures
   - Standard four parts—Fig. 11.9a, b
      - Indication—displaced fracture in young patient or physiologically young/active, elderly amenable to surgical intervention

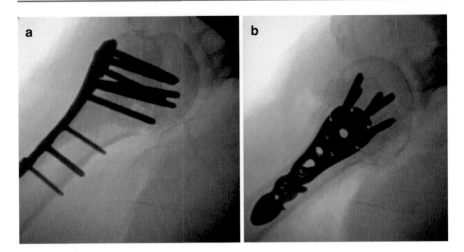

**Fig. 11.10** (**a, b**) 4 Part—ORIF

- Techniques—ORIF w/ locked plating in young/physiologically young (Fig. 11.10a, b), hemiarthroplasty in Young, RSA in elderly (Fig. 11.11)
  - Valgus impacted
    - Indications—displaced fracture in young patient or physiologically young/active, elderly amenable to surgical intervention
    - Techniques—ORIF with locked plating, CRPP (if within 10 days), IM nailing in select fractures, hemiarthroplasty in young patient with unstable medial hinge
  - Head split—Fig. 11.12
    - Indications—displaced fracture in young patient or physiologically young/active, elderly amenable to surgical intervention
    - Techniques—ORIF (Fig. 11.13) versus hemiarthroplasty in young patients, physiologically young/active, RSA in elderly
  (d) Complex proximal 1/3 fractures with shaft extension (Fig. 11.14a, b), segmental
    - Indication—displaced fracture in young patient or physiologically young/active, elderly amenable to surgical intervention
    - Techniques—ORIF with locked plating, orthogonal plating (Fig. 11.15), IM nail
7. **Treatment algorithm based on diagnosis**—based less now on classification due to poor correlation with outcome and poor intraobserver reliability
  (a) Nonoperative—**majority** of patients
    - 80–85%—minimally displaced, high rate of union, low rate of future displacement or complications compared to ORIF

**Fig. 11.11** RSA for
fracture

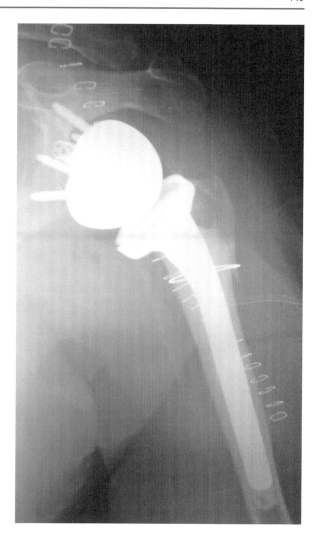

- Sling immobilization and serial radiographs
  - Every 2 × 6 weeks
  - Progressive PROM when fracture "sticky" (2–3 weeks)
  - AROM at 6 weeks, strengthening at 3 months. Maximum improvement at 1 year
- Will result in some malunion and stiffness, well tolerated usually
(b) Operative treatment—goal to restore anatomy, allow for early motion and union and maximize function in patients with displaced fractures
  - Surgical Options—CRPP, suture osteosynthesis, ORIF with plates/screws, intramedullary fixation and arthroplasty options (hemiarthroplasty/RSA), ARIF

**Fig. 11.12** 3 Part head split

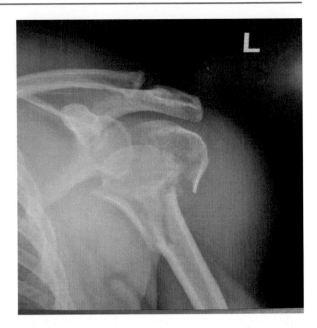

**Fig. 11.13** 3 Part head split—ORIF

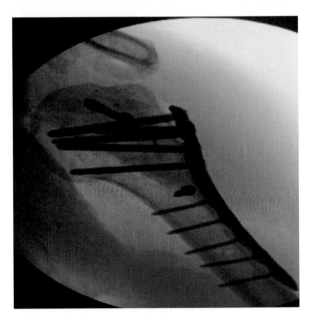

- CRPP—closed reduction percutaneous pinning
    - Indications—two-part surgical neck, select three-part/four-part valgus impacted fractures: usually young patients, good bone, no comminution, and adequate closed reduction

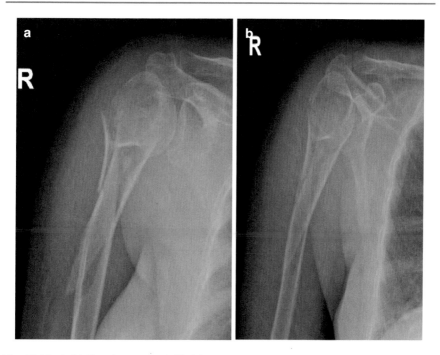

**Fig. 11.14** (**a**, **b**) Complex proximal 1/3rd fracture w/shaft extension

**Fig. 11.15** Complex
proximal 1/3rd—ORIF w/
orthogonal plating

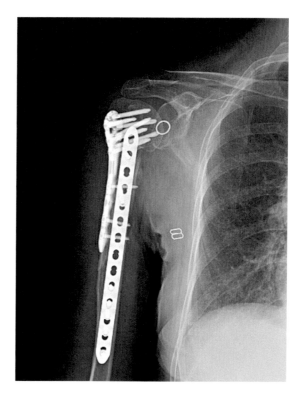

- Suture osteosynthesis
  - Indications—isolated greater tuberosity fractures, surgical neck fractures in elderly (parachute technique)
  - Avoids implant-related complications—multiple heavy sutures in cuff/bone to offset deforming forces
- ORIF—open reduction internal fixation with plates/screws
  - Locking technology and specific implants have improved healing rates and outcomes
  - Indications—greater tuberosity fractures >5 mm displaced, two-, three-, and four-part fractures, head split, combined shaft/proximal humerus
       Need good bone
       Need good medial calcar reduction, at least five screws in head and appropriate calcar screws of sufficient length
       Augment with sutures in cuff, through plate
       Plate placed lateral to bicipital groove, appropriate height of plate (avoid impingement, proper placement of screws in head)
- Intramedullary nail
  - Indications—surgical neck, select three-/four-part, combined shaft/proximal humerus, pathologic fractures
       Inserted percutaneously, insertion point more along articular surface
       Weaker in torsional stress than plates
- Hemiarthroplasty
  - Indications—younger patient with unreconstructible articular surface (complex fracture dislocation, head split) with good tuberosities
  - Good results with:
       Anatomic tuberosity reduction and healing
       Restoration of humeral height and version
            5.6 cm from superior aspect of pectoralis major
- Reverse shoulder arthroplasty
  - Indications—elderly, lower demand individuals with three-/four-part fractures, fracture dislocations (Fig. 11.16a–c), comminuted tuberosities, poor bone stock, preexisting rotator cuff disease, underlying degenerative disease of glenohumeral joint with poor function and fracture displacement
  - Function can be adequate despite tuberosity malposition, nonunion
  - Need adequate glenoid bone stock and deltoid function
  - Tuberosity repair needed for improved function, rotation, tension, and stability of prosthesis
- ARIF—arthroscopic-assisted internal fixation
  - Indications—isolated greater tuberosity fractures (3–5 mm displacement or greater in select fractures/patients)
       ARIF with screws
       ARIF with cuff repair constructs (transosseous-equivalent techniques)

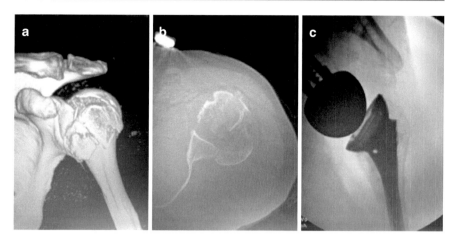

**Fig. 11.16** (a–c) 4 Part fracture dislocation

(c)  Augmentation
- Structural and biologic
    - Suture augment to plate (increased strength of construct, tuberosity fixation, and rotational stability)
    - Bone graft (auto/allograft)—fill void in metaphyseal region; give structural and biologic support for stability and healing of fracture
    - Cement
    - Endosteal bone peg—can aid in stability of unstable fractures
        Loss of posteromedial calcar support, varus
(d)  Surgical approaches
- Deltopectoral (anterior)
    - Workhorse of the shoulder—ORIF, suture osteosynthesis, arthroplasty for all fracture types
- Lateral deltoid split
    - Indications
        Isolated greater tuberosity fractures (rotator cuff repair approach)
        ORIF
            Increased incidence of axillary nerve injury (3–7 cm from lateral border of acromion)
- Percutaneous
    - CRPP
        Axillary, musculocutaneous nerve, biceps tendon, and cephalic vein at risk
    - IM nailing
    - Four-part valgus impacted fractures (within 10 days)
        Technically difficult
- Extended deltopectoral/anterolateral
    - Complex fracture patterns with shaft extension, segmental

(e) Surgical risks and complications
- Screw cut-out
  - Most common after ORIF, increased risk due to increased age and osteoporosis
- Fracture displacement, tuberosity escape
- Malunion
- Articular perforation
  - Fracture settling, loss of calcar support
- Infection
- Nerve Injury
- Posttraumatic stiffness/capsulitis
- Rotator cuff dysfunction
  - Tuberosity malposition, subacromial scarring, cuff injury
- AVN
- Posttraumatic DJD
- Nonunion
  - Increased in elderly and tobacco use

## Bibliography

1. Gupta AK, Harris JD, Erickson BJ, et al. Surgical management of complex proximal humerus fractures: a systematic review of 92 studies including 4500 patients. J Orthop Trauma. 2015;29(1):54–9.
2. Maier D, Jaeger M, Izadpahanah K, Strohm PC, Suedkamp NP. Proximal humeral fracture treatment in adults. J Bone Joint Surg Am. 2014;96(3):251–61.
3. Bernstein J, Adler LM, Blank JF, Dalsey RM, Williams GR, Iannotti JP. Evaluation of the Neer system of classification of proximal humerus fractures with computerized tomographic scans and plain radiographs. J Bone Joint Surg Am. 1996;78(9):1371–5.
4. Platzker P, Kutscha-Ilsberg F, Lehr S, Vecsei V, Gaebler C. The influence of displacement on shoulder function in patients with minimally displaced fractures of the greater tuberosity. Injury. 2005;36(10):1185–9.
5. Tejwani NC, Liporace F, Walsh M, France MA, Zuckerman JD, Egol KA. Functional outcome following one-part proximal humeral fractures. A prospective study. J Shoulder Elb Surg. 2008;17(2):216–9.
6. Park TS, Choi IY, Kim YH, Park MR, Shon JH, Kim SI. A new suggestion for the treatment of minimally displaced fractures of the greater tuberosity of the proximal humerus. Bull Hosp Jt Dis. 1997;56(3):171–6.
7. Court-Brown CM, Cattermole H, McQueen MM. Impacted valgus fractures (B1.1) of the proximal humerus: the results of nonoperative treatment. J Bone Joint Surg Br. 2002;84(4):504–8.
8. Matassi F, Angeloni R, Carulli C, et al. Locking plate and fibular allograft augmentation in unstable fractures of the proximal humerus. Injury. 2012;43(11):1939–42.
9. Gradl G, Dietze A, Kaab M, Hopfenmuller W, Mittlemeier T. Is locking nailing of humeral head fractures superior to locking plate fixation? Clin Orthop Relat Res. 2009;467(11):2986–93.
10. Edwards SL, Wilson NA, Zhang LQ, Flores S, Merk BR. Two-part surgical neck fractures of the proximal part of the humerus: A biomechanical evaluation of two fixation techniques. J Bone Joint Surg Am. 2006;89(10):2258–64.
11. Boileau P, Krishnan SG, Tinsi L, Walch G, Coste JS, Mole D. Tuberosity malposition and migration: Reasons for poor outcomes after hemiarthroplasty for displaced fractures of the proximal humerus. J Shoulder Elb Surg. 2002;11(5):401–12.

12. Murachovsky J, Ikemoto RY, Nascimento LG, Fujiki EN, Milani C, Warner JJ. Pectoralis major tendon reference (PMT): A new method for accurate restoration of humeral length with hemiarthroplasty for fracture. J Shoulder Elb Surg. 2006;15(6):675–8.

13. Gallinet D, Clappaz P, Garbuio P, Troper Y, Obert L. Three or four parts complex proximal humerus fractures: Hemiarthroplasty versus reverse prosthesis. A comparative study of 40 cases. Orthop Traumatol Surg Res. 2009;95(1):48–55.

14. Anakwenze OA, Zoller S, Ahmad CS, Levine WN. Reverse shoulder arthroplasty for acute proximal humerus fractures: a systematic review. J Shoulder Elb Surg. 2014;23(4):e73–80.

15. Ferrel JR, Trinh TQ, Fischer RA. Reverse total shoulder arthroplasty versus hemiarthroplasty for proximal humerus fractures: a systematic review. J Orthop Trauma. 2015;29(1):60–8.

16. Schnetzke M, Bockmeyer J, Porschke F, Studier-Fischer F, Grutzner PA, Guehring T. Quality of reduction influences outcome after locked plate fixation of proximal humeral Type C fractures. J Bone Joint Surg Am. 2016;98:1777–85.

17. Hettrich CM, Boraiah S, Dyke JP, Neviaser A, Helfet DL, Lorich DG. Quantitative assessment of the vascularity of the proximal part of the humerus. J Bone Joint Surg Am. 2010;92(4):943–8.

18. Robinson CM, Seah M, Marder RA. The epidemiology, risk of recurrence, and functional outcome after an acute traumatic posterior dislocation of the shoulder. J Bone Joint Surg Am. 2011;93(17):1605–13.

19. Court-Brown CM, Garg A, McQueen MM. The translated two-part fracture of the proximal humerus. Epidemiology and outcome in the older patient. J Bone Jt Surg B. 2001;83(6):799–804.

20. Yuksel HY, Yimaz S, Akshalin E, Celebi L, Muratli HH, Bicimoglu A. The results of non-operative treatment for three and four part fractures of the proximal humerus in low demand patients. J Orthop Trauma. 2011;25(10):588–95.

21. Calvo E, de Miguel I, de la Cruz JJ, Lopez-Martin N. Percutaneous fixation of displaced proximal humeral fractures: indications based on the correlation between clinical and radiographic results. J Shoulder Elb Surg. 2007;16(6):774–81.

22. Keener JD, Parsons BO, Flatow EL, Rogers K, Williams GR, Galatz LM. Outcomes after percutaneous reduction and fixation of proximal humeral fractures. J Shoulder Elb Surg. 2007;16(3):330–8.

23. Konrad G, Audige L, Lambert S, Hertel R. Similar outcomes for nail versus plate fixation of three-part proximal humerus fractures. Clin Orthop Relat Res. 2012;470(2):602–9.

24. Zhu Y, Lu Y, Shen J, Zhang J, Jiang C. Locking intramedullary nails and locking plates in the treatment of two-part proximal humeral surgical neck fractures: a prospective randomized trial with a minimum of three years of follow up. J Bone Joint Surg Am. 2011;93(2):159–68.

25. Olerud P, Ahrengart L, Ponzer S, Saving J, Tidemark J. Internal fixation versus nonoperative treatment of displaced 3-part proximal humeral fractures in elderly patients: a randomized controlled trial. J Shoulder Elb Surg. 2011;20(5): 26(2):747–55.

26. Fjalstead T, Hole M, Hovden A, Blucher J, Stromsoe K. Surgical treatment with an angular stable plate for complex displaced proximal humeral fractures in elderly patients: a randomized controlled trial. J Orthop Trauma. 2012;26(2):98–106.

27. Robinson CM, Page RS. Severely impacted valgus proximal humerus fractures. J Bone Joint Surg. 2004;86(2):143–55.

28. Gardner MJ, Weil Y, Barker JU, Kelly BT, Helfet DL, Lorich DG. The importance of medial support in locked plating of proximal humerus fractures. J Orthop Trauma. 2007;21(3):185–91.

29. Thanasas C, Kontakis G, Angoules A, Limb D, Giannoudis P. Treatment of proximal humerus frcatures with locking plates: a systematic review. J Shoulder Elb Surg. 2009;18(6):837–44.

30. Hettrich CM, Neviaser A, Beamer BS, Paul O, Helfet DL, Lorich DG. Locked plating of the proximal humerus using an endosteal implant. J Orthop Trauma. 2012;26(4):212–5.

31. Garrigues GE, Johnston PS, Pepe MD, Tucker BS, Ramsey ML, Austin LS. Hemiarthroplasty versus reverse total shoulder arthroplasty for acute proximal humerus fractures in elderly patients. Orthopedics. 2012;35(5):703–8.

32. Boyle MJ, Youn SM, Frampton CM, Ball CM. Functional outcomes of reverse shoulder arthroplasty compared with hemiarthroplasty for acute proximal humeral fractures. J Shoulder Elb Surg. 2013;22(1):32–7.

33. Fjalestad T, Hole MO, Blucher J, et al. Rotator cuff tears in proximal humeral fractures: an MRI cohort study in 76 patients. Arch Orthop Trauma Surg. 2010;130(5):575–81.
34. Gallo RA, Sciulli R, Daffner RH, et al. Defining the relationship between rotator cuff injury and proximal humerus fractures. Clin Orthop Relat Res. 2007;458:70–7.
35. Neer CS. Displaced proximal humeral fractures. I. Classification and evaluation. J Bone Joint Surg Am. 1970;52(6):1077–89.
36. Court-Brown CM, Bugler KE, Clement ND, Duckworth AD, McQueen MM. The epidemiology of open fractures in adults. A 15 year review. Injury. 2012;43(6):891–7.
37. Sidor ML, Zuckerman JD, Lyon T, et al. The Neer Classification system for proximal humeral frcatures. An assessment of interobserver reliability and intraobserver reproducibility. J Bone Joint Surg Am. 1993;75(12):1745–50.
38. Murray IR, Amin AK, White TO, Robinson CM. Proximal humeral fractures: current concepts in classification, treatment and outcomes. J Bone Joint Surg Br. 2011;93(1):1–11.
39. Solberg BD, Moon CN, Franco DP, Paiement GD. Surgical treatment of three and four-part proximal humeral fractures. J Bone Joint Surg Am. 2009;91(7):1689–97.
40. Hertel R, Hempfing A, Stiehler M, Leunig M. Predictors of humeral head ischemia after intracapsular fracture of the proximal humerus. J Shoulder Elb Surg. 2004;13(4):427–33.
41. Bahrs C, Rolauffs B, Stuby F, et al. Effect of proximal humeral fractures on the age specific prevalence of rotator cuff tears. J Trauma. 2010;69(4):901–6.
42. Koval KJ, Gallagher MA, Marsicano JG, et al. Functional outcome after minimally displaced fractures of the proximal part of the humerus. J Bone Joint Surg Am. 1997;79(2):203–7.
43. Rowles DJ, McGrory JE. Percutaneous pinning of the proximal part of the humerus. An anatomic study. J Bone Joint Surg Am. 2001;83(11):1695–9.
44. Dimakopoulos P, Panagopulos A, Kasimatis G. Transosseous suture fixation of proximal humeral fractures. J Bone Joint Surg Am. 2007;89(8):1700–9.
45. Park JY, Pandher DS, Chun JY, et al. Antegrade humeral nailing through the rotator cuff interval: a new entry portal. J Orthop Trauma. 2008;22(6):419–25.
46. Gardner MJ, Griffith MH, Dines JS, et al. The extended anterolateral acromial approach allows minimally invasive access to the proximal humerus. Clin Orthop Relat Res. 2005;434:123–9.
47. Gerber C, Werner CM, Vienne P. Internal fixation of complex fractures of the proximal humerus. J Bone Joint Surg Br. 2004;86(6):848–55.
48. Robinson CM, Wylie JR, Ray AG, et al. Proximal humeral fractures with a severe varus deformity treated by fixation with a locking plate. J Bone Joint Surg Br. 2010;92(5):672–8.
49. Gardner MJ, Boraiah S, Helfet DL, Lorich DG. Indirect medial reduction and strut support of proximal humerus fractures using an endosteal implant. J Orthop Trauma. 2008;22(3):195–200.
50. Frankle MA, Greenwald DP, Markee BA, et al. Biomechanical effects of malposition of tuberosity fragments on the humeral prosthetic reconstruction for four-part proximal humerus fractures. J Shoulder Elb Surg. 2001;10(4):321–6.
51. Banco S, Andrisani D, Ramsey M, Friedman B, Fenlin JM. The parachute technique: valgus impaction osteotomy for two-part fractures of the surgical neck of the humerus. J Bone Joint Surg Am. 2001;2:38–42.
52. Tamai K, Hamada J, Ohno W, Saotome K. Surgical anatomy of multipart fractures of the proximal humerus. J Shoulder Elb Surg. 2002;11:421–7.
53. Visser CP, Coene LN, Brand R, Tavy DL. Nerve lesions in proximal humerus fractures. J Shoulder Elb Surg. 2001;10:421–7.

# Clavicle Fractures (Medial, Midshaft, Lateral)

**12**

Andrew Boltuch and Jonathan Levy

## Introduction

(a) Clavicle fractures are common injuries of the shoulder girdle, which can be separated into medial, midshaft, and lateral fracture types.

(b) This chapter will review the history, physical exam findings, radiographs, and treatment algorithms separated by fracture location.

1. History
   (a) Mechanism of injury and associated injuries
      - Low energy mechanism
         - Elderly fall from standing
      - High energy mechanism
         - Mortality rate of 32% in high energy clavicle fractures in the setting of poly trauma commonly due to head and chest injuries [1]
         - Traction versus compression mechanism of failure
         - Associated injuries include closed head injury, pulmonary injury, rib fractures, scapula fracture (floating shoulder), neurologic injury, and scapulothoracic dissociation
   (b) Patient activity level and expectations for shoulder strength, endurance, and need for speedy recovery
   (c) Modifiable risk factors including patient smoking status
   (d) Risk factors for patient noncompliance including alcohol abuse, psychiatric conditions, or poor social conditions
2. Physical exam
   (a) Midshaft clavicle fracture
      - Inspect for skin tenting and complete a thorough distal neurovascular exam

A. Boltuch (✉) · J. Levy
Holy Cross Orthopedic Institute, Oakland Park, FL, USA

© The Author(s), under exclusive license to Springer Nature Switzerland AG 2022
C. M. Chebli, A. M. Murthi (eds.), *The Resident's Guide to Shoulder and Elbow Surgery*, https://doi.org/10.1007/978-3-031-12255-2_12

- Typical deformity includes:
  - Medial fragment displaced posterosuperior (sternocleidomastoid muscle)
  - Lateral fragment displaced inferomedial (weight of the arm and the pull of the pectoralis muscle)
  - "Shoulder ptosis" where the upper extremity droops forward
(b) Lateral clavicle fracture
  - Mimics acromioclavicular joint separations with inferior translation of extremity
  - Increased clavicular prominence with CC ligament disruption
(c) Medial clavicle fracture
  - Ensure no posterior sternoclavicular displacement
    - May lead to:
      Stridor from tracheal compression
      Dysphagia from esophageal compression
      Vascular compromise due to compression of aortic arch, carotid, or subclavian arteries
3. Radiographs
  (a) Midshaft clavicle fracture
    - Upright AP clavicle
    - Upright 20° cephalic tilt for displacement
      - Good for Z-type fractures
    - AP incorporating both clavicles to evaluate shortening
      - A line may be drawn connecting the medial and lateral clavicle through its midportion
  (b) Lateral clavicle fracture
    - Zanca view: centered on AC joint with 15° cephalic tilt for improved imaging of lateral clavicle fractures
  (c) Medial clavicle fracture
    - Often best characterized with CT scan
    - Serendipity view determines anteroposterior displacement
      - X-ray beam centered on sternum with 40° cephalic tilt of the beam
  (d) CT scan provides a more accurate measurement of displacement and shortening but not required in most situations
4. Treatment
  (a) Midshaft clavicle fracture (Fig. 12.1)
    - Nonoperative: <2 cm of shortening and <100% displacement
      - 0–2 Weeks: Simple sling immobilization. Simple sling immobilization for 4 weeks
      - 2–4 Weeks: May begin passive shoulder range of motion to 90° of forward elevation with continued use of sling Active and active assisted motion week 4–6
      - 4–6 Weeks: Increase passive and active assisted ROM to 120° of forward flexion
      - 6–8 Weeks: May begin unrestricted shoulder ROM and strengthening if radiographic union present Strengthening at 6 weeks if evidence of union on radiographs

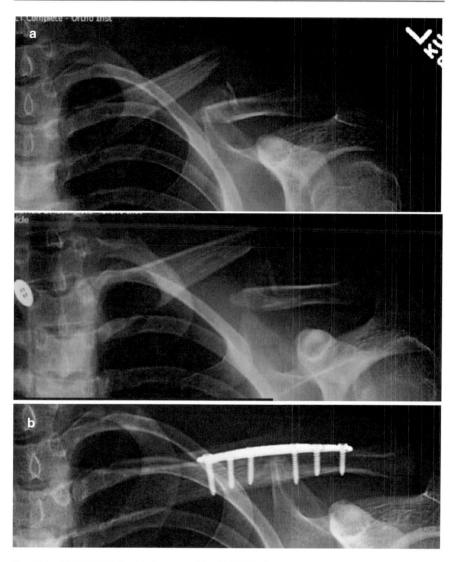

**Fig. 12.1** (**a**) Midshaft clavicle fracture with >100% displacement and Z-type fracture pattern. (**b**) Midshaft clavicle fracture status post open reduction with internal fixation

- Operative
  - Absolute indications: open or impending open injury (i.e., tenting of skin), associated vascular injury
  - Relative indications: bilateral clavicle fracture, polytrauma, need for rapid return to function, >2 cm of shortening, >100% displacement, Z-type fractures, floating shoulder [2, 3]
- Fixation options: superior plating, anteroinferior plating, dual plating, intramedullary fixation
  - Superior plating
     Benefits: tension side of fracture, less deltoid dissection, more resistant to axial bending [4]

- Anteroinferior plating
    Benefits: larger screw length, avoidance of neurovascular structures, less prominence for shoulder load bearing patients, increased bending rigidity [5]
- No difference in complication rates or nonunion between superior and anteroinferior plating [6]
- Intramedullary fixation
    Benefits: less soft tissue stripping, less hardware prominence, decreased risk of peri-incisional numbness
    Drawbacks: limited ability to withstand axial load and torsional forces
        Generally avoided in comminuted or segmental fractures [7]
        Second-generation implants include all intramedullary variable pitch designs (dual track; acumed) as well as a lockable nail with deployable medial "grippers" to improve rotational stability (Sonoma CRx; Sonoma Orthopedic Products)
            Further investigation needed to determine clinical benefits of these products
  (b) Lateral clavicle fracture
      • Neer classification (Fig. 12.2)

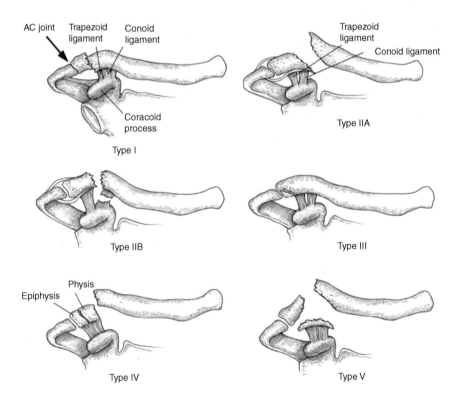

**Fig. 12.2** Neer classification of lateral clavicle fractures. (Journal of the American Academy of Orthopaedic Surgeons19 [7]:392–401, July 2011)

- Decision to operate based on integrity of CC ligaments (Figs. 12.3 and 12.4)
  - Nonoperative: Neer type I, III, and IV
  - Operative: Neer type II and V
- Fixation options—locking plate, hook plate, suture fixation, or combination
  - Large lateral fragment: plate with multiple lateral locking screw option
  - Small lateral fragment: hook plate spanning the AC joint vs. locking plate with lateral locking screw options

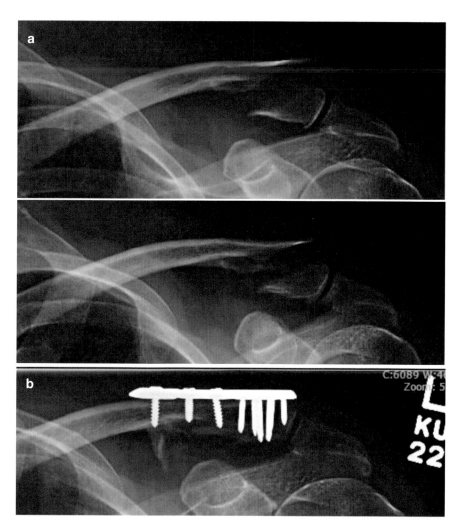

**Fig. 12.3** (**a**) Neer type IIA lateral clavicle fracture. (**b**) Neer type IIA lateral clavicle fracture status post open reduction with internal fixation utilizing distal screw cluster locking plate

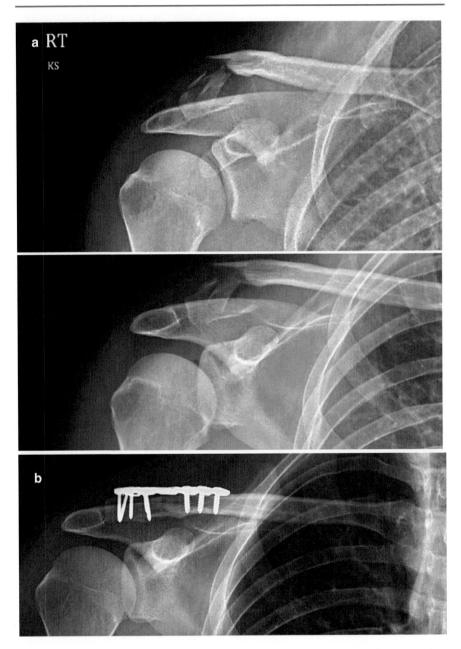

**Fig. 12.4** (**a**) Neer type V lateral clavicle fracture. (**b**) Neer type V lateral clavicle fracture s/p ORIF with suture augmentation for CC ligament reconstruction

Supplement with screw fixation or suture fixation to the coracoid
   (c) Medial clavicle fracture
   - Nonoperative: typically treated nonoperatively with low rates of nonunion
   - Operative: significant displacement with posterior displacement into the mediastinum, open fracture, and segmental fracture
   - Fixation options: plate with distal screw cluster
5. Surgical approach
   (a) Positioning
   - Supine with reverse Trendelenburg on radiolucent table (Fig. 12.5)
     - C-arm positioned at patient's head versus from contralateral side
     - May be favored for anteroinferior approach
   - Beach chair position (Fig. 12.6)
     - Favored for lateral fracture fixation
     - Bump under ipsilateral scapula
     - Care taken to turn head away to allow drill trajectory and unencumbered radiographs
        Confirm radiographs prior to draping
     - C-arm positioned at patient's head versus from contralateral side
   (b) Approach
   - Anterosuperior and anteroinferior approach for plating
     - Longitudinal incision in line or at inferior border of clavicle
     - Avoid transection of suprascapular nerves
     - Limited soft tissue dissection
        Anteroinferior approach includes limited deltoid stripping off the clavicle
     - Two-layered closure
   - Lateral approach vs. retrograde technique through fracture site for intramedullary fixation
6. Risks and complications
   (a) Nonunion
   - 15% nonunion rate in nonoperative treatment of completely displaced fractures, 1–5% following surgical intervention [8]
   - Symptomatic nonunion treated with ORIF and bone grafting
   (b) Malunion
   - More symptomatic in younger population
   - Loss of shoulder strength and endurance, particularly abduction endurance [9]
   (c) Hardware failure
   - Avoid use of one-third tubular and reconstruction plates
   (d) Neurovascular injury
   - At risk when drilling anterior to posterior at medial clavicle
   - At risk when drilling superior to inferior at middle clavicle

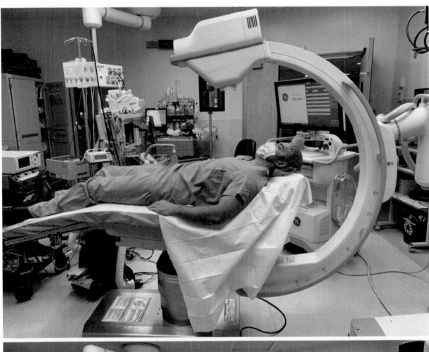

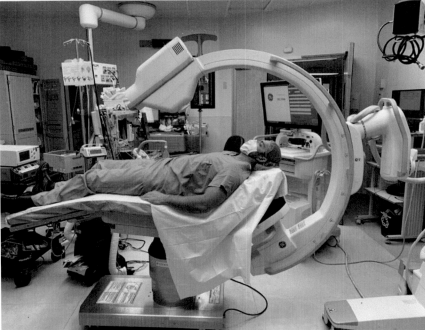

**Fig. 12.5** Caudal and cranial (inlet and outlet) clavicle views for supine positioning with reverse Trendelenburg on radiolucent table

**Fig. 12.6** Beach chair position with C-arm positioning for clavicle ORIF

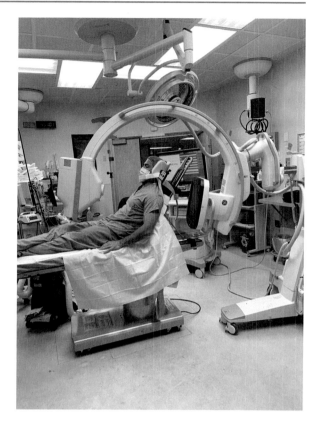

(e) Infection
  • Overall rate of 2–5%
  • Decreased by careful soft tissue handling and two-layered closure incorporating muscular layer

## References

1. Mckee MD, Stephen DJ, Kreder HJ, et al. Functional outcome following clavicle fractures in polytrauma patients. J Trauma. 2000;47(3):616.
2. Fuglesang HFS, Flugsrud GB, Randsborg P-H, Stavem K, Utvåg SE. Radiological and functional outcomes 2.7 years following conservatively treated completely displaced midshaft clavicle fractures. Arch Orthop Trauma Surg. 2016;136(1):17–25.
3. Hill JM, McGuire MH, Crosby LA. Closed treatment of displaced middle-third fractures of the clavicle gives poor results. J Bone Jt Surg Br. 1997;79(4):537–9.
4. Favre P, Kloen P, Helfet DL, Werner CML. Superior versus anteroinferior plating of the clavicle: a finite element study. J Orthop Trauma. 2011;25(11):661–5.
5. Partal G, Meyers KN, Sama N, et al. Superior versus anteroinferior plating of the clavicle revisited: a mechanical study. J Orthop Trauma. 2010;24(7):420–5.
6. Ai J, Kan S-L, Li H-L, et al. Anterior inferior plating versus superior plating for clavicle fracture: a meta-analysis. BMC Musculoskelet Disord. 2017;18:159.

7. Eichinger JK, Balog TP, Grassbaugh JA. Intramedullary fixation of clavicle fractures: anatomy, indications, advantages, and disadvantages. J Am Acad Orthop Surg. 2016;24(7):10.
8. Zlowodzki M, Zelle BA, Cole PA, Jeray K, McKee MD. Treatment of acute midshaft clavicle fractures: systematic review of 2144 fractures: on behalf of the Evidence-Based Orthopaedic Trauma Working Group. J Orthop Trauma. 2005;19(7):504–7.
9. Mckee MD, Pedersen EM, Jones C, et al. Deficits following nonoperative treatment of displaced midshaft clavicular fractures. JBJS. 2006;88(1):35–40.

# Acromioclavicular Joint Injuries

# 13

Trenton Sprenkle and Steven Klepps

## Introduction

Acromioclavicular joint injuries are common in young athletes and trauma patients. While the majority are treated conservatively, several factors including type/grade of injury, association with fracture, and patient level of function guide operative treatment.

1. History (how to ask directed questions)
   (a) Prevalence
      - Common in young athletes and trauma patients. Males > females
      - Accounts for 40–50% of shoulder injuries in contact sports
   (b) Mechanism of injury
      - Often direct injury to superior shoulder, forceful contact with the ground
      - Direct blow to the shoulder in contact sports especially into wall/structure
   (c) Presenting symptoms
      - Pain and swelling in the superior aspect of the shoulder
      - Deformity to superior shoulder
      - Loss of motion
      - Unable to continue sports/activity
      - There may be associated neck pain or numbness and tingling

T. Sprenkle
Sanford Orthopedics and Sports Medicine—Sanford Health, Fargo, ND, USA

School of Medicine and Health Sciences, University of North Dakota, Grand Forks, ND, USA

S. Klepps (✉)
Department of Orthopedics, St. Vincent's Hospital, Billings, MT, USA
e-mail: sjklepps@montanabones.com

© The Author(s), under exclusive license to Springer Nature Switzerland AG 2022
C. M. Chebli, A. M. Murthi (eds.), *The Resident's Guide to Shoulder and Elbow Surgery*, https://doi.org/10.1007/978-3-031-12255-2_13

(d) Important related information
   • Investigate regular activity of the patient before injury
   • Dominant hand
   • Occupation
   • History of previous shoulder problems
   • Assess for possible associated distal clavicle fracture, SC joint dislocation, periosteal sleeve injury in the pediatric population, and coracoid fracture based on location of pain
2. Physical exam (which correlate to the complaint)
   (a) Gross inspection of the shoulder for deformity
      • Palpation at AC joint, coracoid, scapula body, sternoclavicular joint, and clavicle
      • Access stability of the AC joint in anterior/posterior and superior/inferior planes. Reducible with taking weight off the arm?
   (b) Active and passive range of motion at the shoulder
      • Muscle strength testing
   (c) Neurovascular exam, cervical evaluation
   (d) Physical exam useful in determining Rockwood classification [1, 2]
      • Type I or II injury—injury to the AC joint capsule only
         – Pain with palpation of the AC joint
         – Cross-body adduction testing is painful
         – The only deformity is slight swelling
      • Type III—injury to the coracoclavicular (CC) ligaments as well as the capsule
      • Type V—injury CC ligaments, capsule, and perforation of deltotrapezial fascia
         – Type III and V—pain and deformity in the AC joint and increased CC space
            Clavicle superior to the acromion because of the downward force of the arm
            Type III injury *reducible* when the arm pushed upward while the distal clavicle is held down or when the patient shrugs their shoulders
            Type V injury *not reducible* as the clavicle is trapped within the trapezius [1, 2]. This distinction is helpful in initial surgical decision making [3, 4]
      • Type IV injury
         – Posterior protrusion of the clavicle. Horizontal instability?
      • Type VI injury
         – Rare injury. The clavicle is displaced inferior into the subcoracoid position. This allows the medial acromion to be easily palpated. Assessment of neurovascular status is extremely important due to displacement of clavicle towards the brachial plexus and axillary vascular structures

3. Imaging (what to order and when) (need high quality imaging)
   (a) Injury to the AC joint generally can be definitively diagnosed through plain radiographs
      - AP of bilateral shoulders
        - Assess coracoclavicular distance and AC widening
          Compare to contralateral side
          AC width index—described to assist with assessing horizontal instability [6, 7]
      - The AC joint view (also called the Zanca view) (Fig. 13.1a)
        - Reduced radiation, X-ray beam directed 15° cephalad
          Avoids overlap between the spine of the scapula and the AC joint
      - An axillary view is utilized to detect posterior displacement in a type IV injury (Fig. 13.1b)
        - The treating physician cannot solely rely on this X-ray as the acromion is noted to overhang the clavicle in up to 30% of axillary views
        - Must correlate with physical exam [5]
      - Clavicle and scapular radiographs if suspicious of other areas of concern
        - Rule out associated fractures—distal clavicle, sternoclavicular injury (bipolar clavicle), scapula fracture (floating shoulder), coracoid fracture, and periosteal sleeve fracture
        - Periosteal sleeve fractures can be identified by a thin line of calcification from the periosteum inferior to the displaced distal clavicle
      - Weighted radiographs generally are not helpful and have fallen out of favor
   (b) Finding based on classification
      - Type I—No evidence of separation on plain radiographs
      - Type II—Slight widening or superior elevation of AC joint
      - Type III—Increase in CC distance 25–100%

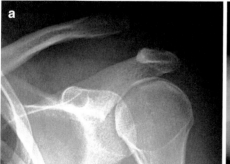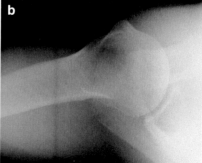

**Fig. 13.1** (a) AP (Zanca) radiograph of the AC joint showing a type III separation with 100% displacement of the clavicle superior to the acromion. (b) Axillary radiograph of the shoulder showing the clavicle posteriorly displaced relative to the anterior edge of the acromion

- Type IV—Axillary view shows clavicle posterior to the anterior acromion
- Type V—Increase in CC distance 100–300%
- Type VI—Distal clavicle displaced inferior to the coracoid

(c) Ultrasound
  - Has been used to further assess instability, especially horizontal, which may be helpful in borderline cases [8]

4. Treatment algorithm based on diagnosis

(a) Nonoperative treatment
  - Usually reserved for types I–III injuries
    - Treatment strategies consist of a short period of immobilization with a sling, followed by staged therapy from gentle ROM to eventual strengthening exercises and return to sport or work
    - Type I or II injuries typically require 2–3 weeks of nonsurgical treatment followed by gradual return to sport; type III injuries typically require 4–6 weeks
    - Return to sport criteria
        Full range of motion and strength
        Minimally tender AC joint
    - Nonsurgical treatment is considered unsuccessful if the patient is unable to return to sport or work at 3 months
        Surgery considered [9]
    - Patients who do not fully recover after 6 weeks of nonsurgical treatment are more likely to require surgery
  - A recently developed program of progressive rehabilitation is organized into four phases based on return of function [10]
    - Phase I
        Ice, NSAIDs—reduce pain and swelling
        Scapula stabilization treatment and lower extremity strengthening
        Sling for comfort only
            Patients having a type III injury typically require a longer period in sling
    - Phase II
        Considered when patient at 75% of normal range of motion
        Focus on restoring full range of motion. Strengthening exercises are allowed
    - Phase III
        Considered when 75% of strength returns
        The goal is to regain full strength; power and endurance are emphasized
    - Phase IV
        Strength of the injured arm equal to that of the contralateral arm
        Sport-specific training initiated—return to sport
  - Treatment based on type of injury
    - Type I and II
        Treated nonoperatively to achieve symptom relief and return to activity

Type II separations have been associated with persistent pain, and degenerative changes have been reported to develop 5–10 years after injury [11]

Distal clavicle resection and meniscus removal can be considered for a patient with type II separations that remain symptomatic

If instability is noted at the time of surgery, AC joint stabilization should be performed

Distal clavicle resection alone in setting of instability associated with persistent pain is believed to be due to underlying instability [9]. Therefore, open resection should be considered for distal clavicle resection of type II separations because it allows manual evaluation for subtle instability

- Type III separations

Controversial, but in the United States, they are usually treated nonsurgically, with some exceptions. More commonly treated surgically in Europe [4]

Patients who are overhead athletes or do heavy manual labor have been considered for early repair, but studies have reported good results with nonsurgical treatment even in these patients [4, 12]

No definitive data to show functional superiority of surgical vs. nonsurgical treatment [13]

92% success rate with 21 year f/u in patients treated nonoperatively

Up to 3 months may be needed for return to full function and return to sport or work. Typically longer than type I or II injuries

For this reason, there is some question about the advisability of acute repair in athletes injured near the end of the season because a full course of nonsurgical treatment followed by surgery might not provide adequate time for recovery before the next season begins

- IV, V, and VI separations are initially treated surgically in healthy patients because these injuries tend to remain symptomatic if treated nonsurgically

(b) Operative treatment
- Many surgical techniques have been described making it difficult to determine the best surgical option
- Surgeons should be aware of the various techniques to make an informed decision on the best option for the individual patient
- Regardless of the surgical technique, the surgeon must decide whether the distal clavicle needs to be resected as part of the reconstruction
  - In general, the distal clavicle can be left in place during an acute repair because it has not developed significant hypertrophy or irregularity. Some authors describe removing the intra-articular disk if it is torn [14]
  - There is some risk of long-term pain or osteoarthritis at the AC joint if the distal clavicle is not resected but none short term

- Removing the distal clavicle may add to horizontal instability after repair [6, 14]
- For chronic separations, the distal clavicle is typically resected due to distal clavicle irregularity/hypertrophy which can lead to pain
• Several important technical points apply to all AC joint reconstruction techniques; these were developed based on biomechanical and clinical studies
  - To avoid slippage, it is important to place the sutures or graft around the coracoid at the base rather than at the tip to avoid graft slippage
      Placing suture anchors into the coracoid or a hole through the coracoid has been proposed as a means of avoiding slippage. This comes with added cost for anchor placement and risk of coracoid fracture [15, 16]
  - When placing sutures or graft around the coracoid, it is important to pass them from medial to lateral to reduce the risk of neurologic injury to the brachial plexus [17]
  - Augmentation with tape (rather than suture fixation) has become common due to its strength but can lead to coracoid or clavicle fracture
  - The clavicle holes for suture augmentation should not be placed too distally within the clavicle. Leads to widened distal clavicle position after repair
  - The same clavicle drill hole locations should be used for both Weaver–Dunn and anatomic reconstruction. Weaver–Dunn only has sutures/tapes placed
  - Over reduction of the clavicle assists with stretching of the reconstruction as the patient recovers from surgery
  - Wide stripping of the clavicle periosteum with débridement of any scar tissue below the clavicle is essential to allow mobilization and over-reduction before the repair
  - The deltotrapezial fascia is oversewn as part of the repair. Therefore, large, thick flaps of tissue are mobilized during the exposure.
• Most common surgical techniques
  - The modified Weaver–Dunn reconstruction
      Standard procedure for many years
      This method involves transferring the coracoacromial (CA) ligament from the acromion to the distal clavicle, with supplementation placed between the coracoid and the clavicle using heavy sutures or tapes (Fig. 13.2)
      The modified Weaver–Dunn reconstruction has been performed well, but postoperative loosening and high rate of reoperation are described [18]. Multiple modifications have been developed leading to a lower prevalence of Weaver–Dunn being performed
          Chuinard reconstruction
              Transfer of the acromion bone fragment with the CA ligament
          Various suture augmentation techniques

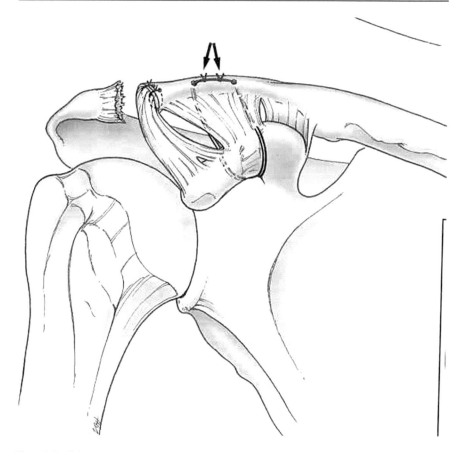

**Fig. 13.2** Schematic drawing of the Weaver–Dunn reconstruction, showing the CA ligament transferred to the distal end of the clavicle, with suture augmentation beneath the coracoid and through drill holes in the clavicle (arrows)

There are potential advantages to performing reconstructions using local tissue as with the modified Weaver–Dunn

Local vascular supply for the graft may maximize the healing potential. The use of local tissue also avoids the risk of reaction and the cost of using foreign material

The effect of taking down the CA ligament is minimal. It is often taken down to treat impingement without significant effect

– The anatomic reconstruction

Has become popular during the past 15 years, primarily as a reaction to the risk of loosening after the modified Weaver–Dunn reconstruction

Anatomic reconstruction involves transferring a tendinous graft, such as the semitendinosus or gracilis, around the coracoid and through drill holes in the clavicle or more recently around the clavicle (nonanatomic) (Fig. 13.3a)

Can be allograft or autograft per patient/physician preference
The main advantage of graft placement is that it provides a stronger biomechanical construct than a CA ligament transfer [1, 2, 19, 21]. Mobilizing the CA ligament in the Weaver–Dunn reconstruction often leaves inadequate tissue for the reconstruction [19, 20].
The graft can be fixed with either sutures placed across the graft or with interference screws in the clavicle

The graft can be woven onto itself to avoid screw placement
Screws have been shown to provide the biomechanically strongest fixation, but the use of absorbable screws can lead to a reaction (osteolysis) and subsequent fracture

This factor has led some surgeons to use only sutures for fixation of the graft tissue or to even avoid clavicle tunnels altogether referred to as a "nonanatomic" reconstruction. This can lead to sawing through the graft along the clavicle after reconstruction [15, 21]

Based on anatomic studies, the entire clavicle length is measured as a straight line to determine drill hole placement

The holes are placed at 20% and 30% of the clavicle length from the distal end of the clavicle usually centered over the coracoid
Tunnels are drilled at least 15 mm apart to decrease risk of fracture [15]

Single-tunnel reconstructions have been used to minimize the effects of multiple tunnels with good results [22]
As with the Weaver–Dunn reconstruction, clavicle screw holes should not be placed too distally to avoid a widened AC joint after repair

One prospective study observed a slightly higher clinical score for anatomic reconstruction vs. Weaver–Dunn [20]. The question remains as to whether the clinical benefit of anatomic reconstruction justifies the cost of graft and screws, donor site morbidity, and a possible foreign tissue reaction

Addressing horizontal instability

The reconstruction of coracoclavicular ligaments has been shown to provide good superior–inferior stability but leaves anterior–posterior instability
Recently, more focus on horizontal stabilization techniques has occurred

The tendon auto/allograft can be extended over the AC joint and attached to the acromion (Fig. 13.3b) [23].
Intramedullary graft can be placed [21].
Cerclage sutures can be placed around the AC joint

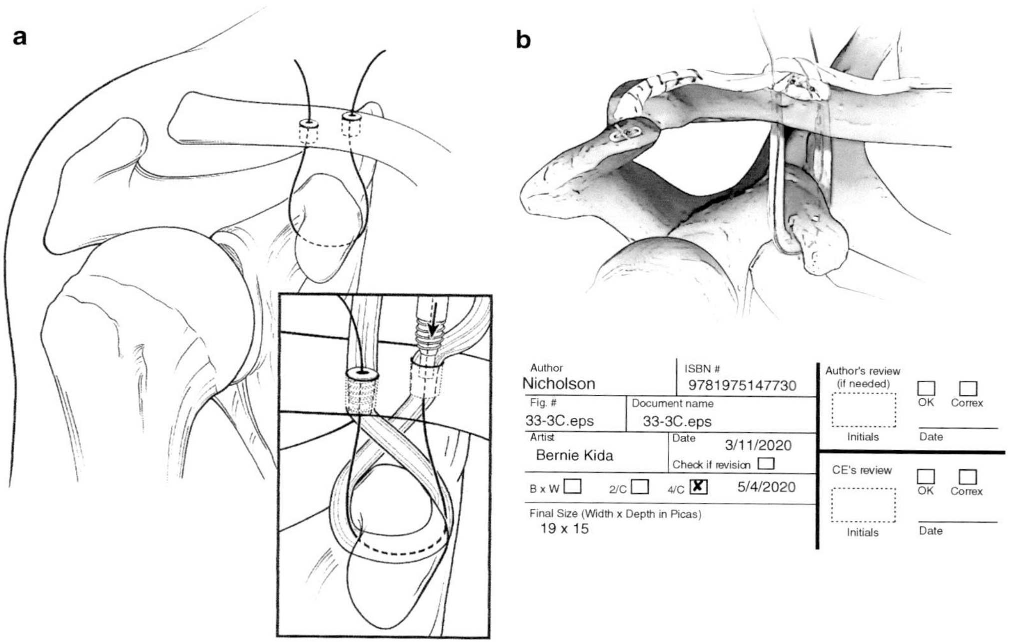

**Fig. 13.3** (**a**) Schematic drawing of the anatomic reconstruction, showing the tendon graft and sutures passed beneath the coracoid and transferred through drill holes in the distal clavicle. Fixation is accomplished with interference screw fixation as shown (**b**) More recently, this author usually ties the graft to itself as shown to avoid screw fixation. If horizontal instability noted, the graft is advanced to the acromion as shown

An additional button extending to the acromion from the coracoid can be added arthroscopically (triple button) with suture augment [24–26]

Several studies have evaluated these various supplemental horizontal techniques with no clear advantage to one technique [7, 27, 28]

Studies have not shown a clear clinical benefit to treating horizontal instability, but there appears to be a movement toward more horizontal stabilization nonetheless [7, 27, 28]

– Arthroscopic reconstruction

Arthroscopic techniques have increased in popularity over the last 10 years [24]

Tends to work best for acute repairs

No difference noted when comparing open and arthroscopic techniques in terms of level of reduction, complications, and rate of revision

Arthroscopic methods may lead to reduced pain and better cosmesis

Arthroscopic techniques involve placing heavy sutures and locking metal clips, i.e., TightRope device (Arthrex, Naples, FL), between the clavicle and coracoid

This fixation device allows motion through the sutures; unlike screw fixation, it is not rigid, and device removal therefore is not required

The principle of this technique is to place the clavicle in its native position in the hope that the CC ligaments will reconstitute themselves

Concept is similar to that of Bosworth screw or Kirschner wire fixation, which are left in place for 6 weeks before removal, but with the advantage of not requiring a second surgery

The Bosworth screw and Kirschner wire fixation methods also carried a risk of screw failure, pin migration, infection, or pullout

Disruption of TightRope-like devices has been reported [17]

"Dogbone" modifications were made to correct this, but there was reported higher failure rate and more symptomatic hardware with the dogbone modification [29]

Single, double, and triple buttons have also been developed with good results reported [22, 25, 26]

No consensus as to the best arthroscopic construct

Arthroscopic methods for reconstructing chronic separations have also been developed

Technique includes combining TightRope device with a CA ligament transfer (with or without a fleck of acromion) [26, 30]

Arthroscopic Weaver–Dunn procedure for chronic instability has been reported to have a high success rate (88%) [30]

The technical challenges of the arthroscopic techniques for chronic instability have likely prevented them from being more widely used

There is concern that arthroscopic surgery is inferior to open surgery in the ability to mobilize the distal clavicle or to oversew the deltotrapezial fascia which is believed to be a key surgical component of reconstructions

An advantage of the arthroscopic technique is that it allows the shoulder to be evaluated for intra-articular pathology at the time of the AC joint repair or reconstruction

In evaluating for intra-articular pathology, studies have found a 15–48% rate of pathology, such as rotator cuff and labral tearing, which can be corrected at the time of AC joint surgery [30, 31]

- Hook plates

  In the United States, more commonly used for distal clavicle fractures or complex injuries

  The hook plate is placed along the distal clavicle and under acromion (for 3–4 months typically)

  As with Bosworth screw fixation, short-term placement allows the CC ligaments and other structures to stabilize [18, 31]

  The role of hook plate placement in primary AC joint separations has been called into question due to high incidence of complications (pain, reoperation) and inferior functional outcomes. However, the hook plate is commonly utilized in Europe for AC separation [18, 25, 32]

  May be useful for AC separations associated with coracoid or scapula fractures in which fixation cannot be placed between the coracoid and the clavicle (Fig. 13.4)

  Hook plates also have been used for revision AC reconstruction, especially if excess distal clavicle was previously resected and poor soft-tissue quality remains

- Surgical approach

  AC reconstruction

  Typical incision extends vertically from AC joint toward coracoid

  Hook plate

  Horizontal incision tracking along the clavicle

  No internervous plane either approach

  Dangers—coracoacromial artery, brachial plexus, axillary artery

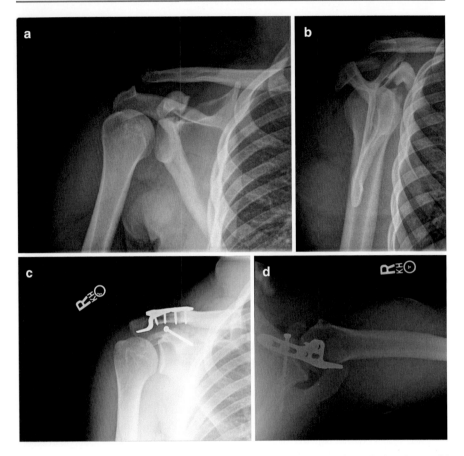

**Fig. 13.4** AP (**a**) and outlet (**b**) radiographs of a type III AC separation with a displaced coracoid fracture. AP (**c**) and axillary (**d**) radiographs of the hook plate placed for stabilizing the AC joint and a single screw placed into the coracoid for fixation. Interval healing of the fracture can be seen

5. Postoperative rehab
   (a) Many different postoperative rehabilitation protocols have been proposed
   (b) Typically, the shoulder is immobilized for the first 6 weeks. During the next 6 weeks, full active and passive range of motion is pursued, with limited lifting
   (c) Strengthening is initiated at 3 months
   (d) Full activity, weight-lifting, and throwing begin at 4 months, with return to contact sports at 6 months
   (e) Overall, patients have a fairly high return to sports with 92–100% returning to some sports and 62% returning to their previous sports [33]

# References

1. Johansen JA, Grutter PW, McFarland EG, Petersen SA. Acromioclavicular joint injuries: indications for treatment and treatment options. J Shoulder Elbow Surg. 2011;20(2 suppl):S70–82.
2. Frank RM, Cotter EJ, Leroux TS, Romeo AA. Acromioclavicular joint injuries: evidence-based treatment. J Am Acad Orthop Surg. 2019;27(17):e775–88. https://doi.org/10.5435/JAAOS-D-17-00105.
3. Nissen CW, Chatterjee A. Type III acromioclavicular separation: results of a recent survey on its management. Am J Orthop (Belle Mead NJ). 2007;36(2):89–93.
4. Schlegel TF, Burks RT, Marcus RL, Dunn HK. A prospective evaluation of untreated acute grade III acromioclavicular separations. Am J Sports Med. 2001;29(6):699–703.
5. Barth J, Boutsiadis A, Narbona P, Lädermann A, Arrigoni P, Adams CR, Burkhart SS, Denard PJ. The anterior borders of the clavicle and the acromion are not always aligned in the intact acromioclavicular joint: a cadaveric study. J Shoulder Elbow Surg. 2017;26:1121–7.
6. Aliberti GM, Kraeutler MJ, Trojan JD, Mulcahey MK. Horizontal instability of the acromioclavicular joint: a systematic review. Am J Sports Med. 2019;48:363546519831013. https://doi.org/10.1177/0363546519831013.
7. Vaisman A, Villalón Montenegro IE, Tuca De Diego MJ, Valderrama Ronco J. A novel radiographic index for the diagnosis of posterior acromioclavicular joint dislocations. Am J Sports Med. 2014;42:112–6.
8. Hobusch GM, Fellinger K, Schoster T, Lang S, Windhager R, Sabeti-Aschraf M. Ultrasound of horizontal instability of the acromioclavicular joint: a simple and reliable test based on a cadaveric study. Wien Klin Wochenschr. 2019;131:81–6.
9. Trainer G, Arciero RA, Mazzocca AD. Practical management of grade III acromioclavicular separations. Clin J Sport Med. 2008;18(2):162–6.
10. Cote MP, Wojcik KE, Gomlinski G, Mazzocca AD. Rehabilitation of acromioclavicular joint separations: operative and nonoperative considerations. Clin Sports Med. 2010;29(2):213–28.
11. Mouhsine E, Garofalo R, Crevoisier X, Farron A. Grade I and II acromioclavicular dislocations: results of conservative treatment. J Shoulder Elbow Surg. 2003;12(6):599–602.
12. Lizaur A, Sanz-Reig J, Gonzalez-Parreño S. Long-term results of the surgical treatment of type III acromioclavicular dislocations: an update of a previous report. J Bone Jt Surg Br. 2011;93(8):1088–92.
13. Smith TO, Chester R, Pearse EO, Hing CB. Operative versus non-operative management following Rockwood grade III acromioclavicular separation: a meta-analysis of the current evidence base. J Orthop Traumatol. 2011;12(1):19–27.
14. Lädermann A, Grosclaude M, Lübbeke A, et al. Acromioclavicular and coracoclavicular cerclage reconstruction for acute acromioclavicular joint dislocations. J Shoulder Elbow Surg. 2011;20(3):401–8.
15. Turman KA, Miller CD, Miller MD. Clavicular fractures following coracoclavicular ligament reconstruction with tendon graft: a report of three cases. J Bone Jt Surg Am. 2010;92(6):1526–32.
16. Gerhardt DC, VanDerWerf JD, Rylander LS, McCarty EC. Postoperative coracoid fracture after transcoracoid acromioclavicular joint reconstruction. J Shoulder Elbow Surg. 2011;20(5):e6–e10.
17. Motta P, Maderni A, Bruno L, Mariotti U. Suture rupture in acromioclavicular joint dislocations treated with flip buttons. Arthroscopy. 2011;27(2):294–8.
18. Moatshe G, Kruckeberg B, Chahla J, Provencher M, Laprade R. Acromioclavicular and coracoclavicular ligament reconstruction for acromioclavicular joint instability: a systematic review of clinical and radiographic outcomes. Athrosc J Arthrosc Relat Surg. 2018;34:1979–95.
19. Thomas K, Litsky A, Jones G, Bishop JY. Biomechanical comparison of coracoclavicular reconstructive techniques. Am J Sports Med. 2011;39(4):804–10.

20. Tauber M, Gordon K, Koller H, Fox M, Resch H. Semitendinosus tendon graft versus a modified Weaver–Dunn procedure for acromioclavicular joint reconstruction in chronic cases: a prospective comparative study. Am J Sports Med. 2009;37(1):181–90.

21. Gonzalez-Lomas G, Javidan P, Lin T, Adamson GJ, Limpisvasti O, Lee TQ. Intramedullary acromioclavicular ligament reconstruction strengthens isolated coracoclavicular ligament reconstruction in acromioclavicular dislocations. Am J Sports Med. 2010;38(10):2113–22.

22. Banffy MB, van Eck CF, ElAttrache NS. Clinical outcomes of a single-tunnel technique for coracoclavicular and acromioclavicular ligament reconstruction. J Shoulder Elbow Surg. 2018;27:S70–5.

23. Kibler WB, Sciascia AD, Morris BJ, Dome DC. Treatment of symptomatic acromioclavicular joint instability by a docking technique: clinical indications, surgical technique, and outcomes. Arthrosc J Arthrosc Relat Surg. 2017;33:696–708.e2.

24. Hann C, Kraus N, Minkus M, Maziak N, Scheibel M. Combined arthroscopically assisted coraco- and acromioclavicular stabilization of acute high-grade acromioclavicular joint separations. Knee Surg Sports Traumatol Arthrosc. 2018;26:212–20.

25. Qi W, Xu Y, Yan Z, Zhan J, Lin J, Pan X, Xue X. The tight-rope technique versus clavicular hook plate for treatment of acute acromioclavicular joint dislocation: a systematic review and meta-analysis. J Invest Surg. 2019;34:1–10. https://doi.org/10.1080/08941939.2019.1593558.

26. Tauber M, Valler D, Lichtenberg S, Magosch P, Moroder P, Habermeyer P. Arthroscopic stabilization of chronic acromioclavicular joint dislocations. Am J Sports Med. 2016;44:482–9.

27. Jordan RW, Malik S, Bentick K, Saithna A. Acromioclavicular joint augmentation at the time of coracoclavicular ligament reconstruction fails to improve functional outcomes despite significantly improved horizontal stability. Knee Surg Sports Traumatol Arthrosc. 2018;27:3747–63. https://doi.org/10.1007/s00167-018-5152-7.

28. Dyrna F, Imhoff FB, Haller B, Braun S, Obopilwe E, Apostolakos JM, Morikawa D, Imhoff AB, Mazzocca AD, Beitzel K. Primary stability of an acromioclavicular joint repair is affected by the type of additional reconstruction of the acromioclavicular capsule. Am J Sports Med. 2018;46:3471–9.

29. Vulliet P, Le Hanneur M, Cladiere V, Loriaut P, Boyer P. A comparison between two double-button endoscopically assisted surgical techniques for the treatment acute acromioclavicular dislocations. Musculoskelet Surg. 2017;102:73–9.

30. Boileau P, Gastaud O, Wilson A, Trojani C, Bronsard N. All-arthroscopic reconstruction of severe chronic acromioclavicular joint dislocations. Arthrosc J Arthrosc Relat Surg. 2019;35:1324–35.

31. Arrigoni P, Brady PC, Zottarelli L, Barth J, Narbona P, Huberty D, Koo SS, Adams CR, Parten P, Denard P, et al. Associated lesions requiring additional surgical treatment in grade 3 acromioclavicular joint dislocations. Arthrosc J Arthrosc Relat Surg. 2014;30:6–10.

32. Stein T, Müller D, Blank M, Reinig Y, Saier T, Hoffmann R, Welsch F, Schweigkofler U. Stabilization of acute high-grade acromioclavicular joint separation: a prospective assessment of the clavicular hook plate versus the double double-button suture procedure. Am J Sports Med. 2018;46:2725–34.

33. Kay J, Memon M, Alolabi B. Return to sport and clinical outcomes after surgical management of acromioclavicular joint dislocation: a systematic review. Arthrosc J Arthrosc Relat Surg. 2018;34:2910–2924.e1.

# Sternoclavicular Joint Dislocation and Instability

# 14

Eitan M. Kohan and Charles L. Getz

## Introduction

- Sternoclavicular injuries range from capsular sprains to dislocations with mediastinal compromise.
- Posterior sternoclavicular dislocations are important to recognize as they put the mediastinal structures at risk. Assume that pain following trauma over the medial clavicle is a posterior dislocation until proven otherwise and rule out any potential devastating mediastinal injuries.

1. History
   *Directed questions to ask*:
   (a) How old is the patient?
      - The medial clavicle is the last epiphysis to ossify (~18–20 years) and last physis to close (~23–25 years)
      - Younger patients are more likely to present with physeal fractures that may be misinterpreted as sternoclavicular dislocations
   (b) What was the mechanism of injury?
      - Often high-energy mechanism (motor vehicle collision, contact sports, etc.) [1]
      - Think about the direction of force that caused the dislocation
         - The direction of force on the sternoclavicular joint can help guide whether an anterior or posterior dislocation is present (i.e., direct blow to anterior clavicle will more likely lead to a posterior dislocation; indirect force from a lateral blow to the shoulder can lead to an anterior or posterior dislocation) [2]

E. M. Kohan (✉) · C. L. Getz
Department of Orthopaedic Surgery, The Rothman Orthopaedic Institute,
Philadelphia, PA, USA
e-mail: Eitan.kohan@rothmanortho.com; Charlie.Getz@rothmanortho.com

© The Author(s), under exclusive license to Springer Nature Switzerland AG 2022
C. M. Chebli, A. M. Murthi (eds.), *The Resident's Guide to Shoulder and Elbow Surgery*, https://doi.org/10.1007/978-3-031-12255-2_14

- Absence of a specific incident points towards atraumatic instability
(c) Is this an initial dislocation or recurring instability?
(d) Is there associated pain?
  - Acute dislocations are painful
  - Chronic, atraumatic dislocations may have minimal or no pain
  - Hypermobility of the SC joints are painless
(e) Posterior dislocations may compress or injure the mediastinum up to 30% of the time [3]. Ask questions to assess mediastinal structures at risk.
  - Chest pain?
  - Difficulty breathing?
  - Hoarseness?
  - Difficulty swallowing?
  - Neurologic abnormalities in the extremities?
(f) Are there any other injuries?
  - Due to the typical high energy mechanism, concomitant injuries are common
2. Physical exam
  (a) Inspection/palpation
    - Head/neck position
      – May tilt towards injured side to lessen tension of sternocleidomastoid on the clavicle
    - Swelling/fullness
      – May represent anteriorly displaced medial clavicle or a swollen capsule overlying a posteriorly displaced joint
      – Posterior dislocations may be missed if anterior fullness is assumed to represent an anterior dislocation
  (b) Range of motion (ROM)
    - In acute injury, shoulder ROM is often painful and difficult to assess
    - In atraumatic instability, overhead elevation may reproduce subluxation and lowering arm may reduce joint
  (c) Directed tests based on history or mechanism
    - Look for signs of mediastinal compression
      – Venous congestion of neck vessels
      – Unequal pulses
      – Abnormal neurologic exam
3. Imaging
  (a) X-rays (views)
    - AP chest
      – Good visualization often difficult due to overlapping structures (vertebrae, ribs)
    - "Serendipity" view [4]
      – X-ray beam centered on SC joints with 40° cephalic tilt
      – Anteriorly, displaced clavicle will appear higher than the normal side
      – Posteriorly, displaced clavicle will appear lower than the normal side (Fig. 14.1)

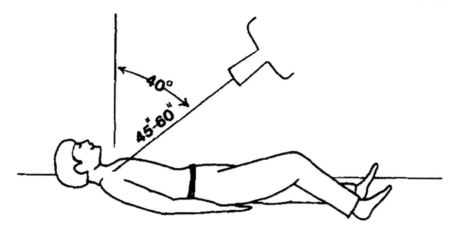

**Fig. 14.1**  "Serendipity" view. The X-ray beam is centered on the sternoclavicular joints and angled 40° towards the head. (*Image reproduced with permission from Cope R: Dislocations of the sternoclavicular joint. Skeletal Radiol. 1993;22(4):233–238*)

**Fig. 14.2**  Hobbs view. The patient leans over the X-ray cassette so that the lower thorax is against the cassette, and the flexed neck is almost parallel to the table. The X-ray beam is vertical and centered on the manubrium. (*Image reproduced with permission from Cope R: Dislocations of the sternoclavicular joint. Skeletal Radiol. 1993;22(4):233–238*)

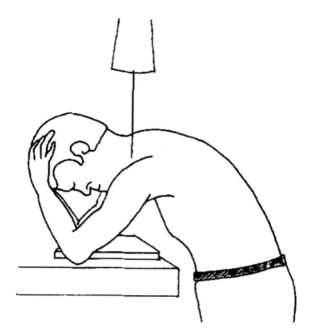

- Less commonly used radiographs include the Hobbs view
    - Patient sits leaning over cassette, and X-ray is shot from posterior-to-anterior centered on SC joint [5] (Fig. 14.2)
- (b) Ultrasound
    - Ultrasound has been proposed as a tool to make the initial diagnosis of sternoclavicular dislocation, although it should be confirmed with CT scan [6]

   (c) CT scan
- Gold standard for diagnosing sternoclavicular dislocation
  - CT scan should include both sternoclavicular joints for comparison
  - Definitively identifies direction of dislocation
  - Can differentiate between dislocation and medial clavicle fractures
- If there is any concern for mediastinal compromise, intravenous contrast can be used to assess for injury to the great vessels

   (d) MRI
- In young children in whom the medial clavicle epiphysis has not ossified, MRI can be useful to differentiate a physeal fracture from sternoclavicular dislocation

4. Classification

   (a) Four factors can help define injury and guide treatment:
- Degree of instability (mild subluxation, moderate subluxation, dislocation) [7]
- Timing (acute, chronic, recurrent)
- Direction (anterior, posterior)
- Mechanism (traumatic, atraumatic)

5. Treatment algorithm based on diagnosis

   (a) *Mild/moderate subluxation (grade 1 and grade 2 sprain)*
- Joint is stable but painful
- Treat symptomatically with analgesia and sling or figure-of-eight brace until pain resolves [8]
  - 1–2 weeks for Grade 1 injuries
  - 3–6 weeks for Grade 2 injuries

   (b) *Acute, traumatic anterior dislocation*
- Attempt closed reduction
  - Technique [8]

         Position patient supine on table with bump between scapulae

         Hold affected arm in 90° abduction and 10°–15° extension

         Apply traction to arm while applying gentle posterolaterally directed pressure over medial clavicle

         Stabilize in figure-of-eight brace
  - Often unstable and may redislocate after traction is released

         Reduction is more likely to succeed if performed within the first 48–72 h [2]

   (c) *Chronic, traumatic anterior dislocation*
- Patients with delayed presentation, or even some after attempted closed reduction, may remain unstable and develop chronic anterior dislocations
  - Chronic anterior dislocations often become asymptomatic and typically have good results, especially in low-demand patients [1, 9]
- In rare cases of patients with chronic instability with associated pain, operative reconstruction can be considered [10]

   (d) *Acute, traumatic posterior dislocation*

- Attempt closed reduction
  - Technique is similar to that for anterior dislocation [8]
      Position patient supine on table with bump between scapulae
      Hold affected arm in 90° abduction and 10°–15° extension
      Apply traction to arm while assistant applies countertraction
      Successful reduction often indicated by audible snap (Fig. 14.3)
  - If traction in abduction is unsuccessful, may attempt reduction by applying traction to the adducted arm while applying posterior pressure to the shoulder [11]
      This attempts to lever the clavicle over the first rib
  - If reduction with traction alone is unsuccessful, may attempt to manipulate the medial clavicle
      Pushing down gently on the medial clavicle may dislodge it from behind the sternum
      Grasping the medial clavicle percutaneously with a sterile towel clip allows direct anterior and lateral traction to be placed on the medial clavicle
  - If closed reduction is successful, joint is often stable [11, 12]
      Immobilize in sling or figure-of-eight splint for 4–6 weeks
      Closed reduction more likely to be successful within 10 days from injury [12]
  - If closed reduction fails, open reduction is indicated [13]
      Posterior dislocation left unreduced risks thoracic outlet syndrome or injury to the vascular mediastinal structures
- Open reduction and sternoclavicular stabilization
  - Technique for open reduction [13]
      Incision made over superior border of medial clavicle, extending to sternum
      Expose SC joint, preserving as much anterior capsule as possible

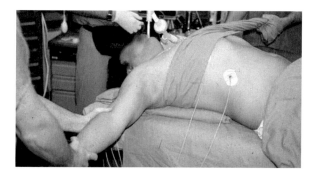

**Fig. 14.3** Intraoperative photograph demonstrating technique for a closed reduction of a posterior sternoclavicular dislocation. (*Image reproduced with permission from Groh GI, Wirth MA. Management of traumatic sternoclavicular joint injuries. J Am Acad Orthop Surg. 2011;19(1):1–7*)

Reduce SC joint with combination of traction on the abducted arm and direct traction on the medial clavicle

In acute setting, repair of ligaments to the medial clavicle after reduction restores stability

- Multiple operative techniques exist for sternoclavicular joint stabilization for continued instability after reduction [10]

Figure-of-eight reconstruction with semitendinosus graft provides biomechanical stability close to that of the intact SC joint [14] (Fig. 14.4)

Do not stabilize SC joint with Kirschner wires due to risk of migration, proximity to mediastinum, and potentially devastating complications [15, 16]

Joint stabilization with cannulated screws or plates has been described, but is currently not favored due to the risk of implant migration [17, 18]

Does not reconstruct the joint, but aims to immobilize the joint long enough for surrounding soft tissues to scar and stabilize the joint

Implants must be removed (typically around 3 months) to minimize risk of breakage and migration

(e) *Chronic posterior dislocation (over 1 week)*
- Attempt closed reduction, but less likely to be successful than acute dislocations [12]
- Open reduction and sternoclavicular stabilization techniques similar to that for acute dislocation

(f) *Atraumatic/recurrent anterior instability*
- Often occurs with anterior elevation of the arm, typically in ligamentously lax females in the second or third decade of life [19]
  - Subluxation typically reproducible with overhead arm elevation and reduces with lowering the arm
  - Patients often have initial pain and are concerned about potential harm [19]

    Given that atraumatic subluxation is typically anterior, there is no risk to the posterior mediastinal structures

  - Patients may have recurrent instability, but typically becomes asymptomatic over time [20]
- Nonsurgical management consists mainly of patient education, shoulder strengthening, and activity restriction [21]
- Surgical stabilization using similar techniques described earlier are utilized for patients who fail conservative treatment [22]

6. Operative Complications
   (a) Nonoperative complications
   - Anterior dislocation
     - Complications are most commonly cosmetic (bump at medial end of clavicle), although patients may develop late osteoarthritis [8]

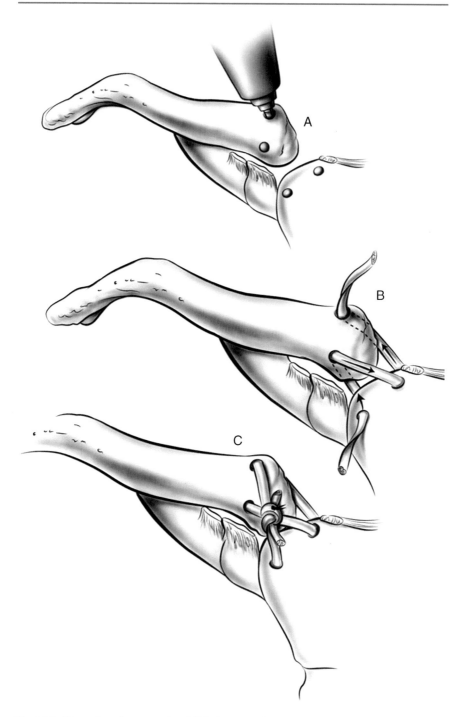

**Fig. 14.4** Illustrations demonstrating drill holes placed in the clavicle and manubrium. The graft is weaved through the holes in a figure-of-eight fashion and sutured into position. (*Image reproduced with permission from Spencer EE, Jr., Kuhn JE. Biomechanical analysis of reconstructions for sternoclavicular joint instability. J Bone Joint Surg Am. 2004;86(1):98–105*)

- Posterior dislocation
  - If left unreduced, posterior dislocation puts the mediastinal structures at risk and can lead to thoracic outlet syndrome, vascular compromise, brachial plexus injury, and tracheoesophageal fistula [12]
  (b) Operative complications [13, 23, 24]
    - Infection
    - Recurrent instability
    - Sternoclavicular osteoarthritis
    - Implant migration
      - Biggest risk is with the use of Kirschner wires that cross the sternoclavicular joint [15, 16]

## References

1. de Jong KP, Sukul DM. Anterior sternoclavicular dislocation: a long-term follow-up study. J Orthop Trauma. 1990;4(4):420–3.
2. Jaggard MK, Gupte CM, Gulati V, Reilly P. A comprehensive review of trauma and disruption to the sternoclavicular joint with the proposal of a new classification system. J Trauma. 2009;66(2):576–84.
3. Ono K, Inagawa H, Kiyota K, Terada T, Suzuki S, Maekawa K. Posterior dislocation of the sternoclavicular joint with obstruction of the innominate vein: case report. J Trauma. 1998;44(2):381–3.
4. Wirth MA, Rockwood CA. Disorders of the sternoclavicular joint. In: Rockwood CAJ, Matsen FA, Wirth MA, Lippitt SB, editors. The shoulder. 4th ed. Philadelphia: Saunders; 2009. p. 527–60.
5. Hobbs DW. Sternoclavicular joint: a new axial radiographic view. Radiology. 1968;90(4):801.
6. Blakeley CJ, Harrison HL, Siow S, Hashemi K. The use of bedside ultrasound to diagnose posterior sterno-clavicular dislocation. Emerg Med J. 2011;28(6):542.
7. Allman FL Jr. Fractures and ligamentous injuries of the clavicle and its articulation. J Bone Jt Surg Am. 1967;49(4):774–84.
8. Yeh GL, Williams GR Jr. Conservative management of sternoclavicular injuries. Orthop Clin N Am. 2000;31(2):189–203.
9. Nettles JL, Linscheid RL. Sternoclavicular dislocations. J Trauma. 1968;8(2):158–64.
10. Sernandez H, Riehl J. Sternoclavicular joint dislocation: a systematic review and meta-analysis. J Orthop Trauma. 2019;33(7):e251–e5.
11. Buckerfield CT, Castle ME. Acute traumatic retrosternal dislocation of the clavicle. J Bone Jt Surg Am. 1984;66(3):379–85.
12. Groh GI, Wirth MA, Rockwood CA Jr. Treatment of traumatic posterior sternoclavicular dislocations. J Shoulder Elbow Surg. 2011;20(1):107–13.
13. Groh GI, Wirth MA. Management of traumatic sternoclavicular joint injuries. J Am Acad Orthop Surg. 2011;19(1):1–7.
14. Spencer EE Jr, Kuhn JE. Biomechanical analysis of reconstructions for sternoclavicular joint instability. J Bone Jt Surg Am. 2004;86(1):98–105.
15. Clark RL, Milgram JW, Yawn DH. Fatal aortic perforation and cardiac tamponade due to a Kirschner wire migrating from the right sternoclavicular joint. South Med J. 1974;67(3):316–8.
16. Smolle-Juettner FM, Hofer PH, Pinter H, Friehs G, Szyskowitz R. Intracardiac malpositioning of a sternoclavicular fixation wire. J Orthop Trauma. 1992;6(1):102–5.

17. Brinker MR, Bartz RL, Reardon PR, Reardon MJ. A method for open reduction and internal fixation of the unstable posterior sternoclavicular joint dislocation. J Orthop Trauma. 1997;11(5):378–81.
18. Franck WM, Jannasch O, Siassi M, Hennig FF. Balser plate stabilization: an alternate therapy for traumatic sternoclavicular instability. J Shoulder Elbow Surg. 2003;12(3):276–81.
19. Higginbotham TO, Kuhn JE. Atraumatic disorders of the sternoclavicular joint. J Am Acad Orthop Surg. 2005;13(2):138–45.
20. Lemos MJ, Tolo ET. Complications of the treatment of the acromioclavicular and sternoclavicular joint injuries, including instability. Clin Sports Med. 2003;22(2):371–85.
21. Rockwood CA Jr, Odor JM. Spontaneous atraumatic anterior subluxation of the sternoclavicular joint. J Bone Jt Surg Am. 1989;71(9):1280–8.
22. Guan JJ, Wolf BR. Reconstruction for anterior sternoclavicular joint dislocation and instability. J Shoulder Elbow Surg. 2013;22(6):775–81.
23. Lunseth PA, Chapman KW, Frankel VH. Surgical treatment of chronic dislocation of the sterno-clavicular joint. J Bone Jt Surg Br. 1975;57(2):193–6.
24. Eskola A, Vainionpaa S, Vastamaki M, Slatis P, Rokkanen P. Operation for old sternoclavicular dislocation. Results in 12 cases. J Bone Jt Surg Br. 1989;71(1):63–5.

# Scapula Fractures

# 15

Joseph T. Labrum IV and Ian R. Byram

1. History
   (a) Mechanism of injury
      - High energy trauma most common (MVC)
      - Pathological fracture (tumor, osteoporosis)
      - Stress fracture (i.e., post reverse shoulder arthroplasty)
   (b) Handedness
   (c) Location/character/quality of pain, exacerbating factors, associated symptoms (numbness, tingling)
   (d) Associated injuries [1, 2]
      - Rib fractures
      - Spine fractures
      - Clavicle fractures
      - Pulmonary contusion
      - Head injury
      - Pneumothorax
      - Sternal fractures
   (e) Baseline activity level
   (f) Antecedent shoulder pain
   (g) Pertinent past medical history, past surgical history, and social history (occupation, tobacco use, prior shoulder arthroplasty)
2. Physical exam
   (a) Inspection/palpation

J. T. Labrum IV (✉)
Department of Orthopaedic Surgery, Vanderbilt Medical Center, Nashville, TN, USA

I. R. Byram
Shoulder, Elbow and Sports Medicine, Bone and Joint Institute of Tennessee,
Franklin, TN, USA
e-mail: ibyram@bjit.org

- Assess for overlying soft tissue injuries involving the scapula/shoulder girdle
- Inspect lacerations and wounds for open fractures
- Evaluate back/thorax for associated injuries/overlying hematoma
  - *Comolli sign*: Triangular swelling over scapula secondary to fracture hematoma
- Evaluate for symmetric chest rise during breathing/flail chest
- Palpate scapular spine, acromion, coracoid, and clavicle

(b) Vascular examination
- The injured extremity should always be checked for palpable pulses. When faint or absent, Doppler should be used to identify a pulse and a brachial brachial index (BBI) should be performed
- If BBI <0.9, consider CTA of the affected extremity
- Scapulothoracic dissociation can be present in the setting of scapula fractures and should be considered in any scapula fracture that presents with a vascular or neurologic injury

(c) Neurologic examination
- The injured extremity should be evaluated for intact distal neurologic function
- Upper extremity sensation: sensation to light touch should be evaluated in the axillary nerve ("regimental badge area"), musculocutaneous (lateral antebrachium), median nerve (thenar eminence), radial nerve ("snuff box"), and ulnar nerve (hypothenar eminence) distributions
- Upper extremity motor function: deltoid muscle (axillary n.), biceps (musculocutaneous n), FPL, FDP2 (median n.), EPL (radial n.), and dorsal interossei (ulnar n.)

(d) ROM/strength testing
- Active/passive glenohumeral ROM and strength testing typically causes severe pain
- Pain with rotator cuff strength testing may indicate occult fracture
- Evaluation of the ipsilateral elbow, wrist, and hand for ROM and signs of associated injury

3. Imaging
   (a) *X-rays*
   - A standard shoulder trauma series should be obtained including:
     - AP Grashey view, axillary view, scapular Y view (true scapular lateral) (Fig. 15.1)
   - Chest radiographs should be obtained to aid in identifying associated injuries
   - Non-rotated CXR to evaluate for lateral scapular displacement (scapulothoracic dissociation)
   (b) Computed tomography (CT) scan
   - CT imaging of the scapula can be helpful in appreciating fracture pattern, fracture displacement, and intra-articular fracture extension into the glenoid [1] (Fig. 15.2)

**Fig. 15.1** AP radiograph of the right shoulder illustrating a comminuted, intra-articular scapular fracture with significant displacement. Associated injuries, including a distal clavicle fracture (asterisk) and rib fracture (arrow) are highlighted

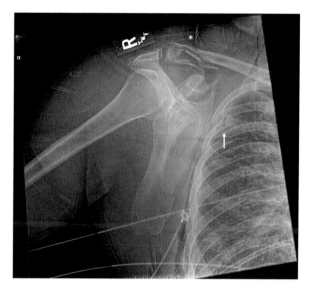

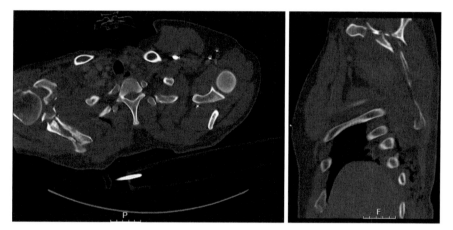

**Fig. 15.2** Axial and sagittal CT reconstructions revealing the complex intra-articular scapular fracture highlighted in Fig. 15.1 radiograph

- Many trauma patients who undergo standard evaluation will often have a CT of the chest abdomen and pelvis, which will include the scapula; however, dedicated scapular CT may be necessary
- In complex scapula fracture patterns, three-dimensional CT image reconstruction can aid in visualization of the injury pattern [3] (Fig. 15.3)
- The glenopolar angle (Fig. 15.4) derived from three-dimensional reconstructions can be utilized to accurately determine degree of scapular neck fracture displacement and can aid in determination of optimal scapula fracture management

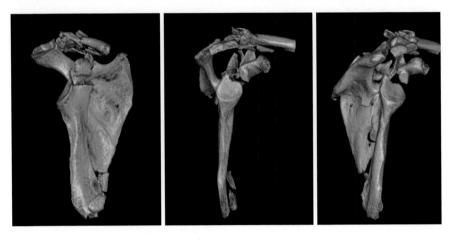

**Fig. 15.3** Three-dimensional CT reconstructions highlighting multiple views of a highly comminuted, intra-articular scapular fracture with fractures of the coracoid, acromion, scapular body, glenoid vault, and distal clavicle. This injury pattern represents a "floating shoulder," with multiple injuries to the shoulder suspensory complex

**Fig. 15.4** Three-dimensional CT reconstruction of an intact scapula demonstrating measurement of the glenopolar angle (GPA). A normal glenopolar angle was previously defined by Bestard et al. as 30°–45°. A GPA of <20° is considered pathologic and should cause consideration of surgical intervention

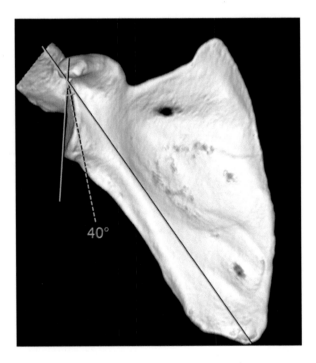

(c) Magnetic resonance imaging (MRI)
  • MRI is useful at evaluating the soft tissue structures around the scapula and glenohumeral joint, namely the rotator cuff and glenoid labrum

- Not typically used in the acute evaluation of scapula fractures, but may be a useful adjunct in the evaluation of other associated injuries (i.e., glenohumeral dislocation) or in the recovery period in the setting of continued pain or weakness
- Useful adjunct for assessing occult or pathological fractures of the scapula

4. Classification

Fracture classifications exist to aid in the description and management of scapula fractures.

(a) Coracoid fracture classification
- Eyres classification system [4]
  - Classification system for coracoid fractures based on location, with five defined injury patterns
  - Type 1 injuries involve the tip of the coracoid, Type 2 injuries involve the midportion of the coracoid, Type 3 injuries involve the base of the coracoid, Type 4 injuries involve fracture propagation into the superior body of the scapula, and Type 5 injuries involve fracture extension into the glenoid fossa
- Ogawa classification system [5]
  - Classification system for coracoid fractures based on fracture location and relation to the coracoclavicular (CC) ligament origin, with two defined injury patterns
  - Type 1 injuries involve fractures of the coracoid that are proximal to the CC ligament origin and Type II injuries involve fractures of the coracoid that are distal to the CC ligament origin

(b) Acromial fracture classification
- Kuhn classification system [6]
  - Classification system for acromial fractures in the native shoulder based on displacement and preservation of the subacromial space
  - See Fig. 15.5 for illustration of this classification system
- Levy classification system [7]
  - Classification system for acromial fractures in the setting of previous reverse shoulder arthroplasty (RSA) with classification based on fracture location in relation to deltoid muscle origin
    Acromial stress has been shown to be related to RSA implant positioning and glenosphere lateralization [8]
  - See Fig. 15.6 for illustration of this classification system

(c) Glenoid fracture classification
- Ideberg classification system [9]
  - Classification system for glenoid fractures based on fracture morphology and location of fracture propagation into the scapular body
  - See Fig. 15.7 for illustration of this classification system
- OTA classification system [10]
  - Broad classification system for scapula fractures that focuses on glenoid involvement but also includes scapular body fractures as well as fractures of the scapular processes

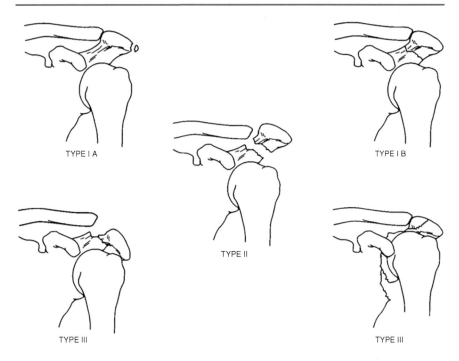

**Fig. 15.5** Kuhn classification system for acromial fractures is depicted. Type 1 injuries are minimally displaced, Type 2 injuries are displaced but do not reduce the subacromial space, and Type 3 injuries are displaced and cause a reduction in the subacromial space. (Reprinted with permission from Kuhn JE, Blasier RB, Carpenter JE. Fracture of the Acromion Process: a proposed classification system. Journal of Orthopedic Trauma. 1994;8(1):6–13)

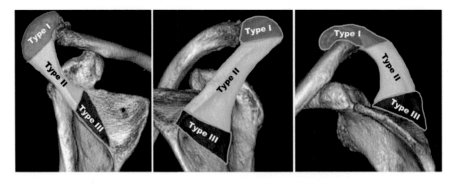

**Fig. 15.6** Levy classification system of acromial fractures in the setting of previous reverse shoulder arthroplasty (RSA) is depicted. Type I injuries involve a portion of the anterior and middle deltoid origin, Type II injuries involve at least the entire middle deltoid origin with a portion but not all of the posterior deltoid origin, and Type III injuries involve the entire middle and posterior deltoid origin. (Reprinted with permission from Levy JC, Anderson C, Samson A. Classification of postoperative acromial fractures following reverse shoulder arthroplasty. J Bone Joint Surg Am 2013; 95: E104–E104)

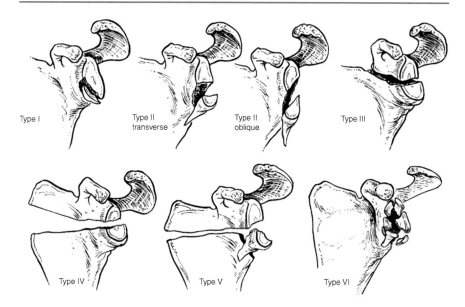

**Fig. 15.7** Ideberg classification system of glenoid fractures is depicted. Type I injuries involve anterior (1a) or posterior (1b) glenoid rim fractures; Type II injuries involve fracture through the glenoid fossa exiting the lateral scapula; Type III injuries involve fracture through the glenoid fossa exiting the superior scapula; Type IV injuries involve fracture through the glenoid fossa exiting the medial scapula; Type Va injuries are a combination of type II and IV injuries; Type Vb injuries are a combination of Type III and IV injuries; Type Vc injuries are a combination of types II, III, and IV; and Type VI injuries are fractures with severe comminution. (Reprinted with permission from Jeong GK, Zuckerman JD. 11. Scapula Fractures. Musculoskeletal Key, 2016, https://musculo-skeletalkey.com/scapula-fractures-2/. Accessed 12/20/20)

5. Treatment algorithm

When contemplating operative vs. nonoperative treatment, surgeons should consider patient age, activity level, scapula fracture severity, associated pathology, shoulder function, and prognosis to determine optimal management. Other than open fractures, operative indications are not absolute and all patient/injury factors must be considered.

(a) Nonoperative treatment

Nonoperative management represents the mainstay of treatment for the vast majority of scapula fractures as most heal without complication due to the rich blood supply and surrounding musculature [1].

• Indications for nonoperative management
  – Isolated fractures of the scapular body or spine
  – Non- or minimally displaced scapular neck fractures
  – Non- or minimally displaced glenoid fractures with intra-articular extension
  – Some acromial and coracoid fractures (see operative indications below)
  – Low-demand elderly or medically ill patients

- Nonoperative management protocol: acute scapular fractures
  - Sling, initial non-weight bearing with affected extremity
  - Encourage ROM exercises for ipsilateral elbow, forearm, wrist, and hand
  - Begin therapy 2 weeks after injury and with passive range of motion
  - Wean from sling at 4–6 weeks and begin active motion
  - Approximately 80% of patients with isolated scapular body, scapular spine, acromion, or coracoid fractures treated nonoperatively obtain good or excellent results [11]
- Nonoperative management protocol: acromial/scapular spine stress fractures following RSA
  - Sling immobilization with abduction pillow 6 weeks—no physical therapy
  - Gentle progressive ROM following 6 weeks of immobilization
  - Nonoperative management of acromial fractures following RSA can result in significant functional deficits depending on fracture morphology and displacement [7]
      Levy I acromial fractures treated operatively did not result in any significant changes in pre- and post-operative range of motion or PROs
      Levy II acromial fractures treated operatively were noted to have significant improvements in pain scores, postoperative range of motion, strength, and all PROs
      Levy III acromial fractures treated operatively were observed to have significantly improved external rotation strength and improved SANE score postoperatively
      Postoperative scapular fractures lead to inferior clinical results following RSA [12, 13]

(a) Operative treatment
- Indications for surgery
  - Open scapula fracture or bony prominence resulting in skin tenting
  - Double disruption of the shoulder suspensory complex (SSC) [14]
      SSC is a ring within the shoulder girdle that is composed of the glenoid fossa, coracoid process, coracoclavicular ligaments, distal clavicle, acromioclavicular joint, and acromial process
      Disruption can result in a "floating shoulder"
  - Concomitant scapular and clavicular fractures (Fig. 15.8a, b)
  - Glenohumeral instability (glenoid fractures)
      Double row suture anchor "bony Bankart bridge" technique [15]
      Arthroscopic-assisted cannulated screw fixation (Fig. 15.9)
  - Scapular neck fracture with >40° angulation or >1 cm of translation, glenopolar angle <22°, lateral border offset >20 mm [2, 16, 17]
      Posterior plating with Judet approach

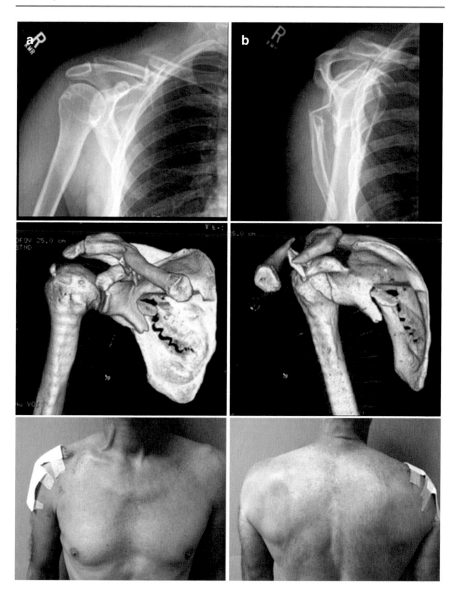

**Fig. 15.8** (a) Radiographs, three-dimensional reconstructions and clinical photos revealing a patient with displaced fractures of the right scapula and clavicle and clinically evident shoulder girdle deformity. (**b**) Postoperative radiographs and clinical photo from the injury depicted in Fig. 15.9a status post open reduction internal fixation. Clinical photo reveals a well-healed Judet approach utilized for scapular plating

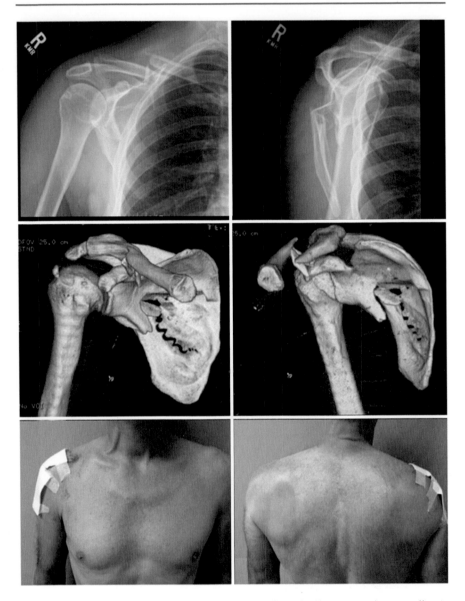

**Fig. 15.9** Radiographs, sagittal CT imaging, and three-dimensional reconstructions revealing an Ideberg type II fracture with associated glenohumeral instability. This injury was treated surgically with cannulated screw placement

  – >2 mm articular incongruity within glenoid fossa
    Surgical approach and technique are fracture dependent
    Posterior, anterior, or arthroscopic approach may be utilized
  – Displaced acromial fractures with symptomatic subacromial impinge-
    ment [18]

Cannulated screws

Tension band technique

Superior plating

- Acromial and scapular spine fractures s/p RSA resulting in instability or failure to respond to nonoperative treatment (Fig. 15.10a)

Superior and/or posterior plating has been described (Fig. 15.10b) [19]

Limited clinical outcome data exist

• Surgical approaches

- Judet approach [20]

Posterior approach to the scapula (Fig. 15.11)

Utilizes the internervous plane between infraspinatus (suprascapular n.) and teres minor (axillary n.)

Access to scapular neck, posterior glenoid rim, and inferior scapular pillar

Structures at risk: posterior branch of the axillary nerve (deltoid innervation), suprascapular artery and nerve (infraspinatus innervation)

Extensile approach: elevate the infraspinatus origin to expose the superior/medial borders and body of the scapula

- Modified Judet approach [20, 21]

Windowed approach to spare infraspinatus origin

May be utilized for lateral border or posterior glenoid exposure

- Deltopectoral approach

Anterior approach to the scapula

Utilizes the internervous plane between deltoid (axillary n.) and pectoralis major (medial and lateral pec n.)

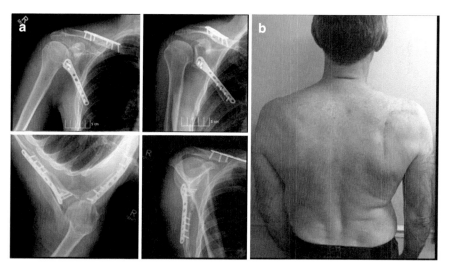

**Fig. 15.10** (**a**) Radiographs and CT imaging revealing a Levy Type II scapula fracture status post RSA. (**b**) Intra-operative picture and postoperative radiographs showing locked orthogonal plating of a scapular spine fracture in the setting of previous RSA

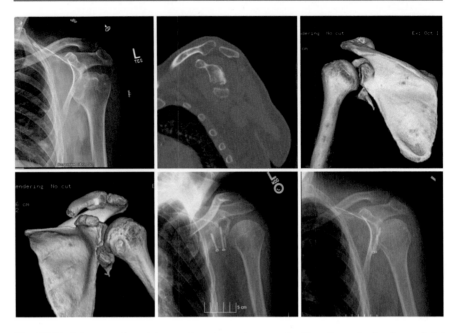

**Fig. 15.11** Intra-operative picture and postoperative scapular Y radiograph showing a Judet approach utilized for ORIF of a scapular body fracture in the setting of previous RSA

Rotator interval split: access to coracoid

Subscapularis management: subscapularis peel vs. subscapularis tenotomy vs. lesser tuberosity osteotomy to gain access to glenohumeral joint

Allows access to glenoid fossa, anterior glenoid rim, and coracoid

Structures at risk: axillary nerve and artery

– Superior approach

Interval between trapezius and deltoid to expose subcutaneous bone

Utilized for scapular spine and acromial fractures

• Risks and complications

– Infection

Incidence of infection after scapula ORIF is estimated to range 1–3.5% [11]

– Malunion

Symptomatic malunion following nonoperative management is uncommon. Symptomatic malunions are typically seen in patients with scapula fracture patterns that meet surgical indications but are managed conservatively

Malunion is rare following ORIF, but can result from inadequate reduction or loss of stable fixation

- Nonunion
  Scapular fracture nonunion following both nonoperative and operative treatment is extremely rare secondary to a rich osseous blood supply and stabilizing soft tissue structures
- Iatrogenic nerve injury
- Hardware failure, intra-articular hardware

## References

1. Cole PA, Gauger EM, Schroder LK. Management of scapular fractures. J Am Acad Orthop Surg. 2012;20(3):130–41.
2. Cole PA, Freeman G, Dubin JR. Scapula fractures. Curr Rev Musculoskelet Med. 2013;6(1):79–87.
3. Armitage BM, Wijdicks CA, Tarkin IS, et al. Mapping of scapular fractures with three-dimensional computed tomography. J Bone Jt Surg Am. 2009;91(9):2222–8.
4. Eyres KS, Brooks A, Stanley D. Fractures of the coracoid process. J Bone Jt Surg Br. 1995;77(3):425–8.
5. Ogawa K, Yoshida A, Takahashi M, Ui M. Fractures of the coracoid process. J Bone Jt Surg Br. 1997;79(1):17–9.
6. Kuhn JE, Blasier RB, Carpenter JE. Fractures of the acromion process: a proposed classification system. J Orthop Trauma. 1994;8(1):6–13.
7. Levy JC, Anderson C, Samson A. Classification of postoperative acromial fractures following reverse shoulder arthroplasty. J Bone Jt Surg Am. 2013;95(15):e104.
8. Wong MT, Langohr GDG, Athwal GS, Johnson JA. Implant positioning in reverse shoulder arthroplasty has an impact on acromial stresses. J Shoulder Elbow Surg. 2016;25(11):1889–95.
9. Ideberg R, Grevsten S, Larsson S. Epidemiology of scapular fractures. Incidence and classification of 338 fractures. Acta Orthop Scand. 1995;66(5):395–7.
10. Jaeger M, Lambert S, Südkamp NP, et al. The AO Foundation and Orthopaedic Trauma Association (AO/OTA) scapula fracture classification system: focus on glenoid fossa involvement. J Shoulder Elbow Surg. 2013;22(4):512–20.
11. Zlowodzki M, Bhandari M, Zelle BA, et al. Treatment of scapula fractures: systematic review of 520 fractures in 22 case series. J Orthop Trauma. 2006;20(3):230–3.
12. Teusink MJ, Otto RJ, Cottrell BJ, Frankle MA. What is the effect of postoperative scapular fracture on outcomes of reverse shoulder arthroplasty? J Shoulder Elbow Surg. 2014;23(6):782–90.
13. Hattrup SJ. The influence of postoperative acromial and scapular spine fractures on the results of reverse shoulder arthroplasty. Orthopedics. 2010;33(5):329.
14. Goss TP. Double disruption of the superior shoulder suspensory complex. J Orthop Trauma. 1993;7(2):99–106.
15. Millet PJ, Braun S. The "bony Bankart bridge" procedure: a new arthroscopic technique for reduction and internal fixation of a bony Bankart lesion. Arthroscopy. 2009;25(1):102–5.
16. Bestard EA, Schvene HR, Bestard EH. Glenoplasty in management of recurrent shoulder dislocation. Contemp Orthop. 1986;12(1):47–55.
17. Romero J, Schai P, Imhoff AB. Scapular neck fracture—the influence of permanent malalignment of the glenoid neck on clinical outcome. Arch Orthop Trauma Surg. 2001;121(6):313–6.
18. Hill BW, Anavian J, Jacobson AR, Cole PA. Surgical management of isolated acromion fractures: technical tricks and clinical experience. J Orthop Trauma. 2014;28(5):e107–13.

19. Bauer S, Traverso A, Walch G. Locked 90°-double plating of scapular spine fracture after reverse shoulder arthroplasty with union and good outcome despite plate adjacent acromion fracture. BMJ Case Rep. 2020;13(9):e234727.
20. Cole PA, Dugarte AJ. Posterior scapula approaches: extensile and modified Judet. J Orthop Trauma. 2018;32(Suppl 1):S10–1.
21. Obremskey WT, Lyman JR. A modified Judet approach to the scapula. J Orthop Trauma. 2004;18(10):696–9.

# Distal Biceps Rupture

**16**

Paul Sethi, Thomas Evely, and Jade Cohen

## Introduction

Complete or partial rupture of the distal biceps tendon most commonly occurs in the dominant arm of active middle-aged men as a result of eccentric force exerted on a flexed forearm. The incidence of distal biceps ruptures is estimated to be 1.2 ruptures per 100,000 people per year [1]. Diagnosis is often made clinically by detailed history and physical exam; however, MRI is often helpful.

1. History
   - (a) The most common mechanism of injury is a sudden eccentric load against a flexed elbow during an event such as heavy lifting, a fall, or sporting activity [2–4]. An audible pop is heard in approximately 35% of cases [3, 4].
   - (b) The patients may complain of weakness with elbow flexion and supination. Partial ruptures can present the same as complete ruptures with a history of an injury or may present with more insidious onset.
   - (c) Female patients most commonly have a history of prodromal symptoms and present at older ages [2].
   - (d) Increased risk of distal biceps rupture in those with history of smoking and increased body mass index [5].

P. Sethi (✉)
The ONS Sports and Shoulder Service, The ONS Foundation for Clinical Research and Education, Greenwich, CT, USA
e-mail: sethi@onsmd.com

T. Evely
Plancher Orthopaedics and Sports Medicine, New York, NY, USA

J. Cohen
Orthopaedic and Neurosurgery Specialist, Greenwich, CT, USA
e-mail: jadecohen@wustl.edu

2. Physical exam
   (a) Inspection/palpation: With a distal biceps rupture, the patients can develop swelling and ecchymosis on inspection. The degree of swelling and ecchymosis is dependent on the amount of disruption of the bicipital aponeurosis [2]. One should observe for a "Popeye deformity" and observe the biceps contour [3]. On palpation, the patient may exhibit tenderness along the antecubital fossa elbow on the anterior surface from the antecubital fossa extending down to the proximal radius [2]. The examiner should attempt to palpate the biceps tendon with the elbow flexed: however, they must also discriminate between the lacertus fibrosus, which is often intact, and the biceps tendon.
   (b) ROM: Typically preserved in these injuries but may be limited secondary to pain [2].
   (c) Strength: There may be loss of supination and elbow flexion strength [3].
   (d) Special test:
      • Biceps hook test: Patient's arm is held in 90° of flexion with supination, and the examiner attempts to hook the distal biceps tendon from lateral to medial. With an intact tendon, the examiner is able to hook the tendon and pull it forward. A partially ruptured tendon may show an intact hook test but with pain present [6].
      • Biceps squeeze test [7]: Examiner squeezes the relaxed biceps muscle with the elbow held in 90° of flexion. If the tendon is intact, then the examiner should see forearm supination versus when the tendon is ruptured, no supination is observed.
      • Biceps aponeurosis flex test: Used to detect if the bicipital aponeurosis (lacertus fibrosus) is intact or ruptured with the distal biceps tendon. The elbow is held in 75° of flexion, and the patient is instructed to make a fist and then flex and supinate the wrist. The examiner palpates in the antecubital fossa to detect the sharp edge of the tensioned bicipital aponeurosis that is medial and distal to the biceps tendon [8].
3. Imaging
   (a) Diagnosis of a distal biceps tendon rupture can often be made on history and physical exam alone. However, there are times when the diagnosis is not so clear and imaging is needed.
   (b) X-ray: routinely obtained first; however, they are typically normal since bony avulsion is relatively rare with distal biceps rupture.
   (c) Magnetic resonance imaging (MRI): MRI is useful when history and physical are not conclusive for distal biceps rupture. The absence of the tendon insertion or a fluid-filled sheath is suggestive of complete rupture (Fig. 16.1):
      • Partial ruptures typically have high signal intensity, fluid within the tendon sheath, or either thickening or thinning of the tendon insertion [9]. MRI has been found to be 100% sensitive and 82.8% specific for complete ruptures and 59.1% sensitive and 100% specific for partial ruptures [10]. MRI is useful for the evaluation of complete and partial injuries as well as the amount of retraction of the tendon in complete rupture [5].

**Fig. 16.1** MRI scan showing a biceps tendon of insufficient length for a primary repair. The biceps tendon can sometimes be found invaginated upon itself in the biceps muscle belly

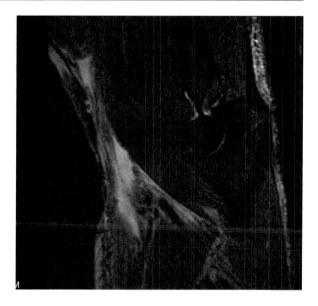

**Fig. 16.2** Biceps tendon insertion site on the radial tuberosity. The far ulnar insertion may be important for supination and is not easy to recreate through a single anterior incision. Surgeons may choose a posterior incision, if anterior approach uses ulnar-based anchors or a screw to push the tendon to the ulnar side of the tuberosity

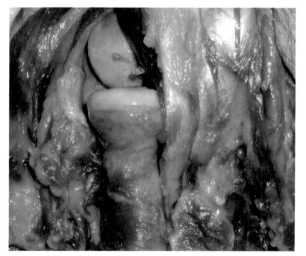

- FABS view has been described to increase the accuracy of MRI for distal biceps ruptures, perhaps best for assessing partial tears. The patient is positioned prone, and the shoulder is abducted to 180°, and then the elbow is flexed to 90°.
- Ruptures can be further categorized into severity of injury with the first being complete rupture of the tendinous attachment on the radial tuberosity (Fig. 16.2). Partial ruptures can be divided into low-grade partial ruptures (<50% of the tendinous attachment) and high-grade partial ruptures (>50% of the tendinous attachment).

(d) Ultrasound is a cost-effective alternative to MRI and more convenient for patients when conducted in the office. This operator-dependent test is more useful for detecting complete versus partial ruptures. US examination has been found to have 95% sensitivity and 71% specificity in differentiating complete tears from intact tendons [11].

4. Nonoperative treatment

(a) Biomechanical studies on nonoperative treatment have shown a 40% loss of supination strength, 79% loss in supination endurance, 30% loss of flexion strength, and 30% loss in flexion endurance [12].

(b) Freeman et al. [13] compared a group of nonoperatively treated patients and compared them with operative group. They found a significant difference of mean supination strength in those treated operatively, but no difference in elbow flexion strength.

(c) Physical therapy should be started to work on improving strength [5, 14]. The supinator and brachioradialis muscles are the remaining supinator muscles after a distal biceps rupture, and their moment arms are longer when the forearm is pronated [15, 16].

(d) The brachioradialis is a supinator of the forearm until neutral rotation, then it becomes a pronator and also an elbow flexor [15, 16].

(e) Therapeutic exercise targeted at strengthening the brachioradialis could decrease the subjective fatigue with elbow supination and flexion [5].

5. Operative treatment

(a) In 1985, Baker and Bierwagen [17] and Morrey et al. [12] changed the current thought and demonstrated better supination strength, flexion strength, and endurance with operative treatment.

(b) Ideal surgical candidate for operative treatment has a symptomatic complete biceps tear in a patient that desires maximum supination strength and endurance or a patient with high-grade partial tear failing to improve with nonoperative measures [2]. Biomechanical studies have confirmed increased strength and endurance [18] and restored function in forearm supination and elbow flexion in patients after distal biceps repair [19].

(c) Surgical repair reliably decreased pain and improved supination and elbow flexion strength compared with nonoperative management: it rarely restored full supination strength: [20]

- Single-incision technique: Performed either through transverse incision 3–4 cm distal to the antecubital crease or can be done through a more extensile "S"-shaped incision for a more chronic tear (Fig. 16.3). The surgeon must have good visualization using the single-incision technique. A tourniquet may be needed to aid in exposure, but is not used routinely. The recurrent radial vessels are well visualized without a tourniquet. The forearm should be in hyper-supination at the time of incision and throughout the procedure. Hyper-supination moves the posterior interosseous nerve away from the surgical wound and protects it from injury:

**Fig. 16.3** Transverse incision has excellent cosmesis but is hard to extend

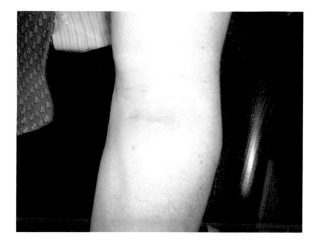

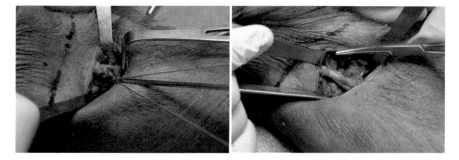

**Fig. 16.4** Anatomical repair of the distal biceps tendon through single anterior incision. (Left) In a deep forearm, an arthroscopic knot pusher device can help tie down the sutures. (Right) Repaired distal biceps tendon. The interference screw is placed on the radial side of the bone tunnel to recreate the ulnar-sided attachment [21]

- The surgeon should be well aware of the position of the lateral antebrachial cutaneous nerve (LABC), but it does not need to be distinctly identified on approach but rather protected. The LABC nerve is a branch of the musculocutaneous nerve and enters the forearm between the biceps and brachialis laterally. The interval between the brachioradialis and pronator teres should be identified leading the surgeon to the torn tendon stump and a seroma or a small hematoma. Another more proximal transverse incision may be made if the tendon stump is retracted too proximal. Usually, the biceps tendon stump can be delivered into the field using a milking type maneuver on the biceps muscle belly and adding elbow flexion.
- The tendon stump should be debrided and release of any adhesions that may prohibit excursion (Fig. 16.4). There are significant neurovascular structures, particularly on medial aspect of the antebrachial

area. The median nerve and brachial artery can be palpated medial to the biceps tendon. The radial nerve is more lateral and typically out of the surgical field, but only by a few centimeters. Dissection is carried down using prono-supination to aid in finding the radial tuberosity. Through the anterior incision, fixation techniques include cortical button with or without interference-interosseous screw or suture anchors.

- The advantages of this technique include single-incision exposure with decreased risk of heterotopic ossification seen with classic two-incision technique [2]. Critics of the single-incision technique suggest that this is a nonanatomic repair with loss of strength and endurance in supination. Schmidt et al. found that the single-incision technique moved the reattachment site 6 mm more anterior on the radial tuberosity, which leads to average supination strength loss of 10% in neutral rotation and 33% loss going from neutral to 60° of supination [20, 22]

• Two-incision technique: Involves a similar, but generally smaller, anterior incision close to the antecubital fossa. When dissecting, care must be taken to avoid injury to the LABC nerve that is lateral to the biceps tendon. The tendon is retrieved, debrided, and prepared in the same manner as with single incision. A Krakow stitch or looped suture is used to secure the tendon:

- A second posterolateral incision is made with the arm in pronation (Fig. 16.5). It is important to perform a muscle-splitting approach at extensor carpi ulnaris and supinator. Care must be taken to avoid exposing the ulna and to decrease the risk of synostosis [5]. The tendon may be secured to the bone through bone tunnels, cortical button, or suture anchors.

- The most significant advantage to this technique is placing the distal biceps stump in more anatomic position on posterior radial tuberosity. Schmidt et al. [20] suggest that this restores the cam effect of the

**Fig. 16.5** Posterior incision approach. Subperiosteal dissection should be avoided. High-grade partial tears may be approached through an isolated posterior approach [5]

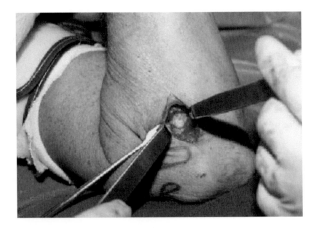

biceps tendon and leads to greater strength in supination. They also found higher load to failure rates with two-incision technique with two EndoButtons (Arthrex, Naples, FL) [20]. The second posterolateral incision involves splitting the supinator, which some suggest may cause loss of supination strength as result [5].

(d) Fixation biomechanics
   - Fixation techniques include bone tunnels, distal biceps buttons, suture anchors, and interference screws. The normal biceps tendon has a mean failure strength of 204 N and maximum strength of 222 N [23].
   - Mazzocca et al. [24] compared these four fixation techniques in biomechanical study:
     – Load to failure:
         Distal biceps button: (440 N)
         Suture anchors (381 N)
         Bone tunnels (310 N)
         Interference screw (232 N)
     – There was no significant tendon displacement comparing the four techniques.
   - Mazzocca et al. [25] went on to propose a technique that included the use of EndoButton (Arthrex, Naples, FL) along with an interference screw. They propose that the biceps button provides the greatest load to failure and the interference helps to provide stability during cyclic loading [25]. The interference screw also pushes the biceps tendon to a more anatomic ulnar position (Fig. 16.6).
   - Sethi et al. [21] proposed the tension-slide technique (TST), which allows for tensioning of the repair through the single anterior incision (Fig. 16.7). The TST eliminates technical concern regarding button flipping, determination of suture length between the button and the biceps, and suture diastasis between button and tendon (Fig. 16.8). They also found that this

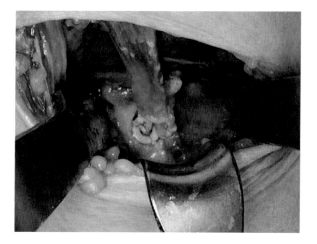

**Fig. 16.6** Interference screw placed on the radial side of the tunnel, forcing the tendon to a more ulnar and anatomic position [26]

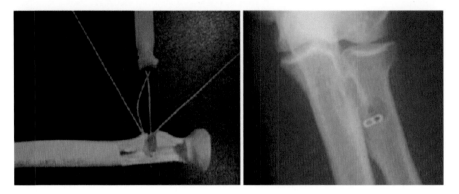

**Fig. 16.7** Tension-slide fixation technique using a cortical button. (Left) Cross-sectional image of diastasis between the biceps and radial tuberosity after cycling. This gapping can result in catastrophic failure of the cortical button construct when the tendon is not well seated in the bone. (Right) Radiograph showing button flipped on tuberosity [21]

**Fig. 16.8** Cross-section of the radius and distal biceps with a tension-slide repair using a cortical button. The biceps tendon is flush against the posterior cortex of the bone, with no suture diastasis [21]

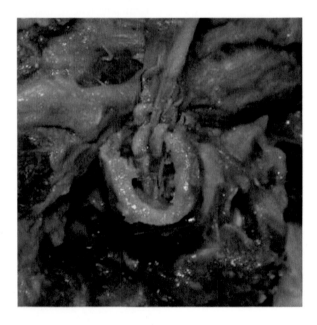

technique significantly reduced gap formation and motion at repair site while maintaining the standard strength of the cortical button [21].

- The surgeon should employ the method they are most comfortable with and use techniques to avoid iatrogenic nerve injury and heterotopic ossification.

(e) Complications
- The overall complication rate of distal biceps tendon has been reported up to 24.5% with slightly higher rates in chronic reconstructions (Table 16.1) [27].

**Table 16.1** Shows the most common complications of distal biceps repair and tips to avoid

| Complications of distal biceps repair | |
|---|---|
| Injury | Tips to avoid injury |
| LABCN injury/ superficial radial nerve palsy | This is the most common complication after single-incision approach and usually resolves. The LABCN does not need to be dissected. Avoid excessive retraction and radial side of wound. A gauze sponge may be placed under the soft tissue retractor on the radial side of the wound |
| PIN injury | Keep forearm supinated during procedure. Limit dissection on the radial side of the tuberosity. Avoid pointed retractors placed on radial side of radial tuberosity. For cortical button fixation, aim drill neutral to 30° ulnar if bi-cortical drilling is done |
| Heterotopic ossification/ synostosis | Use muscle splitting approach for posterolateral incision and avoid exposure of ulna. Thorough irrigation after preparing of radial tuberosity. Meticulous hemostasis with careful attention to recurrent radial vessels. Consider using bone wax to cover cannulated hole of interference screw when used. The use of NSAIDs to prevent HO is not proven |
| Proximal radius fracture | Use fluoroscopy to avoid proximal tunnel. Leave cortical bone on ulnar side radial tuberosity when drilling for biceps tunnel |

- Minor complications include injury to sensory nerves of the LABC and superficial radial nerve that resolve with time. Major complications of this procedure are potentially devastating and include injuries to motor nerves (PIN and median), radioulnar synostosis, re-rupture, vascular injury, compartment syndrome, and deep infection.
- A systematic review [27] examined 3091 surgical repairs of the distal biceps tendon. Overall complication rate was 25% with 20.4% being minor complications and 4.6% major complications. The most common major complications were PIN palsy (1.6%), median nerve palsy (0.3%), and ulnar nerve palsy (0.1%). Most of these motor nerve injuries recovered fully with expectant management.
- Major complications (4.6%):
  - Re-rupture rate was 1.7% overall with no significant difference between fixation mechanism.
  - Symptomatic HO (1.4%).
  - Deep infection (0.2%).
  - Vascular injury (0.06%).
  - Proximal radius fracture (0.1%).
  - Complex regional pain syndrome (0.1%).
- Minor complications (20.4%):
  - Injury to LABC (9.2%).
  - Injury to superficial radial nerve (2.4%).
  - Mild HO (2.4%).

6. Chronic distal biceps ruptures
   (a) Chronic repairs of the distal biceps are generally classified as an injury greater than 4 weeks from time of injury [5, 20, 28]. These may be neglected injuries or patients treated nonoperatively that had continued pain and weakness. Chronic repairs are more difficult to treat due to tendon and muscle adhesions, tendon shortening, and biceps tunnel obliteration [5, 20].

(b) Goal should always be for primary repair when possible due slightly inferior functional outcomes of reconstruction compared with primary repair [5, 20, 28]. Primary repair may require high flexion angles (>60°) to restore the biceps to the radial tuberosity, and up to 100° of flexion has been reported to be safe [29, 30]. Despite repairs requiring high degrees of flexion, the biceps tendon will stretch with time allowing for full return of elbow extension.

(c) The normal mean distal biceps tendon has a length of 4.2 cm [20, 31]. Chronic tendon ruptures may cause attritional loss of the biceps (<2 cm) tendon requiring augmentation [5]. Multiple grafts have been suggested including palmaris longus autograft, semitendinosus autograft, flexor carpi radialis autograft, Achilles tendon allograft (Fig. 16.9), and acellular dermal allograft.

(d) A recent systematic review and meta-analysis [32] on distal biceps reconstructions found no significant difference between graft type and fixation technique for postoperative range of motion, strength, and patient-reported outcomes. There were more complications in the autograft group when graft weave was used compared with onlay technique [32].

(e) Acellular dermal allograft can be used when tendon is attritionally thinned or lacks the elasticity to be repaired back to the radial tuberosity (Fig. 16.10). Mirzayan et al. [26] proposed the use of an acellular dermal allograft wrapped around the tendon as an augmentation (Fig. 16.11). Follow-up biomechanical study showed that acellular dermal allograft augmentation restored the biomechanical properties similar to native tendon with no significant difference in load to failure or gap formation compared with native tendon (Fig. 16.12) [33]

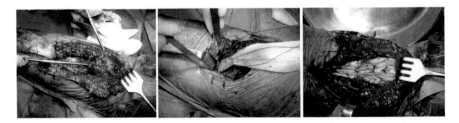

**Fig. 16.9** An Achilles allograft is used to wrap around the muscle belly of the chronic distal biceps with absent or insufficient tendon. A hamstring graft is another suitable option for this delayed reconstruction

**Fig. 16.10** Attritionally thinned biceps tendon with sufficient length. Repair may be augmented using an acellular dermal autograft to restore native biomechanical properties [26]

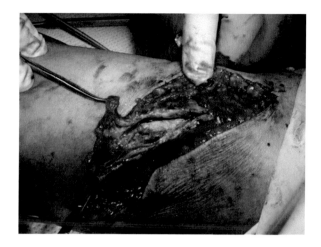

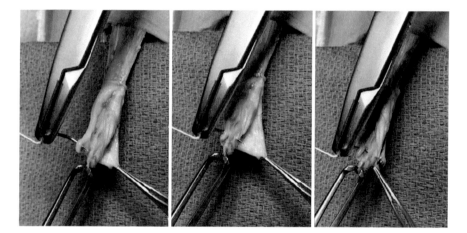

**Fig. 16.11** #0 FiberWire suture (Arthrex, Naples, FL) is passed through the graft, the native tendon, then through the graft again securing the graft to the tendon and preventing it from sliding [26]

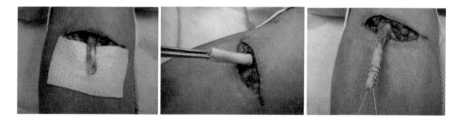

**Fig. 16.12** (Left) Transverse incision is made at or distal to the antecubital crease, and the distal bicep tendon is identified and delivered through the incision. (Middle) The graft is wrapped around the distal end of the bicep tendon. The narrow portion (12 mm) is placed distal, and the wider base (15 mm) is on the proximal end. (Right) #2 FiberWire (Arthrex, Naples, FL) is used to place Krakow sutures through the graft and tendon [26]

# References

1. Safran MR, Graham SM. Distal biceps tendon ruptures: incidence, demographics, and the effect of smoking. Clin Orthop Relat Res. 2002;404:275–83.
2. Haverstock J, Athwal GS, Grewel R. Distal biceps injuries. Hand Clin. 2015;31(4):631–40.
3. Pflederer N, Zitterkopf Z, Saxena S. Bye bye biceps: case report describing presentation, physical examination, diagnostic workup, and treatment of acute distal biceps brachii tendon rupture. J Emerg Med. 2018;55(5):702–6.
4. Rodríguez CG, López CG, Hernández TO, et al. Distal biceps tendon rupture: diagnostic strength of ultrasonography and magnetic resonance. Rev Esp Cir Ortop Traumatol. 2020;64(2):77–82.
5. Srinivasan RC, Pederson WC, Morrey BF. Distal biceps tendon repair and reconstruction. J Hand Surg. 2020;45(1):48–56.
6. O'Driscoll SW, Goncalves LBJ, Dietz P. The hook test for distal biceps tendon avulsion. Am J Sports Med. 2007;35(11):1865–9.
7. Ruland RT, Dunbar RP, Bowen JD. The biceps squeeze test for diagnosis of distal biceps tendon ruptures. Clin Orthop Relat Res. 2005;437:128–31.
8. El Maraghy A, Devereaux M. The "bicipital aponeurosis flex test": evaluating the integrity of the bicipital aponeurosis and its implications for treatment of distal biceps tendon ruptures. J Shoulder Elbow Surg. 2013;22(7):908–14.
9. Falchook FS, Zlatkin MB, Erbacher GE, et al. Rupture of the distal biceps tendon: evaluation with MR imaging. Radiology. 1994;190:659–63.
10. Festa A, Mulieri PJ, Newman JS, et al. Effectiveness of magnetic resonance imaging in detecting partial and complete distal biceps tendon rupture. J Hand Surg Am. 2010;35(1):77–83.
11. Lobo Lda G, Fessell DP, Miller BS, et al. The role of sonography in differentiating full versus partial distal biceps tendon tears: correlation with surgical findings. AJR Am J Roentgenol. 2013;200(1):158–62.
12. Morrey BF, Askew LJ, An KN, et al. Rupture of the distal tendon of the biceps brachii. A biomechanical study. J Bone Jt Surg Am. 1985;67(3):418–21.
13. Freeman CR, McCormick KR, Mahoney D, et al. Nonoperative treatment of distal biceps tendon ruptures compared with a historical control group. J Bone Jt Surg Am. 2009;91(10):2329–34.
14. Parikh P, MacDermid JC, Tuli V, et al. Distal biceps tendon rupture: is surgery the best course of treatment? Two case reports. J Hand Ther. 2020;34:463–8.
15. Bremer AK, Sennwald GR, Favre P, et al. Moment arms of forearm rotators. Clin Biomech (Bristol, Avon). 2006;21(7):683–91.
16. Murray WM, Delp SL, Buchanan TS. Variation of muscle moment arms with elbow and forearm position. J Biomech. 1995;28(5):513–25.
17. Baker BE, Bierwagen D. Rupture of the distal tendon of the biceps brachii. Operative versus non-operative treatment. J Bone Jt Surg Am. 1985;67(3):414–7.
18. Cusick MC, Cottrell BJ, Cain RA, Mighell MA, et al. Low incidence of tendon rerupture after distal biceps repair by cortical button and interference screw. J Shoulder Elbow Surg. 2014;23:1532–6.
19. Sutton KM, Dodds SD, Ahmas CS, et al. Surgical treatment of distal biceps rupture. J Am Acad Orthop Surg. 2010;18(3):139–48.
20. Schmidt CC, Styron JF, Lin EA, et al. Distal biceps tendon anatomical repair. J Bone Jt Surg. 2017;7(4):1–3.
21. Sethi P, Cunningham J, Miller S, et al. Anatomical repair of the distal biceps tendon using the tension-slide technique. Tech Shoulder Elb Surg. 2008;9(4):182–7.
22. Schmidt CC, Weir DM, Wong AS, et al. The effect of biceps reattachment site. J Shoulder Elbow Surg. 2010;19(8):1157–65.
23. Idler CS, Montgomery WH, Lindsey DP, Badua PA, Wynne GF, Yerby SA. Distal biceps tendon repair: a biomechanical comparison of intact tendon and 2 repair techniques. Am J Sports Med. 2006;34(6):968–74.

24. Mazzocca AD, Burton KJ, Romeo AA, Santangelo S, Adams DA, Arciero RA. Biomechanical evaluation of 4 techniques of distal biceps brachii tendon repair. Am J Sports Med. 2007;35(2):252–8.
25. Mazzocca AD, Bicos J, Arciero RA, Romeo AA, Cohen MS, Nicholson G. Repair of distal biceps tendon ruptures using a combined anatomic interference screw and cortical button. Tech Shoulder Elb Surg. 2005;6(2):108–15.
26. Mirzayan R, Conroy C, Sethi PM. Distal biceps repair with acellular dermal graft augmentation. Tech Shoulder Elb Surg. 2015;16:89–93.
27. Watson JN, Moretti VM, Schwindel L, Hutchinson MR. Repair techniques for acute distal biceps tendon ruptures: a systematic review. J Bone Jt Surg Am. 2014;96(24):2086–90.
28. Frank T, Seltser A, Grewal R, et al. Management of chronic distal biceps tendon ruptures: primary repair vs. semitendinosus autograft reconstruction. J Shoulder Elbow Surg. 2019;28:1104–10.
29. Morrey ME, Abdel MP, Sanchez-Sotelo J, Morrey BF. Primary repair of retracted distal biceps tendon ruptures in extreme flexion. J Shoulder Elbow Surg. 2014;23:679–85.
30. Bosman HA, Fincher M, Saw N. Anatomic direct repair of chronic distal biceps brachii tendon rupture without interposition graft. J Shoulder Elbow Surg. 2012;21(10):1342–7.
31. Darlis NA, Sotereanos DG. Distal biceps tendon reconstruction in chronic ruptures. J Shoulder Elbow Surg. 2006;15(5):614–9.
32. Litowski ML, Purnell J, Hildebrand KA, Bois AJ. Surgical outcomes and complications following distal biceps tendon reconstruction: a systematic review and meta-analysis. JSES Int. 2020;5:24–30.
33. Conroy C, Sethi P, Macken C, Wei D, Kowalsky M, Mirzayan R, Pauzenberger L, Dyrna F, Obopilwe E, Mazzocca AD. Augmentation of distal biceps repair with an acellular dermal graft restores native biomechanical properties in a tendon-deficient model. Am J Sports Med. 2017;45(9):2028–33.

# Triceps Rupture

# 17

Jay Keener

## Introduction

Triceps tendon ruptures are rare entity (1% tendon injuries), which are easily misdiagnosed and often require surgical intervention.

1. History
   (a) Mechanism of injury
      - Eccentric phase of heavy pressing exercise [1–3]
      - Forceful elbow extension (i.e., football lineman) [3–5]
      - Fall onto outstretched hand [2, 6, 7]
      - High energy blunt trauma (less common) [1, 2, 6, 7]
      - Laceration (rare) [2, 7]
   (b) Associated symptoms [2, 6–8]
      - Tearing or pop at time of injury
      - Acute onset of sharp pain localized to the posterior elbow (may be diffuse)
      - Swelling and ecchymosis about the posterior elbow
      - Pain and weakness with elbow extension
   (c) Patient factors
      - Gender (male predominance [8–10])
      - Age (30–50 years common [1, 6, 8])
      - Chronic olecranon bursitis [1, 6]
      - Chronic systemic illness: [1, 6, 11, 12]
         – Chronic renal dysfunction, renal osteodystrophy
         – Type 1 diabetes mellitus
         – Rheumatoid arthritis

J. Keener (✉)
Department of Orthopedic Surgery, Washington University, St Louis, MO, USA
e-mail: keenerj@wustl.edu

© The Author(s), under exclusive license to Springer Nature Switzerland AG 2022
C. M. Chebli, A. M. Murthi (eds.), *The Resident's Guide to Shoulder and Elbow Surgery*, https://doi.org/10.1007/978-3-031-12255-2_17

- – Hyperparathyroidism
- – Osteogenesis imperfecta
- – Familial tendinopathy
- Steroid use [1, 6, 13–16]
  - – Anabolic steroids
  - – Oral corticosteroids
  - – Local corticosteroid injections (e.g., triceps tendonitis and olecranon bursitis)
- Fluoroquinolone antibiotic use [17, 18]
  (d) Differential diagnosis [1, 8]
  - Triceps strain
  - Olecranon bursitis
  - Triceps tendinopathy
  - Olecranon fracture
  - Radial head fracture
  (e) Example presentations
  - Forty year-old male bodybuilder reports acute onset of pain, swelling, and ecchymosis on the posterior elbow during the eccentric phase of a bench press
  - Fifty-three year-old male with chronic renal dysfunction reports pain and swelling on the elbow after falling onto an outstretched hand
2. Physical exam
  (a) Inspection and palpation
  - Visually assess elbow for swelling and ecchymosis, particularly at the posterior aspect
  - Palpate for defect (Fig. 17.1)
  - Palpate for tenderness
    - – Tendinous insertion of triceps on olecranon
    - – Musculotendinous junction
    - – Olecranon process
    - – Swelling in olecranon bursa
  (b) Range of motion (ROM)—often normal
  - Flexion–extension arc—normal range 0°–145°. [19]
    - – Loss of terminal flexion
        Limited by pain or swelling
        May suggest intraarticular pathology [19]
  - Pronosupination arc—usually preserved. If limited, rule out associated diagnosis
  (c) Strength testing
  - Elbow extension
    - – Variable degree of extension weakness based on the extent of tendon injury
    - – Should assess extension strength in both extended and flexed elbow positions

**Fig. 17.1** Palpable defect. Lateral view of left elbow showing lateral ulnar skin abrasion and dimple-shaped defect more posteriorly at the triceps insertion. (Yeh et al. [2])

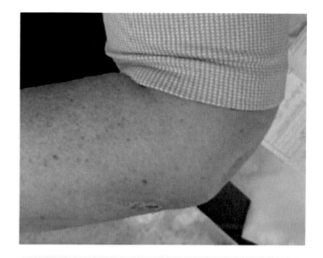

Clinical photograph of a palpable defect proximal to the olecranon in a patient with distal triceps rupture. The abrasion just distal to the olecranon indicates the area of impact during injury.

- Lack of antigravity extension suggests complete rupture of central tendon and lateral triceps expansion (Fig. 17.2)
- Preservation of antigravity extension does not rule out triceps tendon injury:

  Partial rupture—minimal weakness, pain with strength testing
  Complete central rupture with intact lateral triceps expansion
  Compensation by anconeus

(d) Directed tests based on history or mechanism of injury
- Triceps squeeze test [2, 7, 21]
  - Patient lies prone with elbow at edge of table, flexed 90° with forearm suspended
  - With the patient relaxed, examiner firmly squeezes triceps muscle belly
  - *Positive test*: lack of elbow extension

    Important to note that the presence of elbow extension does *not* exclude partial ruptures or complete central ruptures with intact lateral triceps expansion
- Focused motor and sensory examination proximal and distal to the elbow to rule out neurologic injury

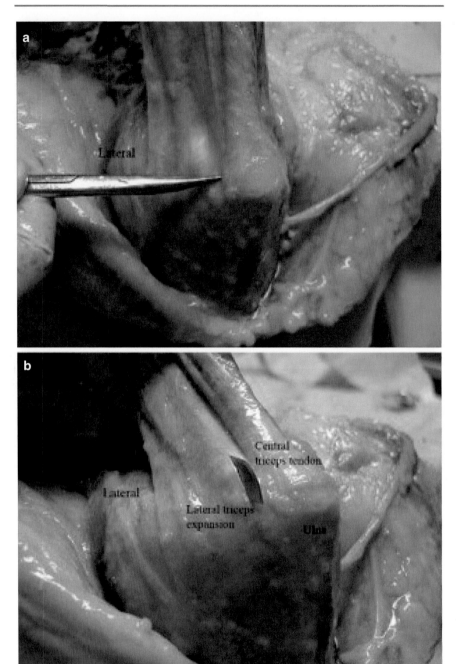

**Fig. 17.2** Lateral triceps expansion. Posterior view of the lateral aspect of the left elbow. (**a**) Surgical instrument demonstrating the superficial border of the lateral triceps expansion and central triceps tendon. (**b**) The lateral expansion is sharply separated from the central triceps tendon. (Keener et al. [20])

**Fig. 17.3** Dunn-Kusnezov or "flake" sign. Lateral radiograph of the elbow. Note the displaced bone fragment in the posterior elbow indicating avulsed osteophyte from the olecranon tip and triceps injury. (Keener et al. [7])

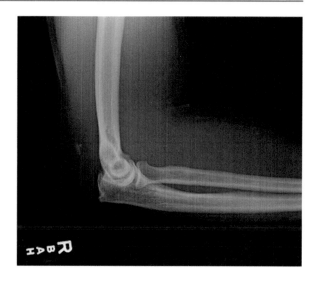

3. Imaging
   (a) X-rays
      - Anteroposterior, oblique, lateral of elbow
         – Dunn–Kusnezov or "flake" sign [1, 2, 6, 7, 12, 22] (Fig. 17.3)
            Thin osseous fragment proximal to olecranon on lateral radiograph
            Present in >60% triceps tendon ruptures, complete or partial
         – Calcification in tendon or olecranon bursa: [23]
            Indicates chronic pathology
   (b) MRI [6, 7, 24–26]
      - Sagittal T2 sequences:
         – Complete rupture (Fig. 17.4)
            Large area of increased signal intensity indicating fluid-filled defect
            Retracted proximal tendon
            Typically at tendon-bone interface
         – Partial rupture (Fig. 17.5)
            Small hyperintense area with surrounding edema
            May occur in superficial or deep layers
            Medial tears may be more common, but lateral tears have also been reported
      - Sagittal T1 or proton density sequences
         – Increased signal within tendon may represent chronic partial tears
   (c) Ultrasound [25, 27]
      - Comparable accuracy to MRI for complete and superficial partial tears
         – Efficacy for deep partial tears and chronic pathology less clear
      - Useful for serial exams to track progression of partial tears
      - Accessible and cost-effective
      - Dependent on skill of operator and quality of available technology

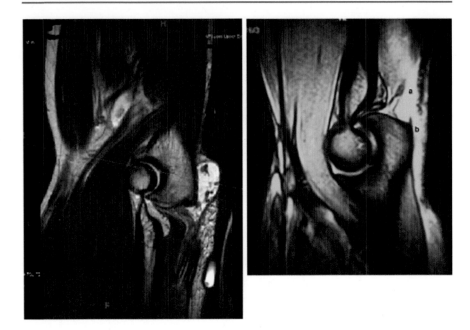

**Fig. 17.4** Complete triceps tendon rupture. MRI sequences from two separate elbows demonstrating disruption of the central triceps tendon from the olecranon. Note on both cases preservation of the insertion of the deeper medial head of the triceps. (Keener et al. [7]; Gaviria et al. [6])

   (d) CT scan [2]
- Limited utility
- Consider for evaluation of occult fractures

4. Treatment Algorithm
   (a) Nonoperative management
- Indications [2, 6, 7, 28, 29] (Fig. 17.6)
  - Partial tear (<50%)
    Preserved extension strength
    Elderly
    Low demand
    High comorbidity burden
    Tear location intramuscular or at musculotendinous junction
  - Complete tear or high-grade partial tear (>50%) in patients unfit for surgery
- Principles [2, 6, 7]
  - Immobilization with elbow in 30° flexion for 3–4 weeks for acute injuries
  - Transition to adjustable brace
    Controlled, gradual increase in flexion over 6–8 weeks
  - Progressive strengthening once full range of motion attained

**Fig. 17.5** Partial triceps tendon rupture. MRI sequence demonstrating a high-grade partial rupture of the triceps tendon where the superficial tendon injury is proximally displaced but the deeper central tendon is intact. (Keener et al. [7])

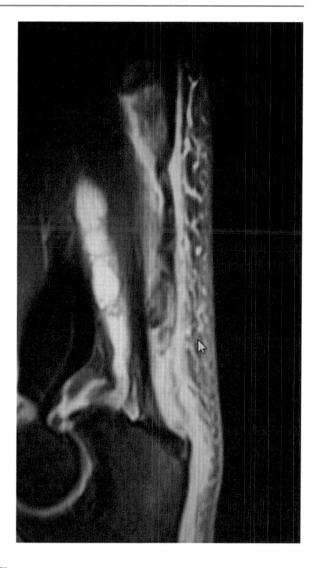

- Monitoring [27]
    - Consider serial ultrasound during first 4 weeks to assess healing and rule out delayed complete rupture
- (b) Operative management
    - Indications [2, 6, 7, 28, 29] (Fig. 17.6)
        - Complete or high-grade partial rupture (>50%)
        - Low-grade partial rupture (<50%)
            Loss of extension strength
            Young
            Athletic, active

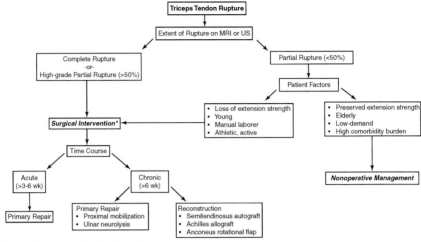

**Fig. 17.6** Algorithm for management of triceps tendon ruptures

Manual laborer

Failure of nonoperative treatment

- Surgical approaches
  - Open

    Positioning

    Lateral decubitus or prone—extremity draped over arm board

    Supine—arm placed across the chest

    Direct posterior approach (Fig. 17.7)

    Eight- to twelve-centimeter longitudinal incision, curved radially over olecranon

    Elevate full-thickness flaps medially and laterally

    Expose distal triceps and proximal ulna

    Gently debride tendon edge

    Debride and lightly decorticate triceps footprint (Fig. 17.8) on olecranon to create bleeding bone bed

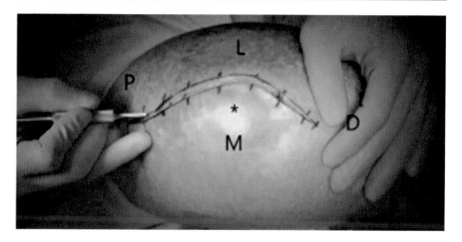

**Fig. 17.7** Posterior approach to the elbow. A 10 cm longitudinal curvilinear incision is made, curving just lateral to the tip of the olecranon. *Olecranon; *D*,distal, *L* lateral, *M* medial, *P* proximal. (Sarokhan et al. [30])

**Fig. 17.8** Triceps tendon insertional footprint. The triceps tendon has been dissected from the olecranon. The footprint insertion of the central triceps tendon is outlined. Note the broad dome-shaped appearance. (Keener et al. [20])

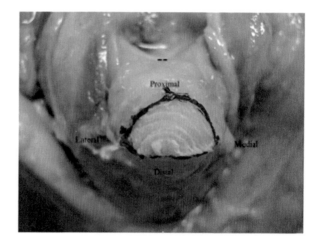

- Surgical options
  - Acute (<3–6 weeks)
    - Open repair
      - Transosseous—single row fixation
        Proximal control of triceps tendon with running locked suture configuration
        Use a 2-mm drill to create tunnels, either cruciate [8] (Fig. 17.9) or parallel (Fig. 17.10) configuration [30]
        Shuttle sutures through tunnels, and tie over bone bridge
      - Double-row repair [7, 31]—better recreation of footprint anatomy and superior fixation strength

**Fig. 17.9** Cruciate transosseous repair. The cruciate repair consists of a Bunnell-type suture through the triceps tendon secured in the olecranon through crossing diagonal tunnels. (van Riet et al. [8])

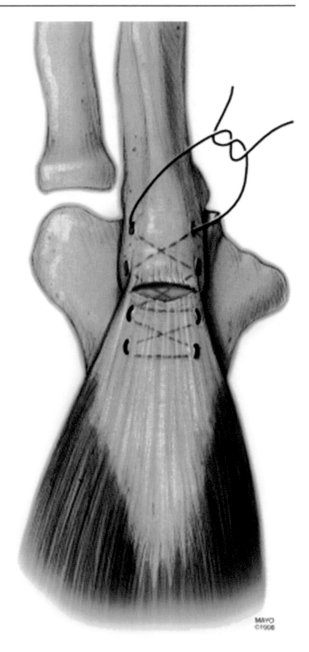

Standard (Fig. 17.11)

Place two double-loaded anchors ~12 mm from olec-ranon tip

Pass sutures from anchors through tendon (proximal to tendon edge), and tie in horizontal mattress configuration

**Fig. 17.10** Parallel transosseous repair. A parallel repair consists of heavy sutures braided into the triceps tendon and secured with parallel tunnels placed within the olecranon and then passed back through the tendon. (Sarokhan et al. [30])

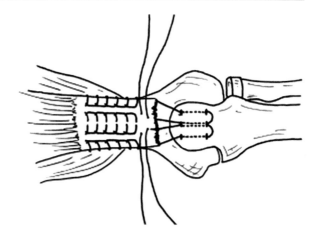

Secure sutures distally in dorsal ulna using additional anchors [31, 33], or intramedullary button [34]
Other
Can reinforce edges of tendon with running locked suture, and secure limbs in distal row [7, 31]
Addition of suture tape can augment tendon compression [32]
Knotless (preferred for acute injuries)
Knotless double-row configurations have been described [35, 36]
Combination of Krackow type configuration through transosseous tunnels combined with single anchor fixation on dorsal ulna
Additional considerations [7]
Sizeable bony avulsion attached to the tendon—reduce fragment to olecranon with sutures or anchors
Lateral expansion disruption—incorporate in the repair construct
–   Chronic (>6 weeks)
Repair [6]
Extensive release from posterior humerus to spiral groove, protecting radial nerve
Neurolysis of ulnar nerve
Direct repair favorable when tendon can be reduced with elbow flexed <45°
Reconstruction
Options for augmentation [2, 7, 37, 38]
Semitendinosus tendon autograft
Achilles tendon allograft
Anconeus rotational flap

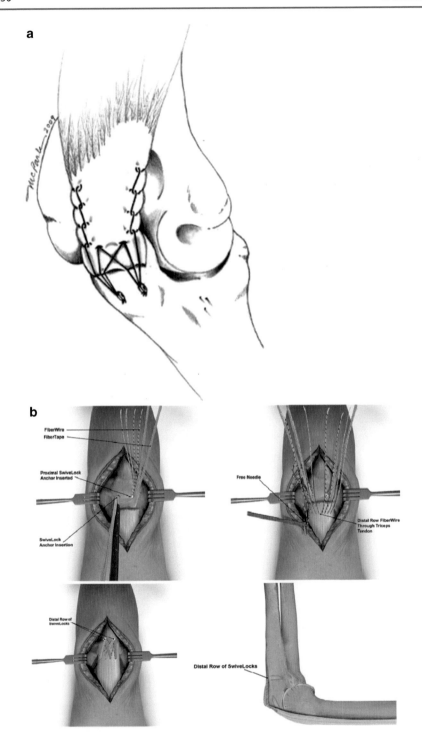

**Fig. 17.11** Double-row repair. (**a**) Knotted double-row repair. A running suture is secured along the medial and lateral aspect of the tendon. One suture anchor is placed at the olecranon tip. The anchor sutures are passed through the central tendon, knots are tied, and then the sutures are secured along with the running sutures to two interference anchors placed on the dorsum of the olecranon. (**b**) Knotless double-row repair. The technique shown uses two anchors at the olecranon tip loaded with three sutures. Each suture is passed through the tendon in mattress configurations, separated and secured to two anchors placed on the dorsum of the olecranon. (Yeh et al. [31]; Caldwell et al. [32])

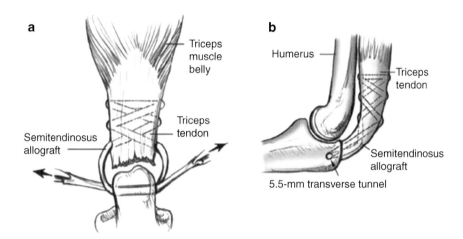

**Fig. 17.12** Semitendinosus graft augmentation. In chronic cases where a tendon graft is needed, a hamstring graft is passed multiple times transversely and obliquely through the triceps tendon and then secured in the olecranon through a transverse bone tunnel. (Yeh et al. [2])

> Semitendinosus augmentation [2, 7] (Fig. 17.12)
> > Weave graft through remaining triceps tendon in Bunnell fashion
> > Secure free limbs in olecranon through transverse bone tunnel using interference screw
> – Postoperative protocol [6, 7, 29]
> > Immobilization with elbow in 30°–45° of flexion for 1–2 weeks
> > Initiate active elbow flexion, passive elbow extension at 2 weeks
> > Progress to active elbow extension at 4 weeks (or once full range of motion achieved)
> > Gentle strengthening at 6 weeks and gradual progression over several months
> > No heavy resistance until 4–6 months postoperatively
> • Risks and complications [1, 3, 6–8, 29, 39–42]
> > – Olecranon fracture or articular breach during drilling to create transosseous tunnels or in preparation for suture anchors

- Inflammatory response to suture material
- Olecranon bursitis
- Persistent pain, numbness, and swelling
- Extension weakness (typically mild)
- Flexion contracture (typically minimal)
- Re-rupture (professional athletes, military personnel, manual laborers, and poor tissue quality)
- Less common: superficial infection, heterotopic ossification, anterior arm pain, ulnar nerve entrapment, posterior interosseous nerve palsy, lateral antebrachial cutaneous nerve paresthesia, and median nerve paresthesia.

## References

1. Dunn JC, Kusnezov N, Fares A, et al. Triceps tendon ruptures: a systematic review. Hand. 2017;12:431–8. https://doi.org/10.1177/1558944716677338.
2. Yeh PC, Dodds SD, Ryan Smart L, Mazzocca AD, Sethi PM. Distal triceps rupture. J Am Acad Orthop Surg. 2010;18:31–40. https://doi.org/10.5435/00124635-201001000-00005.
3. Giannicola G, Bullitta G, Rotini R, et al. Results of primary repair of distal triceps tendon ruptures in a general population. Bone Jt J. 2018;100:610–6. https://doi.org/10.1302/0301-620X.100B5.BJJ-2017-1057.R2.
4. Rettig AC. Traumatic elbow injuries in the athlete. Orthop Clin North Am. 2002;33:509–22. https://doi.org/10.1016/S0030-5898(01)00017-7.
5. Mair SD, Isbell WM, Gill TJ, Schlegel TF, Hawkins RJ. Triceps tendon ruptures in professional football players. Am J Sports Med. 2004;32:431–4. https://doi.org/10.1177/0095399703258707.
6. Gaviria M, Ren B, Brown SM, McCluskey LC, Savoie FH, Mulcahey MK. Triceps tendon ruptures: risk factors, treatment, and rehabilitation. JBJS Rev. 2020;8:e0172. https://doi.org/10.2106/JBJS.RVW.19.00172.
7. Keener JD, Sethi PM. Distal triceps tendon injuries. Hand Clin. 2015;31:641–50. https://doi.org/10.1016/j.hcl.2015.06.010.
8. Van Riet RP, Morrey BF, Ho E, O'Driscoll SW. Surgical treatment of distal triceps ruptures. J Bone Jt Surg Ser A. 2003;85:1961–7. https://doi.org/10.2106/00004623-200310000-00015.
9. Koplas MC, Schneider E, Sundaram M. Prevalence of triceps tendon tears on MRI of the elbow and clinical correlation. Skelet Radiol. 2011;40:587–94. https://doi.org/10.1007/s00256-010-1043-9.
10. Stucken C, Ciccotti MG. Distal biceps and triceps injuries in athletes. Sports Med Arthrosc. 2014;22:153–63. https://doi.org/10.1097/JSA.0000000000000030.
11. Tsourvakas S, Gouvalas K, Gimtsas C, Tsianas N, Founta P, Ameridis N. Bilateral and simultaneous rupture of the triceps tendons in chronic renal failure and secondary hyperparathyroidism. Arch Orthop Trauma Surg. 2004;124:278–80. https://doi.org/10.1007/s00402-003-0628-3.
12. Gupta RR, Murthi AM. Distal humeral fracture with associated triceps tendon avulsion in a renal transplant recipient. Orthopedics. 2010;33:26. https://doi.org/10.3928/01477447-20100129-26.
13. Mirzayan R, Singh A, Acevedo DC, Sodl JF, Yian E, Navarro RA. Surgical treatment of 150 acute distal triceps tendon ruptures. J Shoulder Elb Surg. 2015;24:e120–1. https://doi.org/10.1016/j.jse.2014.11.027.

14. Lambert MI, St Clair Gibson A, Noakes TD. Rupture of the triceps tendon associated with steroid injections. Am J Sports Med. 1995;23:776.
15. Stannard JP, Bucknell AL. Rupture of the triceps tendon associated with steroid injections. Am J Sports Med. 1993;21:482–5. https://doi.org/10.1177/036354659302100327.
16. Sollender JL, Rayan GM, Barden GA. Triceps tendon rupture in weight lifters. J Shoulder Elb Surg. 1998;7:151–3. https://doi.org/10.1016/S1058-2746(98)90227-0.
17. Shybut TB, Puckett ER. Triceps ruptures after fluoroquinolone antibiotics: a report of 2 cases. Sports Health. 2017;9:474–6. https://doi.org/10.1177/1941738117713686.
18. Khaliq Y, Zhanel GG. Fluoroquinolone-associated tendinopathy: a critical review of the literature. Clin Infect Dis. 2003;36:1404–11. https://doi.org/10.1086/375078.
19. Smith MV, Lamplot JD, Wright RW, Brophy RH. Comprehensive review of the elbow physical examination. J Am Acad Orthop Surg. 2018;26:678–87. https://doi.org/10.5435/JAAOS-D-16-00622.
20. Keener JD, Chafik D, Kim HM, Galatz LM, Yamaguchi K. Insertional anatomy of the triceps brachii tendon. J Shoulder Elb Surg. 2010;19:399–405. https://doi.org/10.1016/j.jse.2009.10.008.
21. Viegas SF. Avulsion of the triceps tendon. Orthop Rev. 1990;161:242–6. https://doi.org/10.1136/emj.19.3.271.
22. Weng PW, Wang SJ, Wu SS. Misdiagnosed avulsion fracture of the triceps tendon from the olecranon insertion: case report. Clin J Sport Med. 2006;16:364–5. https://doi.org/10.1097/00042752-200607000-00016.
23. Chan APH, Lo CK, Lam HY, Fung KY. Unusual traumatic triceps tendon avulsion rupture: a word of caution. Hong Kong Med J. 2009;15:294–6.
24. Wenzke DR. MR imaging of the elbow in the injured athlete. Radiol Clin North Am. 2013;51(2):195–213. https://doi.org/10.1016/j.rcl.2012.09.013.
25. Tagliafico A, Gandolfo N, Michaud J, Perez MM, Palmieri F, Martinoli C. Ultrasound demonstration of distal triceps tendon tears. Eur J Radiol. 2012;81:1207–10. https://doi.org/10.1016/j.ejrad.2011.03.012.
26. Sampath SC, Sampath SC, Bredella MA. Magnetic resonance imaging of the elbow: a structured approach. Sports Health. 2013;5:34–49. https://doi.org/10.1177/1941738112467941.
27. Harris PC, Atkinson D, Moorehead JD. Bilateral partial rupture of triceps tendon: case report and quantitative assessment of recovery. Am J Sports Med. 2004;32:787–92. https://doi.org/10.1177/0363546503258903.
28. Thomas JR, Lawton JN. Biceps and triceps ruptures in athletes. Hand Clin. 2017;33:35–46. https://doi.org/10.1016/j.hcl.2016.08.019.
29. Blackmore SM, Jander RM, Culp RW. Management of distal biceps and triceps ruptures. J Hand Ther. 2006;12:485–7. https://doi.org/10.1197/j.jht.2006.02.001.
30. Sarokhan AK, Leung NL. Acute triceps tendon repair: a technique utilizing 3 curved tunnels and proximal knots. Arthrosc Tech. 2019;8:e705. https://doi.org/10.1016/j.eats.2019.03.005.
31. Yeh PC, Stephens KT, Solovyova O, et al. The distal triceps tendon footprint and a biomechanical analysis of 3 repair techniques. Am J Sports Med. 2010;38:1025–33. https://doi.org/10.1177/0363546509358319.
32. Caldwell PE, Evensen CS, Vance NG, Pearson SE. Distal triceps speed bridge repair. Arthrosc Tech. 2018;7(9):e907–13. https://doi.org/10.1016/j.eats.2018.04.013.
33. Dimock RAC, Kontoghiorghe C, Consigliere P, Salamat S, Imam MA, Narvani AA. Distal triceps rupture repair: the triceps pulley-pullover technique. Arthrosc Tech. 2019;8(1):e85–91. https://doi.org/10.1016/j.eats.2018.09.006.
34. Scheiderer B, Imhoff FB, Morikawa D, et al. The V-shaped distal triceps tendon repair: a comparative biomechanical analysis. Am J Sports Med. 2018;46(8):1952–8. https://doi.org/10.1177/0363546518771359.
35. Paci JM, Clark J, Rizzi A. Distal triceps knotless anatomic footprint repair: a new technique. Arthrosc Tech. 2014;3(5):e621–6. https://doi.org/10.1016/j.eats.2014.06.019.

36. Clark J, Obopilwe E, Rizzi A, et al. Distal triceps knotless anatomic footprint repair is superior to transosseous cruciate repair: a biomechanical comparison. Arthrosc J Arthrosc Relat Surg. 2014;30:1254–60. https://doi.org/10.1016/j.arthro.2014.07.005.
37. Sanchez-Sotelo J, Morrey BF. Surgical techniques for reconstruction of chronic insufficiency of the triceps. J Bone Jt Surg Ser B. 2002;84(8):1116–20. https://doi.org/10.1302/0301-620 X.84B8.12902.
38. Weistroffer JK, Mills WJ, Shin AY. Recurrent rupture of the triceps tendon repaired with hamstring tendon autograft augmentation: a case report and repair technique. J Shoulder Elb Surg. 2003;12(2):193–6. https://doi.org/10.1016/S1058-2746(02)00016-2.
39. Horneff JG, Aleem A, Nicholson T, et al. Functional outcomes of distal triceps tendon repair comparing transosseous bone tunnels with suture anchor constructs. J Shoulder Elb Surg. 2017;26(12):2213–9. https://doi.org/10.1016/j.jse.2017.08.006.
40. Kose O, Kilicaslan OF, Guler F, Acar B, Yuksel HY. Functional outcomes and complications after surgical repair of triceps tendon rupture. Eur J Orthop Surg Traumatol. 2015;25(7):1131–9. https://doi.org/10.1007/s00590-015-1669-3.
41. Finstein JL, Cohen SB, Dodson CC, et al. Triceps tendon ruptures requiring surgical repair in national football league players. Orthop J Sports Med. 2015;3(8):2325967115601021. https://doi.org/10.1177/2325967115601021.
42. Balazs GC, Brelin AM, Dworak TC, et al. Outcomes and complications of triceps tendon repair following acute rupture in American military personnel. Injury. 2016;47(10):2247–51. https://doi.org/10.1016/j.injury.2016.07.061.

# Medial and Lateral Epicondylitis

# 18

Jesse McCarron and John Kafrouni

## Introduction

Medial and lateral epicondylitis of the elbow are degenerative tendinopathies affecting a large percent of the population between the ages of 40 and 60. Epicondylitis is self-limited with resolution of symptoms occurring within 1 year of onset for 80% or more of patients and 10% of patients or less requiring surgical intervention.

1. Anatomy
   (a) Lateral epicondylitis
      • Involves the wrist and finger extensors originating on the lateral elbow [1] (Fig. 18.1)
         – Extensor carpi radialis brevis (ECRB)
         – Extensor digitorum communis (EDC)
            The ECRB and EDC have a common tendinous origin when viewed from its superficial surface but can be identified as two distinct structures when viewed from their deep surface [2, 3]
   (b) Medial epicondylitis
      • Involves the flexor/pronator musculature originating off the medial epicondyle of the elbow
         – Pronator teres (PT)
         – Flexor carpi radialis (FCR)
         – Flexor digitorum superficialis (FDS)
         – Flexor carpi ulnaris (FCU)
            Common tendon origin with the inability to distinguish one muscle-tendon unit from the other until individual muscles become distinct more distally in forearm

J. McCarron (✉) · J. Kafrouni
Rebound Orthopedics and Neurosurgery, Vancouver, WA, USA
e-mail: JMcCarron@reboundmd.com; JKafrouni@reboundmd.com

235

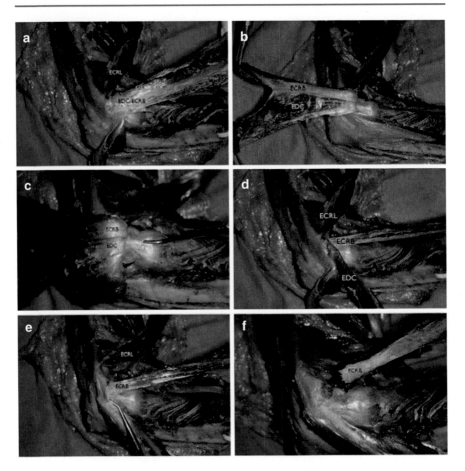

**Fig. 18.1** (a) Lateral view of a cadaveric specimen. The ECRL, which has a muscular origin, has been reflected anteriorly and the extensor carpi ulnaris posteriorly, revealing the common extensor tendon origin of the ECRB and EDC. These are indistinguishable when viewed from the outer surface. (b) The muscles and tendons have been reflected proximally. The origins of the ECRB anteriorly and the EDC posteriorly are identifiable on the undersurface of the extensor origin. (c) Close-up view of the two tendons, which can be separated back to the origins. The underlying lateral collateral ligament (probe) should be noted. (d) By reflecting the EDC posteriorly, the tendinous origin of the ECRB is isolated. (e) The EDC has been removed allowing better visualization of the bony ECRB origin on the humerus. (f) The ECRB footprint has been drawn and measured with evaluation of the tendons from the humerus [2]

2. Pathophysiology and pathogenesis
    (a) Relative absence of classic inflammatory changes/inflammatory cell types within the involved tissues
    (b) Histologically, mixed inflammatory and reactive tissue, described as angio-fibroblastic hyperplasia [4]
    (c) Tendinopathy or epicondylopathy rather than true tendonitis [5, 6]

    (d) Pathogenesis is multifactorial:
- Repetitive over use
- Microtears in the proximal muscle tendon junction
- Incomplete or failed healing/remodeling response

3. History
   (a) Patients between 40 and 60 years of age
   (b) Present with repetitive overuse, direct blunt trauma, or traction injury to arm
   (c) Sharp/burning pain at lateral or medial epicondyle
   (d) Aggravated by gripping, wrist or finger extension (lateral epicondylitis), or wrist flexion and pronation (medial epicondylitis)
   (e) Aching pain at night/worse in AM with initiation off activities (start-up pain)

4. Physical exam
   (a) Absence of swelling, bruising, redness, and warmth
   (b) Motion limited only by pain
   (c) Stability normal
   (d) Sensory normal
   (e) Tenderness/provocative tests
   - Lateral epicondylitis
     - Five millimeters distal to the lateral epicondyle, over the radial head (ECRB origin)
     - Provocative maneuvers: gripping, active or resisted wrist, or finger extension
   - Medial epicondylitis
     - Five millimeters distal to the medial epicondyle
     - Provocative maneuvers: gripping, active or resisted wrist flexion, or pronation

5. Diagnostic studies
   (a) X-rays: typically normal, soft tissue calcifications may be seen adjacent to the epicondyle
   (b) Additional imaging only if symptoms associated with significant trauma, or after failure of conservative treatment (time, rest, medications, and therapy)
   - MRI: high signal intensity on T2 imaging sequences, in the region of the ECRB (lateral epicondylitis) or the common flexor/pronator origin (medial epicondylitis) (Fig. 18.2)
     - Good for identifying concomitant pathology
     - Only 50–69% of patients presenting with chronic epicondylitis have increased signal on T2 imaging [7]
     - Increased signal intensity in the ECRB is present in 11% of the general population with no symptoms [8]
   - High frequency musculoskeletal ultrasound (MSKUS): disruption of the normal hyperechoic tendon architecture, with swollen tendon and hypoechoic areas representing tendon detachment and/or disorganized collagen matrix (Fig. 18.3)
     - Good for both static and dynamic exam of tendon architecture

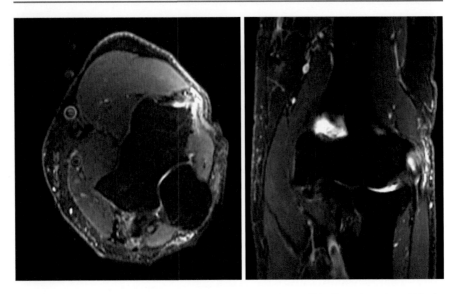

**Fig. 18.2** Axial and coronal MRI of patient with lateral epicondylitis. Hyperintensity within the ECRB origin at the lateral epicondyle. Note the deeper, intact LUCL complex

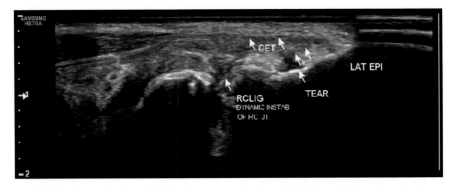

**Fig. 18.3** MSKUS image of lateral elbow in patient with lateral epicondylitis. *CET* common extensor tendon, *RCLIG* radial collateral ligament complex, *LatEpi* lateral epicondyle. Note the hypoechoic dark triangular signal at the site of ECRB tendinopathic changes (TEAR)

- Imaging modality of choice if considering nonsurgical procedural interventions (autologous blood patch, platelet-rich plasma, percutaneous tenotomy, etc.) [9]
6. Differential diagnosis
    (a) Table 18.1.
7. Treatment options
    (a) Rarely require surgery, 80% of patients reporting resolution of symptoms within 1 year of first onset [10]
    (b) Ten percent or less require surgery [11–13]

**Table 18.1**   Differential diagnosis for patients presenting with lateral or medial elbow pain

| Differential diagnosis for epicondylitis | |
| --- | --- |
| Lateral epicondylitis | Medial epicondylitis |
| Lateral/radial collateral ligament injury | Ulnar collateral ligament injury |
| Capitellar OCD | Ulnar neuritis |
| Radial tunnel syndrome | |
| Radiocapitellar plica | |

(c) Initial treatment
- Education and management of expectations
  - Self-limiting nature of diagnosis
  - Ok to work through it
  - Unlikely to need surgery
- NSAIDS
- Physical therapy
  - Early rest and stretching (elbow/wrist/fingers)
  - Concentric strengthening
  - Eccentric strengthening
  - Clinically improved pain score and function as compared with placebo [14]
- Bracing
  - Proximal forearm bracing (counterforce brace)

    Mechanism of action: dissipation of the forces from the muscle distally and/or reducing maximal contractile force generation from the muscle [15]

    Reduced pain severity at 2 weeks and reduced frequency of pain between 6 and 12 weeks with bracing [16]
  - Wrist bracing

    Cock-up for lateral epicondylitis

    Neutral brace for medial epicondylitis

(d) Nonsurgical procedural interventions
- Extracorporeal shock wave therapy (ECSW)
  - Mechanisms of action: stimulates production of growth factors, neovessel formation, and suppression of nociceptors
  - VAS scores and grip strength improved at 12 weeks [17]
  - Meta-analysis shows better overall safety and efficacy versus corticosteroid injection [18]
- Corticosteroid injection (CSI)
  - Current use of corticosteroids in refractory epicondylitis appears contraindicated
  - Provides reduce pain at 2–3 months, but statistically worse outcomes are seen at greater than 2–12 months [19]
- Prolotherapy
  - Injection of a sclerosing injectable solution, most often hypertonic dextrose (10–30%) in local anesthetic

- Mechanism of action: enhancement of the inflammatory response [20] with subsequent proliferation and remodeling
- Slightly greater efficacy over a longer period compared with CSI [21]
- Autologous blood injection (AB)
  - Improve pain and functional outcome scores when compared with corticosteroid injections [22]
  - Efficacy similar to extracorporeal shock wave
- Percutaneous tenotomy
  - Typically performed with an 18–20 gauge needle, under ultrasound guidance
  - Followed by a course of physical or hand therapy
    Eighty percent reports good/excellent outcome [23]
- Platelet-rich plasma (PRP)
  - Platelet concentration 4–6 times greater than whole blood
  - Multiple methods of preparation resulting in either leukocyte-rich (LR) or leukocyte-poor (LP) concentrate
    Insufficient data to develop firm clinical guidelines regarding optimal leukocyte concentration [24]
    Better 1 and 2 year outcomes (VAS, grip strength, and DASH) than corticosteroids or bupivacaine [25–27]
    Followed by course of physical therapy (Table 18.2)
- Stem cell therapy
  - Multiple preparations and sources of stem cell harvest, without sufficient data to support any one technique
  - Small heterogeneous studies show improved imaging findings, VAS, grip strength, quick DASH [28]

(e) Surgical treatment
- Open debridement lateral epicondylitis
  - First described by Nirschl and Pettrone in 1979 [13]
  - The patient is positioned supine, non-sterile tourniquet
  - Four-centimeter skin incision from the lateral epicondyle extended over capitellum and the midline of the radial head
  - The fascia is incised just proximal to the tip of the epicondyle in line with the EDC fibers of the superficial aponeurosis
  - Fascia is released proximally along the lateral supracondylar ridge to the muscular origin of the ECRL (L-shaped incision)
  - Dissection is carried down to bone, releasing EDC/ECRB origin from the lateral epicondyle (Fig. 18.4)
  - Involved pathologic tissue (angiofibroblastic hyperplasia) has a gray, soft, disorganized appearance
  - All pathologic tissue is sharply excised, often resulting in complete removal of the ECRB origin, down to and including capsulectomy
  - Resection distally should not go below the tip of the epicondyle in order to preserve the lateral ligament complex

**Table 18.2** Phases of tissue response following PRP injection and associated progression of rehabilitation time line

| Phase of tendon healing/goal | Duration | Activity level and restrictions | Rehabilitation progression |
|---|---|---|---|
| Inflammatory/ protective beginning of repair phase/early loading | Three days acute, protective up to 14 days, symptom dependent Early repair begins at 4 days, progression to weight bearing variable | – Maybe nonweight bearing if in pain<br>– Avoid NSAIDS<br>– Limited ice<br>– Avoid weights/ resistance training<br>– Static stretching | – Gentle preservation of range of motion may begin<br>– Consider brace for support<br>– Relative rest<br>– Consider pain medication<br>– Ok for aerobic exercise if treated tendon unloaded |
| Repair phase/early strengthening | 2–6 weeks | – Progress to full weight bearing<br>– Static through dynamic stretching progression/ PNF<br>– Avoid eccentrics | – Progress activity<br>– Soft tissue mobilization<br>– Isometric, isotonic exercise<br>– Dumbbells, bands, cables |
| Remodeling phase/ collagen maturation | 6–12 weeks | – Introduction of eccentrics<br>– No restrictions | – Eccentric exercise, if intolerant—heavy isometrics<br>– Power/plyometric training<br>– Progress to sport specific drills |
| Return to sport/ desired activities | Weeks 12 + | – None<br>– Consider re-treating or other modalities at 6 months if not at desired functional level | – Sport conditioning and injury prevention |

**Fig. 18.4** Interoperative photograph showing elevation of CEO (left). Beneath this is the light-gray mucinoid pathologic tissue that is completely excised [29]

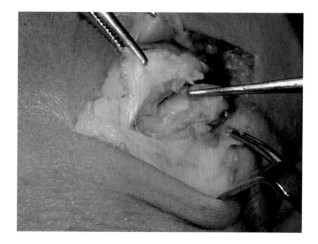

- Decortication of the exposed lateral supracondylar ridge or a more limited abrading of the bone at the ECRB footprint can be performed
- Closure should anatomically repair the superficial muscular fascia of the EDC; complete closure of the deeper defect created by pathologic tissue resection is not required
- Patient is placed into a splint for 1 week, followed by splint removal and initiation of gentle active motion
- Arthroscopic debridement lateral epicondylitis
  - The first arthroscopic debridement of lateral epicondylitis outside of a cadaveric model was reported by Baker et al. in 2000 [30]
  - Lateral decubitus position with a Western arm holder and a tourniquet placed proximally on the upper arm
  - Joint is distended with 20 mL of NS injected through the lateral soft spot
  - Proximal anteromedial portal is established first, 2 cm proximal to the medial epicondyle and 1 cm anterior to the medial intermuscular septum
  - The lateral capsule is visualized, and the proximal anterolateral portal (used for ECRB debridement) is established by an outside to inside technique using a spinal needle (Fig. 18.5)

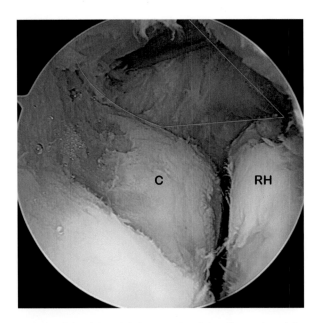

**Fig. 18.5** Arthroscopic view of lateral joint capsule of the elbow, viewed from the proximal anteromedial portal in a patient with concomitant elbow arthritis and chronic lateral epicondylitis. Joint debridement and osteophyte removal has been completed, and ECRB debridement is about to be undertaken. Shaver is coming through the lateral capsule in the area of the common extensor origin. Capsulectomy and ECRB debridement will continue within the area defined by the blue lines, staying above the equator of the radiocapitellar joint to preserve the LUCL. *C* capitellum, *RH* radial head. (Copyright Jesse McCarron, MD)

- A 3.5 mm shaver is inserted through the lateral capsule, and diagnostic arthroscopy is performed
- Debridement of the lateral joint capsule and ECRB is performed staying strictly superior to a line defined by the lateral epicondyle and the equator of the radial head to prevent iatrogenic lateral collateral ligament complex injury [31]
- Resect posteriorly and laterally to the footprint of the ECRB on the bone of the lateral condyle. The upper border of the resection defined by muscular origin of ECRL
- Disorganized, gray, fibrotic tissue resected until shiny, white, tendon fibers are remaining
- Bone at the ECRB footprint should be abraded with an aggressive shaver or bur
- Capsular closure can be performed after completion of debridement, but is not considered necessary
- Splinted for 1 week before return to clinic for splint removal and initiation of motion
- Open debridement medial epicondylitis
  - Positioned supine with the arm abducted and externally rotated on an arm board and a non-sterile tourniquet
  - Five-centimeter curved incision is approximately 1 cm proximal and posterior to the medial epicondyle and extended distally
  - Dissection is carried down to the medial epicondyle and the common flexor origin
  - Fascia is incised longitudinally in line with its fibers starting at the medial epicondyle
  - A T-shaped incision of fascia can be made off of the medial supracondylar ridge to allow visualization of the deeper pathologic tissue
  - Pathologic tissue having a mucinoid, gray appearance is excised, leaving all normal appearing tendon tissue
  - The exposed bone at the medial epicondyle and common origin footprint is rongeured or drilled to promote bleeding at the debridement site
  - Superficial fascia is anatomically closed with absorbable suture, but closure of the deeper defect does not need to be performed
  - Some authors advocated suture anchor at the site of debridement to mitigate risks of postoperative weakness with resisted pronation [32]
  - Standard skin closure and the arm are splinted for 1 week before removal and initiation of gentle active range of motion
- Arthroscopic debridement medial epicondylitis
  - The flexor/pronator origin is on average 20.8 mm (range 14.4–25.1 mm) from the ulnar nerve and 8.3 mm (range 5.9–10.4 mm) from the medial collateral ligament (MCL) [33]
  - Positioning and draping as standard for elbow arthroscopy
  - Joint insufflation and standard proximal anteromedial placement followed by proximal anterolateral portal (see Arthroscopic Debridement of Lateral Epicondylitis)

- – Debridement of pathologic tissue performed via the proximal antero-medial portal using a shaver and RF thermal ablation device
  - – Debridement of the exposed bone on the medial condyle [34]
- • Postsurgical rehabilitation
  - – Similar for all surgical techniques
  - – Splint to rest the elbow/wrist/hand for 1 week
  - – Splint removal and initiation of gentle active motion
  - – Once full active motion is restored, gradual grip strengthening is encouraged
  - – Six weeks resistance exercises for the elbow and wrist:
    - Concentric strengthening
    - Progression to eccentric strengthening
  - – After 12 weeks, return to sports or heavy activity can begin once residual symptoms have dissipated
- • Surgical outcomes
  - – Open and arthroscopic procedures have equivalent efficacy [35–37]
  - – Good to excellent outcomes reported in 70–94% of patients [32, 38–40]
  - – Durable benefits with improved outcomes at mid- and long-term follow-up when compared with first year after surgery [29, 40, 41]
  - – A significant percentage of patients report some degree of residual pain [35, 37, 38, 40–43]
- • Surgical complications
  - – Residual pain is typically reported as the primary complication of surgical treatment
    - Etiology is variable [44]
      - Incorrect/incomplete preoperative diagnoses
        - Concomitant PIN entrapment/radial tunnel syndrome (Fig. 18.6)
        - Unrecognized posterolateral rotatory instability (PLRI) in lateral epicondylitis
        - Incomplete surgical debridement
        - Iatrogenic injuries—over aggressive resection leading to compromise of the lateral ligament complex

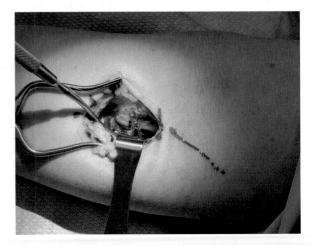

**Fig. 18.6** Vascular leash compressing the radial nerve in the proximal forearm (radial tunnel syndrome) in patient who presented with diagnosis of lateral epicondylitis (Copyright Jesse McCarron, MD)

# References

1. Greenbaum BI, Vangsness J, Tibone CT, Atkinson J, R. Extensor carpi radialis brevis. An anatomical analysis of its origin. J Bone Jt Surg Br. 1999;5(81):926–9.
2. Cohen MS, Romeo AA, Hennigan SP, Gordon M. Lateral epicondylitis: anatomic relationships of the extensor tendon origins and implications for arthroscopic treatment. J Shoulder Elb Surg. 2008;17(6):954–60. https://doi.org/10.1016/j.jse.2008.02.021.
3. Bernholt DL, Rosenberg SI, Brady AW, Storaci HW, Viola RW, Hackett TR. Quantitative and qualitative analyses of the lateral ligamentous complex and extensor tendon origins of the elbow: an anatomic study. Orthop J Sports Med. 2020;8(10):1–7. https://doi.org/10.1177/2325967120961373.
4. Kraushaar BS, Nirschl RP. Tendinosis of the elbow (tennis elbow): clinical features and findings of histological, immunohistochemical, and electron microscopy studies. J Bone Jt Surg Ser A. 1999;81(2):259–78. https://doi.org/10.2106/00004623-199902000-00014.
5. Abat F, Alfredson H, Cucchiarini M, Madry H, Marmotti A, Mouton C, Oliveira JM, et al. Current trends in tendinopathy: consensus of the ESSKA basic science committee. Part I: biology, biomechanics, anatomy and an exercise-based approach. J Exp Orthop. 2017;4(1):18.
6. Khan KM, Cook JL, Kannus P, Maffulli N, B. S. Time to abandon the "tendinitis" myth: painful, overuse tendon conditions have a non-inflammatory pathology. BMJ. 2002;324:626.
7. Aoki M, Wada T, Isogai S, Kanaya K, Aiki H, Yamashita T. Magnetic resonance imaging findings of refractory tennis elbows and their relationship to surgical treatment. J Shoulder Elb Surg. 2005;14(2):172–7. https://doi.org/10.1016/j.jse.2004.07.011.
8. van Leeuwen WF, Janssen SJ, Ring D, Chen N. Incidental magnetic resonance imaging signal changes in the extensor carpi radialis brevis origin are more common with age. J Shoulder Elb Surg. 2016;25(7):1175–81. https://doi.org/10.1016/j.jse.2016.01.033.
9. Jacobson J. Fundamentals of musculoskeletal ultrasound. Amsterdam: Elsevier Health Sciences; 2017.
10. Calfee R, Patel A, DaSilva M, Akelman E. Management of lateral epicondylitis: current concepts. J Am Acad Orthop Surg. 2008;16(1):19–29. https://doi.org/10.1016/j.otsr.2019.09.004.
11. Binder A, Hazleman B. Lateral humeral epicondylitis—a study of natural history and the effect of conservative therapy. Br J Rheumatol. 1983;22(2):73–6.
12. Coonrad R, Hooper W. Tennis elbow: its course, natural history, conservative and surgical management. J Bone Jt Surg Am. 1973;55(6):1177–82.
13. Nirschl R, Pettrone F. Tennis elbow: the surgical treatment of lateral epicondylitis. J Bone Jt Surg Am. 1979a;61:832–9.
14. Kim YJ, Wood SM, Yoon AP, Howard JC, Yang LY, Chung KC. Efficacy of nonoperative treatments for lateral epicondylitis: a systematic review and meta-analysis. Plast Reconstr Surg. 2021;147(1):112–25. https://doi.org/10.1097/PRS.0000000000007440.
15. Nirschl RP, Ashman ES. Elbow tendinopathy: tennis elbow. Clin Sports Med. 2003;22(4):813–36. https://doi.org/10.1016/S0278-5919(03)00051-6.
16. Kroslak M, Pirapakaran K, Murrell GAC. Counterforce bracing of lateral epicondylitis: a prospective, randomized, double-blinded, placebo-controlled clinical trial. J Shoulder Elb Surg. 2019;28(2):288–95. https://doi.org/10.1016/j.jse.2018.10.002.
17. Beyazal MS, Devrimsel G. Comparison of the effectiveness of local corticosteroid injection and extracorporeal shock wave therapy in patients with lateral epicondylitis. J Phys Ther Sci. 2015;27(12):3755–8. https://doi.org/10.1589/jpts.27.3755.
18. Yao G, Chen J, Duan Y, Chen X. Efficacy of extracorporeal shock wave therapy for lateral epicondylitis: a systematic review and meta-analysis. Biomed Res Int. 2020;2020:2064781. https://doi.org/10.1155/2020/2064781.
19. Smidt N, Van Der Windt DAWM, Assendelft WJJ, Devillé WLJM, Korthals-de Bos IBC, Bouter LM. Corticosteroid injections, physiotherapy, or a wait-and-see policy for lateral epicondylitis: a randomised controlled trial. Lancet. 2002;359(9307):657–62. https://doi.org/10.1016/S0140-6736(02)07811-X.
20. Dwivedi S, Sobel AD, DaSilva MF, Akelman E. Utility of prolotherapy for upper extremity pathology. J Hand Surg. 2019;44(3):236–9. https://doi.org/10.1016/j.jhsa.2018.05.021.

21. Bayat M, Raeissadat SA, Babaki MM, Rahimi-Dehgolan S. Is dextrose prolotherapy superior to corticosteroid injection in patients with chronic lateral epicondylitis? A randomized clinical trial. Orthop Res Rev. 2019;11:167. https://doi.org/10.2147/ORR.S218698.

22. Ozturan KE, Yucel I, Cakici H, Guven M, Sungur I. Autologous blood and corticosteroid injection and extracoporeal shock wave therapy in the treatment of lateral epicondylitis. Orthopedics. 2010;33(2):84–91. https://doi.org/10.3928/01477447-20100104-9.

23. McShane JM, Nazarian LN, Harwood MI. Sonographically guided percutaneous needle tenotomy for treatment of common extensor tendinosis in the elbow. J Ultrasound Med. 2006;25(10):1281. https://doi.org/10.7863/jum.2006.25.10.1281.

24. Fitzpatrick J, Bulsara MK, McCrory PR, Richardson MD, Zheng MH. Analysis of platelet-rich plasma extraction: variations in platelet and blood components between 4 common commercial kits. Orthop J Sports Med. 2017;5(1):2325967116675272. https://doi.org/10.1177/2325967116675272.

25. Behera P, Dhillon M, Aggarwal S, Marwaha N, Prakash M. Leukocyte-poor platelet-rich plasma versus bupivacaine for recalcitrant lateral epicondylar tendinopathy. J Orthop Surg. 2015;23(1):6–10. https://doi.org/10.1177/230949901502300102.

26. Gosens T, Peerbooms JC, Van Laar W, Den Oudsten BL. Ongoing positive effect of platelet-rich plasma versus corticosteroid injection in lateral epicondylitis: a double-blind randomized controlled trial with 2-year follow-up. Am J Sports Med. 2011;39(6):1200–8. https://doi.org/10.1177/0363546510397173.

27. Peerbooms JC, Sluimer J, Bruijn DJ, Gosens T. Positive effect of an autologous platelet concentrate in lateral epicondylitis in a double-blind randomized controlled trial: platelet-rich plasma versus corticosteroid injection with a 1-year follow-up. Am J Sports Med. 2010;38(2):255–62. https://doi.org/10.1177/0363546509355445.

28. Dakkak A, Krill ML, Fogarty A, Krill MK. Stem cell therapy for the management of lateral elbow tendinopathy: a systematic literature review. Sci Sports. 2021;36(3):181–92. https://doi.org/10.1016/j.scispo.2020.07.005.

29. Coleman B, Quinlan JF, Matheson JA. Surgical treatment for lateral epicondylitis: a long-term follow-up of results. J Shoulder Elb Surg. 2010;19(3):363–7. https://doi.org/10.1016/j.jse.2009.09.008.

30. Baker CL, Murphy KP, Gottlob CA, Curd DT. Arthroscopic classification and treatment of lateral epicondylitis: two-year clinical results. J Shoulder Elb Surg. 2000;9(6):475–82. https://doi.org/10.1067/mse.2000.108533.

31. Smith AM, Castle JA, Ruch DS. Arthroscopic resection of the common extensor origin: anatomic considerations. J Shoulder Elb Surg. 2003;12(4):375–9. https://doi.org/10.1016/S1058-2746(02)86823-9.

32. Vinod AV, Ross G. An effective approach to diagnosis and surgical repair of refractory medial epicondylitis. J Shoulder Elb Surg. 2015;24(8):1172–7. https://doi.org/10.1016/j.jse.2015.03.017.

33. Zonno A, Manuel J, Merrell G, Ramos P, Akelman E, DaSilva M. Arthroscopic technique for medial epicondylitis: technique and safety analysis. Arthroscopy. 2010;26:610–6.

34. do Nascimento AT, Claudio GK. Arthroscopic surgical treatment of medial epicondylitis. J Shoulder Elb Surg. 2017;26(12):2232–5. https://doi.org/10.1016/j.jse.2017.08.019.

35. Kwon BC, Kim JY, Park KT. The Nirschl procedure versus arthroscopic extensor carpi radialis brevis débridement for lateral epicondylitis. J Shoulder Elb Surg. 2017;26(1):118–24. https://doi.org/10.1016/j.jse.2016.09.022.

36. MacDonald PB, Clark T, McRae S, Leiter J, Dubberley J. Arthroscopic vs. open lateral release for the treatment of lateral epicondylitis: a prospective randomized controlled trial. J Shoulder Elb Surg. 2016;25(10):e324. https://doi.org/10.1016/j.jse.2016.07.048.

37. Szabo SJ, Savoie FH, Field LD, Ramsey JR, Hosemann CD. Tendinosis of the extensor carpi radialis brevis: an evaluation of three methods of operative treatment. J Shoulder Elb Surg. 2006;15(6):721–7. https://doi.org/10.1016/j.jse.2006.01.017.

38. Das D, Maffulli N. Surgical management of tennis elbow. J Sports Med Phys Fitn. 2002;42:190–7.

39. Han SH, Lee JK, Kim HJ, Lee SH, Kim JW, Kim TS. The result of surgical treatment of medial epicondylitis: analysis with more than a 5-year follow-up. J Shoulder Elb Surg. 2016;25(10):1704–9. https://doi.org/10.1016/j.jse.2016.05.010.
40. Verhaar JA. Tennis elbow. Anatomical, epidemiological and therapeutic aspects. Int Orthop. 1994;18(5):263–7. https://doi.org/10.1007/BF00180221.
41. Dunn J, Kim J, Davis L, Nirschl R. Ten- to 14-year follow-up of the Nirschl surgical technique for lateral epicondylitis. Am J Sports Med. 2008;36(2):261–6.
42. Goldberg E, Abraham E, Siegel I. The surgical treatment of chronic lateral humeral epicondylitis by common extensor release. Clin Orthop Relat Res. 1988;233:208–12.
43. Lattermann C, Romeo AA, Anbari A, Meininger AK, McCarty LP, Cole BJ, Cohen MS. Arthroscopic debridement of the extensor carpi radialis brevis for recalcitrant lateral epicondylitis. J Shoulder Elb Surg. 2010;19(5):651–6. https://doi.org/10.1016/j.jse.2010.02.008.
44. Morrey BF. Reoperation for failed surgical treatment of refractory lateral epicondylitis. J Shoulder Elb Surg. 1992;1(1):47–55. https://doi.org/10.1016/S1058-2746(09)80016-5.

# Elbow Dislocation

**19**

Gary F. Updegrove and April D. Armstrong

## Introduction

Simple elbow dislocation is defined as a dislocation of the elbow joint without associated fracture or osseous injury. This is in contrast to complex elbow dislocations in which a fracture is present. Most simple elbow dislocations can be treated with closed reduction and rehabilitation.

1. History
    (a) The elbow is a highly constrained and inherently stable joint [1]
        • Stability is provided by osseous congruence and capsuloligamentous static stabilizers in addition to dynamic muscular stabilizers. The static stabilizers have been described as analogous to a fortress [2, 3] (Fig. 19.1)
        • Primary static stabilizers
            – Ulnohumeral articulation
            – Lateral collateral ligament (LCL) complex
            – Anterior bundle of medial collateral ligament (MCL)
        • Secondary static stabilizers
            – Radiocapitellar articulation
            – Common extensor tendon
            – Common flexor–pronator tendon
        • Dynamic stabilizers
            – Muscles that cross the elbow joint, such as the anconeus, biceps, triceps, and brachialis, provide compressive force and dynamic stability

G. F. Updegrove (✉) · A. D. Armstrong
Department of Orthopaedics and Rehabilitation, Penn State Milton S. Hershey Medical Center, Bone and Joint Institute, Hershey, PA, USA
e-mail: gupdegrove@pennstatehealth.psu.edu; aarmstrong@pennstatehealth.psu.edu

© The Author(s), under exclusive license to Springer Nature Switzerland AG 2022
C. M. Chebli, A. M. Murthi (eds.), *The Resident's Guide to Shoulder and Elbow Surgery*, https://doi.org/10.1007/978-3-031-12255-2_19

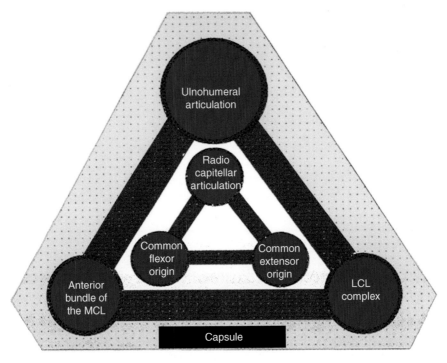

**Fig. 19.1** Algorithm for nonsurgical and surgical treatment of simple elbow dislocation. *LCL* lateral collateral ligament, *MCL* medial collateral ligament. Reprinted with permission from Acute and Recurrent Elbow Instability, in AAOS Comprehensive Orthopaedic Review 3, 2019, American Academy of Orthopaedic Surgeons [3]

(b) Mechanism of injury
- Simple elbow dislocation is most commonly associated with a fall on an outstretched arm
- Posterolateral dislocations (most common)
  – Valgus and axial loading with supination of the forearm
- Posteromedial
  – Varus and axial loading with supination of the forearm
- Posterior
  – Direct posterior force or combination of forces
- In simple elbow dislocation, it is generally accepted that the lateral collateral ligament complex is disrupted. The medial collateral ligament may also be disrupted. The soft tissue injury occurs in a progressive pattern from the lateral side of the elbow, continuing with disruption of the anterior and posterior capsule toward the medial side of the elbow, ultimately with disruption of the medial collateral ligament [2].

2. Physical exam
   (a) Inspection/palpation
      - Inspect skin for open wounds or bruising
      - Evaluate for compartment syndrome. Palpate for compression and firmness in the forearm and assess for pain on passive stretch of the wrist, hand, or fingers
   (b) Neurologic
      - Assess sensory and motor function in radial, median, and ulnar distributions
   (c) Vascular
      - Assessed distal vascular function with radial pulse and/or capillary refill. In rare cases, angiography can be utilized to evaluate for vascular compromise
3. Imaging
   (a) X-rays
      - Anteroposterior and lateral radiographs should be obtained both before and after reduction
      - Radiographs are used to evaluate for direction of dislocation and for fracture or osseous injury
      - Oblique views may be useful at times to evaluate for fracture
      - Postreduction radiographs are obtained weekly during the first 3 weeks to monitor for recurrence of instability and congruency of the joint
   (b) CT scan
      - CT scan may be indicated to provide further osseous detail to evaluate for fracture. CT scan should be attained after reduction and could also be useful to evaluate for congruency of the joint
      - Postreduction CT scan is also useful to evaluate for incarcerated bony fragments
   (c) MRI
      - MRI is not indicated for all simple elbow dislocations despite known or suspected ligamentous injury. It may be of benefit post reduction to classify the extent of soft tissue injury
      - MRI may be utilized if post reduction radiographs do not demonstrate a congruent joint. An osteocartilaginous incarcerated fragment may be better appreciated with MRI study
   (d) Ultrasound
      - Ultrasound may also be used to evaluate for soft tissue injury. This provides the added benefit of the ability to perform a dynamic examination
4. Treatment algorithm based on diagnosis
   (a) Nonoperative treatment
      - For a simple elbow dislocation, closed reduction under appropriate sedation should be attempted. Irreducible elbows are indicated for open

reduction. Those elbows that are able to be reduced should be evaluated for stability while the patient is sedated

- Closed reduction technique
  - Well-sedated patient. Provide inline traction. Correct medial and lateral displacement with gentle manipulation. Supinate the forearm and provide valgus stress to recreate the deformity. Clear the coronoid under the trochlea as the elbow is flexed. Apply pressure to the tip of the olecranon to aid reduction. Flex the elbow while providing varus stress and pronation to complete reduction
  - A concentric joint reduction must be achieved to consider close reduction successful
  - Evaluate for stability of the elbow postreduction. Goal is for stable joint through an arc of motion from 60° to full flexion
- Postreduction
  - Evaluate for joint congruency. If ulnohumeral joint is not congruent, consider possibility of tissue interposition (bone, cartilage, muscle, or nerve)
  - Reassessed neurovascular exam post reduction
  - Consider change of forearm rotation if joint remains incongruent
    Forearm pronation most often renders elbow joint stable in posterolateral elbow dislocation; however, if the medial collateral ligament is torn in addition to the lateral collateral ligament complex, then forearm pronation may cause medial joint gapping. Placing the forearm in neutral is recommended if both medial and lateral ligaments are torn
    Forearm supination most often renders elbow joint stable in the setting of an isolated incompetent medial collateral ligament
- Consider advanced imaging studies such as CT scan or MRI if joint incongruency remains
- A "drop sign" is common after simple elbow dislocation [4]. This is seen as an increase of the ulnohumeral distance on postreduction lateral radiographs. It most often corrects and is likely related to muscle contraction. If this persists past 3 weeks, it is concerning as this may be a warning sign to the presence of instability

(b) Operative treatment

- Though most simple elbow dislocations can be treated nonoperatively, surgical management is indicated in the setting of an irreducible simple elbow dislocation and a reducible elbow with continued instability (Fig. 19.2) [3]
- Surgical options
  - Surgical stabilization is most often performed in a stepwise fashion [5]
    The goal is to achieve concentric reduction with joint stability throughout an arc of motion of 60° to full flexion
    When assessing for stability during operative management, the goal is to achieve stable concentric reduction from 60° to full flexion

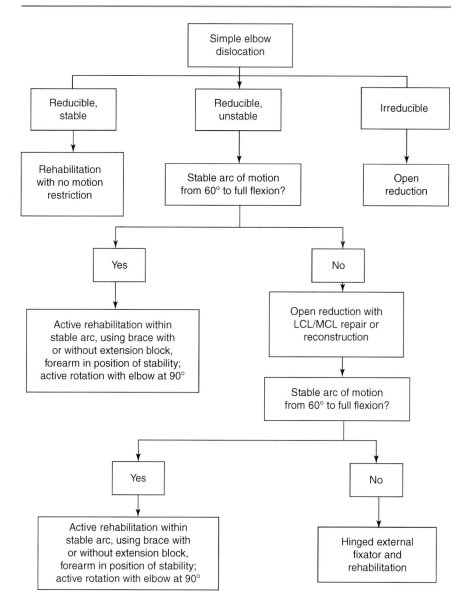

**Fig. 19.2** Illustration demonstrates how the static constraints in the elbow are analogous to the defenses of a fortress. The primary static constraints to elbow instability are the ulnohumeral articulation, the anterior bundle of the medial collateral ligament (MCL), and the lateral collateral ligament (LCL) complex, including the lateral ulnar collateral ligament. The secondary constraints include the capsule, the radiocapitellar articulation, and the common flexor and extensor tendon origins. [(Adapted with permission from the Mayo Foundation for Medical Education and Research, Rochester, MN. All rights reserved.) Reprinted with permission from Acute and Recurrent Elbow Instability, in AAOS Comprehensive Orthopaedic Review 3, 2019, American Academy of Orthopaedic Surgeons [3]]

- The elbow joint is open reduced prior to proceeding with soft tissue repair for stabilization

   It is important to perform an arthrotomy of the joint capsule. This allows for inspection and irrigation of the joint in order to remove any interposed bone or tissue

- Repair, or in rare cases reconstruction, of the lateral ulnar collateral ligament is next performed. The elbow is again reevaluated for stability through the arc of motion

   The lateral collateral ligament complex consists of the lateral ulnar collateral ligament, the annular ligament, the radial collateral ligament, and the accessory collateral ligament

   The lateral ulnar collateral ligament is the primary stabilizer to posterior lateral rotatory instability. The origin of the ligament is just below the lateral epicondyle at the isometric axis of rotation point of the lateral condyle. The ligament inserts on the crista supinatoris of the ulna

   The lateral ulnar collateral ligament is most often avulsed from the origin at the distal humerus. It may also be avulsed from the crista supinatoris in rare cases

   It is important to repair the lateral ulnar collateral ligament to the anatomic origin at the isometric point of the lateral condyle, either through bone tunnels or with anchor fixation

   The common extensor tendon should also be repaired with the ligament to provide additional stability

- If the elbow remains unstable, repair, and in rare cases reconstruction, of the ulnar collateral ligament is performed. The elbow is again assessed for instability

   The medial collateral ligament complex consists of the anterior bundle, the posterior bundle, and the transverse ligament. The anterior bundle is the primary stabilizer to valgus stress. It is often referred to as the ulnar collateral ligament

   The anterior bundle originates from the anteroinferior surface of the medial epicondyle and inserts onto the sublime tubercle at the anteromedial coronoid process

   Similar to the LCL, the MCL is most often avulsed from the origin site at the medial epicondyle. However, avulsion from the sublime tubercle or intrasubstance tear is not uncommon

   The ligament should be repaired with either bone tunnels or suture anchors at the isometric point on the humerus at the anteroinferior portion of the medial epicondyle or at the sublime tubercle on the ulna. Repair of intrasubstance tearing is challenging, and in these cases, ligament reconstruction versus common flexor tendon repair in isolation should be considered

- If medial and lateral ligamentous repair or reconstruction does not provide stability of the elbow, external fixation is utilized. This is either with a static or hinged external fixation construct

  If a hinged external fixator is selected, it is important that the axis of the hinge is in line with the anatomic axis of the elbow joint [6]

- Surgical approaches:
  - A posterior midline skin incision can be used to approach both the medial and lateral elbow. Alternatively, exposure can begin with a lateral skin incision, with the use of a medial skin incision if necessary
  - Deep exposure to the lateral elbow is often through the Kocher interval between the anconeus and extensor carpi ulnaris. This provides direct exposure of the lateral collateral ligament

    In many cases, a traumatic disruption has created exposure through the common extensor tendon. If present, this window can be used to approach the lateral elbow joint

  - Medial exposure of the elbow is often performed between the ulnar and humeral heads of the flexor carpi ulnaris, through the floor the cubital tunnel. Alternatively, an exposure between flexor carpi ulnaris and flexor carpi radialis/palmaris longus may be utilized

    Similar to the lateral side, often a traumatic split in the flexor pronator mass may be visualized and utilized to provide direct exposure of the anterior bundle of the medial collateral ligament

(c) Rehabilitation

- After reduction or operative stabilization, the elbow is mobilized for 5–7 days at 90° of flexion in a position of stable forearm rotation. This will most often be neutral or pronation and very rarely will be stable in supination (isolated MCL injury) [7]
  - One scenario for stability in supination is in the setting of a robust lateral collateral ligament repair while the medial soft tissue injury is not surgically repaired
- At 1 week, active range of motion exercises are started. These are performed in the forearm rotation of elbow stability. Pronation and supination exercises are performed at 90° of elbow flexion only
- Performing elbow range of motion in supine position with arm overhead, referred to as gravity loaded rehabilitation, aids in providing stability. The patient should avoid abducted arm positions as this puts increased strain on the lateral collateral ligament [7]
- Extension is limited to 45° for 3 weeks. At that point, it is progressively advance with a goal of full arc of motion at 6–8 weeks
  - A hinged elbow brace can be utilized to guide progressive motion restriction. Ensure proper forearm rotation in the brace, as many available braces limit the forearm to neutral rotation
  - Thermoplastic splinting may also be helpful to provide stability of the elbow when not performing range of motion exercises

(d) Risks and complications
- Loss of elbow motion is the most common complication after simple elbow dislocation. This is primarily the loss of terminal extension
    - Early active range of motion exercises, most often performed in a supine position with the elbow extended overhead, may help decrease elbow stiffness. Shoulder abduction should be avoided during this rehabilitation to avoid stress on the lateral collateral ligament

        Static progressive splinting may be utilized to regain motion. It is typically started 6 weeks after injury when the elbow is less inflamed
    - Chondral and articular surface injuries may occur during the dislocation or during reduction. This may ultimately lead to posttraumatic degenerative arthritis
    - Heterotopic ossification may form around the elbow joint. Anteriorly, it may form between brachialis and the capsule. Posteriorly, it forms around the triceps and the capsule. Multiple reduction attempts may increase the risk of heterotopic ossification. Indomethacin and local radiation have been suggested by some to decrease the risk of heterotopic ossification
    - Neurovascular injury can occur during injury or reduction maneuver
    - Recurrent or chronic elbow instability after isolated simple elbow dislocation is rare. When present, it is often the result of bony, ligamentous, or combined injuries.

# References

1. Murthi AM, et al. The recurrent unstable elbow: diagnosis and treatment. J Bone Jt Surg Am. 2010;92(8):1794–804.
2. O'Driscoll SW, et al. The unstable elbow. J Bone Jt Surg. 2000;82(5):724–38.
3. Updegrove GF, Getz CL. Acute and recurrent elbow instability. In: Lieberman JR, editor. AAOS comprehensive orthopaedic review. 3rd ed. Rosemont: American Academy of Orthopaedic Surgeons; 2019. p. 824–31.
4. Coonrad RW, et al. The drop sign, a radiographic warning sign of elbow instability. J Shoulder Elbow Surg. 2005;14(3):312–7.
5. Sanchez-Sotelo J, Morrey BF, O'Driscoll SW. Ligamentous repair and reconstruction for posterolateral rotatory instability of the elbow. J Bone Jt Surg. 2005;87:54–61.
6. Tan V, et al. Hinged elbow external fixators: indications and uses. J Am Acad Orthop Surg. 2005;13:503–14.
7. Armstrong A. Simple elbow dislocation. Hand Clin. 2015;31(4):521–31.

# Lateral Ulnar Collateral Ligament Injury

# 20

Nicholas J. Sacksteder and Edward R. Hobgood

## History

*PLRI, first described by O'Driscoll et al. [1] in 1991, is the most common chronic symptomatic elbow instability* [2].

1. Patients most commonly present with a history of trauma.
   (a) Fall on an outstretched arm with axial load, supination, and valgus force.
   (b) Inquire for elbow dislocation.
2. Other causes include iatrogenic and chronic varus positioning.
   (a) Must inquire into patient's surgical history.
      • Open lateral epicondylitis treatment.
      • Open radial head fracture treatment.
      • Elbow arthroscopy.
   (b) Uncommon causes include multiple corticosteroid injections for lateral epicondylitis, crutch walking, and chronic varus deformity [3].
3. Patients frequently present with lateral elbow pain only.
   (a) Inquire as to positions and activities that cause pain.
   (b) Pain with resisted elbow extension, as when rising from a chair.
   (c) Mechanical symptoms such as clicking, catching, or sensations of instability.

N. J. Sacksteder (✉)
Jacksonville Orthopaedic Institute, Jacksonville, FL, USA

E. R. Hobgood
Mississippi Sports Medicine and Orthopaedic Center, Jackson, MS, USA
e-mail: rhetthobgood@msmoc.com

## Anatomy

*The elbow is a complex joint with unique ligamentous restraints and highly congruent osteology.*

1. The lateral elbow consists of four ligaments including the LUCL, radial collateral ligament, annular ligament, and the accessory lateral collateral ligament (see Fig. 20.1).
2. The LUCL functions to prevent varus and external rotation forces.
3. The LUCL's path from the lateral epicondyle to the crista supinatoris on the ulna crosses posterior to the radial head, providing a sling against posterior radial translation.
4. The origin of the LUCL is the lateral epicondyle and shows an average footprint of 26 mm².
5. The center of the LUCL origin is an average of 10.7 mm distal from the lateral epicondyle and 8.2 mm proximal to the capitellar articular margin.
6. The LUCL insertion averages 3.3 mm distal to the crista supinatoris with an average insertional footprint of 22.9 mm² (see Fig. 20.2) [4].

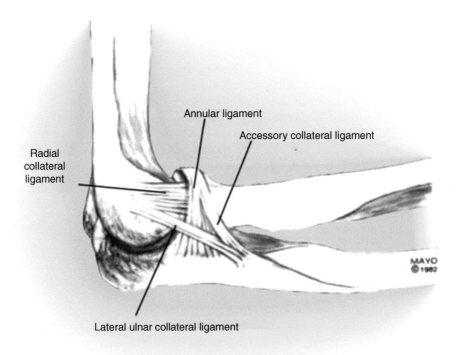

**Fig. 20.1** Lateral elbow ligamentous complex with lateral ulnar collateral ligament (LUCL), radial collateral ligament (RCL), annular ligament (AL), and accessory collateral ligament labeled. (Reprinted with permission by Morrey BF et al. The Elbow and It's Disorders. Elsevier. 2008)

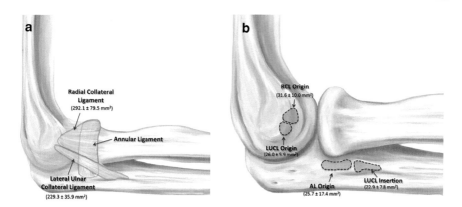

**Fig. 20.2** Diagram demonstrating (**a**) Origin and Insertion of LUCL (**b**) Origin and Insertion of RCL. (Reprinted with permission from Camp CL et al. The lateral collateral ligament complex of the elbow: quantitative anatomic analysis of the lateral ulnar collateral, radial collateral, and annular ligaments. JSES 2019; 2018.09.019)

7. Additional but less significant stability is provided by the radial collateral ligament, accessory collateral ligament, and anterior capsule; however, sectioning of the LUCL alone in cadavers is not enough to produce PLRI [5].

## Physical Exam

*The differential diagnosis for lateral elbow pain includes fracture, lateral epicondylitis, osteochondral defect, plica, radial tunnel syndrome, and PLRI.*

1. Exam should be carried out with the entire arm exposed to assess for alignment, ROM, previous incisions, and scars.
2. Except in a grossly unstable elbow or in cases of acute trauma, inspection will be normal in cases of LUCL injury.
3. Patient's active and passive ROM should be assessed for possible contracture.
   (a) Range of motion may cause catching and clicking.
4. Neurologic exam should be obtained and may demonstrate loss of dynamic stability, although there are no described neurologic deficit patterns specific to LUCL injury.
5. Deep palpation at the LUCL may elicit pain.
6. Specific exam maneuvers for PLRI include assessment for varus instability throughout a range of motion, the lateral pivot shift test, and the chair rise test.
   (a) In the lateral pivot shift test of the elbow, the patient is positioned supine on the exam table with the affected arm overhead. The forearm is fully supinated with the elbow and shoulder flexed to 90°. A valgus and axial stress is applied while moving the elbow from 90° to extension.

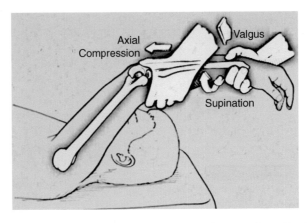

**Fig. 20.3** The lateral pivot shift test. The patient is positioned supine with the elbow fully extended by the examiner. Supination, valgus, and axial load are applied to the extremity as the arm is moved from an extended to flexed position. (Reprinted with permission from Camp CL, Smith J, O'Driscoll SW. Posterolateral Rotatory Instability of the Elbow: Part II. Supplementary Examination and Dynamic Imaging Techniques. Arthroscopy Techniques 2017; 2016.10.012)

- In a relaxed patient, the radial head will sublux at around 30° of elbow flexion but reduce with pronation of elbow and flexion due to increasing triceps tension (see Fig. 20.3).
- The subluxation event is often subtle, whereas the reduction of the radial head is more readily evident.
- This test is also considered positive if the patient exhibits apprehension.
- The sensitivity of the elbow lateral pivot shift is 100% in anesthetized patients but 38% in awake patients [6].

(b) More sensitive in a clinic setting is the chair raise test.
- In this test, the patient is asked to raise themselves from sitting to standing using the arms of their chair.
- This test is considered positive if the patient is reluctant to fully extend the elbow when raising their body weight from sitting to standing exclusively using the upper extremities. Regan et al. report a sensitivity of 88% [7].

(c) In the posterolateral rotatory drawer test, the patient is asked to relax their arm at 90° of flexion. Gentle anterior and posterior force at the radial head may reveal posterior subluxation of the radius on the capitellum. Camp et al. suggest this test to be the most sensitive for evaluation of PLRI [8].

## Imaging

*Physical exam is highly directive toward a diagnosis for PLRI, though imaging is a useful adjunct.*

1. Initial radiographic evaluation should include an AP and lateral view of the elbow:
   (a) AP view should be assessed for previous fracture, carrying angle, and concentric reduction of the radiohumeral and ulnohumeral joints.
   (b) The radial head should direct toward the capitellum in any view.
   (c) The ulnohumeral joint should be assessed for concentric reduction on the trochlea.
   (d) *Isolated LUCL injury often presents with normal radiographs.*
2. MRI may direct care in the case of multiligament elbow injuries:
   (a) Tarallo et al. report good inter- and intra-observer correlation between MRI studies of elbow dislocation and lateral, but not medial, ligamentous injury.
   (b) Indirect markers of lateral ligamentous injury are useful as direct MRI evaluation of ligament competency in the chronic setting is challenging [9]:
       • Additionally, healed injury may demonstrate a signal change, which is indistinguishable from tear.
       • Radiocapitellar subluxation of 1.2 mm is 67% sensitive and 70% specific for PLRI.
       • Radiocapitellar axial incongruity of 0.7 mm offers 63% sensitivity and 70% specificity [10].
3. Fluoroscopic evaluation during pivot shift exam may reveal posterior subluxation of the radial head on a lateral view [11]. AP stress evaluation of the elbow under varus stress and with more than 30° flexion may reveal increased lateral joint space opening.

## Treatment

*Chronicity, quality of reduction, and degree of instability direct LUCL management.*

1. Nonoperative management.
   (a) The treatment of an acute elbow dislocation depends on the quality of closed reduction and the presence of fracture (i.e., simple vs complex).
   (b) Following successful closed reduction of simple elbow dislocation, fluoroscopy can be used to assess the arc of stability, varus and valgus laxity, and concentric reduction.
   (c) The most common pattern of ligamentous injury is posterolateral rotatory instability due to lateral ligamentous injury.
   (d) A successfully reduced elbow is splinted in 90° of flexion with increasing pronation for patients with varus instability and increased supination for patients exhibiting valgus instability.
   (e) If an elbow dislocation is concentrically reduced, initial treatment typically involves static splinting. Postreduction imaging should again be closely assessed for maintenance of reduction.
   (f) Following concentric closed reduction, the splint can be removed in 5–10 days. Radiographs at this time are necessary to verify reduction.

(g) If the radiograph confirms maintenance of reduction, early active ROM in a hinged elbow brace may begin, with most authors suggesting to limit full extension by 30–60.

(h) Ideally, early ROM will be within the stability arc assessed at the time of injury.

(i) Low demand patients, patients with chronic PLRI, and those with excellent stability following reduction can be considered for nonsurgical management.

2. Operative management.

(a) Limited data is available regarding management of subacute PLRI. Although early immobilization of acute injuries may allow satisfactory outcomes, there is minimal evidence to guide the treatment of subacute injury, and subacute injuries may be best treated as if chronic.

(b) *Indications for surgical intervention include chronic injury with symptomatic instability and acute injury with nonconcentric reduction or persistent instability.*

- Although physical therapy with emphasis on strengthening of dynamic stabilizers and bracing may be an appropriate first step for symptomatic management, there is no data to suggest chronic PLRI will resolve with nonsurgical care.

- Surgical approaches include Kocher or posterior midline approach. The Kocher approach allows for facile treatment of concomitant injury, although at a slightly higher risk of neurologic injury. In instances of acute instability, primary repair with fixation of any associated fractures may be undertaken. In cases of subacute or chronic instability, reconstruction with auto- or allograft may be utilized:

  - The patient is positioned in the supine position.
  - The intermuscular plane between the anconeus (radial nerve) and extensor carpi ulnaris (PIN) is utilized.
  - A 5-cm gently curved incision is made from the lateral epicondyle.
  - After identifying the muscular interval, the forearm is pronated to move the PIN away from the dissection.
  - In the event of acute repair, LUCL repair with consideration for internal bracing has been shown to yield satisfactory results [12].
  - In chronic injury, reconstruction of LUCL or both LUCL and RCL may be undertaken, although no clear biomechanical difference has been identified [13].
  - Identifying the isometric point on the lateral epicondyle was once thought critical for graft function. Goren et al. [14] demonstrated in a cadaveric model that ulnar-sided isometry lies across a broad area and may even occur as far as 32 mm from the radial head.

    In effect, there is no true isometric point at the lateral elbow, and the graft is best positioned as close to anatomic footprint as possible.

- – The surgeon may choose auto- or allograft for reconstruction, with plantaris or gracilis allograft and palmaris longus autograft being preferred.
- – Choice of graft configuration is based on surgeon preference, with "Y-tunnels" being the most commonly described.
- – The graft's path must also traverse the posterior radial head, *in* deference to its function as a mechanical block to posterior radial head subluxation.
- – The graft should be secured with interference screws, or it may be docked to bone.
- – Whichever fixation is chosen, tensioning should occur with the arm in 30–60° of flexion and slight pronation to recreate native anatomy.
- – Postoperatively, the arm should be protected from varus stress. The arm is immobilized in 90° of flexion and pronation for 7–10 days postoperatively.
- – Early range of motion is encouraged with the arm kept in pronation as possible to limit stress on the lateral ligamentous complex. A hinged elbow brace is typically used.
- – Full extension is avoided for 3–6 weeks.
- – After 6 weeks, therapy can be progressed in a more aggressive manner.
- Postoperative complications can involve recurrent instability, stiffness, infection, and cutaneous nerve injury.
- Outcomes are found to be satisfactory in 80% with restoration of stability in 90% of patients [15].
- Baghdadi et al. [16] report similar satisfaction and stability with both auto- and allograft. Lin et al. [7] report 93% satisfaction with reconstruction.

LUCL injury is a relatively uncommon problem. Diagnosis is guided strongly by the patient's history and physical exam findings of instability. Imaging, particularly fluoroscopy, is diagnostic in questionable cases. Treatment is directed by timing from injury, with acute injury showing satisfactory results with closed reduction while subacute and chronic insufficiency is best treated surgically. Acute noncentric reduction is best treated with open reduction and fixation of LUCL. Chronic injury is best treated with reconstruction using allo- or autograft. Postoperatively, ROM and supination are limited to allow for graft healing. Full extension is not permitted for at least 3 weeks. Instability may persist postoperatively and is felt to be related to technique.

## References

1. O'Driscoll SW, Bell DF, Morrey BF. Posterolateral rotatory instability of the elbow. J Bone Joint Surg Am. 1991;73(3):440–6.

2. Charalambous CP, Stanley JK. Posterolateral rotatory instability of the elbow. J Bone Joint Surg. 2008;90(3):272–9.
3. Kalainov DM, Cohen MS. Posterolateral rotatory instability of the elbow in association with lateral epicondylitis. A report of three cases. J Bone Joint Surg Am. 2005;87(5):1120–5. https://doi.org/10.2106/JBJS.D.02293.
4. Camp CL, Fu M, Jahandar H, Desai VS, Sinatro AM, Altchek DW, Dines JS. The lateral collateral ligament complex of the elbow: quantitative anatomic analysis of the lateral ulnar collateral, radial collateral, and annular ligaments. J Shoulder Elb Surg. 2019;28(4):665–70. https://doi.org/10.1016/j.jse.2018.09.019; Epub 2018 Dec 6.
5. McAdams TR, Masters GW, Srivastava S. The effect of arthroscopic sectioning of the lateral ligament complex of the elbow on posterolateral rotatory stability. J Shoulder Elb Surg. 2005;14(3):298–301.
6. Regan W, Lapner PC. Prospective evaluation of two diagnostic apprehension signs for posterolateral instability of the elbow. J Shoulder Elb Surg. 2006;15(3):344–6. https://doi.org/10.1016/j.jse.2005.03.009.
7. Lin KY, Shen PH, Lee CH, Pan RY, Lin LC, Shen HC. Functional outcomes of surgical reconstruction for posterolateral rotatory instability of the elbow. Injury. 2012;43(10):1657–61.
8. Camp CL, Smith J, O'Driscoll SW. Posterolateral rotatory instability of the elbow: part I. Mechanism of injury and the posterolateral rotatory drawer test. Arthrosc Tech. 2017;6(2):e401–5; Published 2017 Apr 3. https://doi.org/10.1016/j.eats.2016.10.016.
9. Grafe MW, McAdams TR, Beaulieu CF, Ladd AL. Magnetic resonance imaging in diagnosis of chronic posterolateral rotatory instability of the elbow. Am J Orthop (Belle Mead NJ). 2003;32(10):501–3; discussion 504
10. Hackl M, Wegmann K, Ries C, Leschinger T, Burkhart KJ, Müller LP. Reliability of magnetic resonance imaging signs of posterolateral rotatory instability of the elbow. J Hand Surg Am. 2015;40(7):1428–33. https://doi.org/10.1016/j.jhsa.2015.04.029.
11. Camp CL, O'Driscoll SW, Wempe MK, Smith J. The sonographic posterolateral rotatory stress test for elbow instability: a cadaveric validation study. PM R. 2017;9(3):275–82. https://doi.org/10.1016/j.pmrj.2016.06.014; Epub 2016 Jun 16.
12. Scheiderer B, Imhoff FB, Kia C, Aglio J, Morikawa D, Obopilwe E, Cote MP, Lacheta L, Imhoff AB, Mazzocca AD, Siebenlist S. LUCL internal bracing restores posterolateral rotatory stability of the elbow. Knee Surg Sports Traumatol Arthrosc. 2020;28(4):1195–201. https://doi.org/10.1007/s00167-019-05632-x; Epub 2019 Jul 27.
13. Dargel J, Boomkamp E, Wegmann K, Eysel P, Müller LP, Hackl M. Reconstruction of the lateral ulnar collateral ligament of the elbow: a comparative biomechanical study. Knee Surg Sports Traumatol Arthrosc. 2017;25(3):943–8. https://doi.org/10.1007/s00167-015-3627-3; Epub 2015 May 10.
14. Goren D, Budoff JE, Hipp JA. Isometric placement of lateral ulnar collateral ligament reconstructions: a biomechanical study. Am J Sports Med. 2010;38(1):153–9. https://doi.org/10.1177/0363546509346049; Epub 2009 Oct 1.
15. Sanchez-Sotelo J, Morrey BF, O'Driscoll SW. Ligamentous repair and reconstruction for posterolateral rotatory instability of the elbow. J Bone Joint Surg Br. 2005;87(1):54–61.
16. Baghdadi YM, Morrey BF, O'Driscoll SW, Steinmann SP, Sanchez-Sotelo J. Revision allograft reconstruction of the lateral collateral ligament complex in elbows with previous failed reconstruction and persistent posterolateral rotatory instability. Clin Orthop Relat Res. 2014;472(7):2061–7. https://doi.org/10.1007/s11999-014-3611-0.

# Medial Collateral Ligament Tears

# 21

Meaghan A. Tranovich and Brian R. Wolf

## Introduction

The medial ulnar collateral ligament complex (Fig. 21.1), together with the radial head and the flexor-pronator mass, acts as restraints to valgus instability of the elbow and may become damaged by repetitive microtrauma in overhead athletes [1–3]. UCL reconstruction has become the gold standard of treatment for UCL rupture or partial tears in throwing athletes while new surgical techniques have demonstrated increasingly promising outcomes for UCL repair.

**Fig. 21.1** Anatomy of the medial ulnar collateral ligament complex. (Reprinted by permission from Springer Nature: Springer Operative Treatment of Elbow Injuries by Breazeale NM and Altcheck DW 2002)

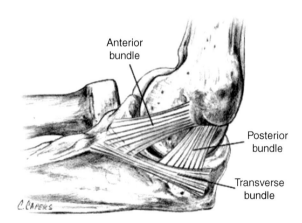

Anterior bundle

Posterior bundle

Transverse bundle

C. CAPERS

M. A. Tranovich · B. R. Wolf (✉)
University of Iowa Hospitals and Clinics, Iowa City, IA, USA
e-mail: meaghan-tranovich@uiowa.edu; brian-wolf@uiowa.edu

1. History
    (a) Classic patient—overhead throwing athlete, especially baseball pitchers [4]
        • Acute injury—may feel sudden medial pain with single pitch or hit
        • Acute-on-chronic injury—antecedent elbow pain that acutely worsens during play
        • Chronic injury—decreased velocity and pitch accuracy [5]
    (b) Level of play (recreational, professional, collegiate, etc.)
    (c) Frequency of play—days/week and weeks/year
        • Pitch count and velocity
    (d) Hand dominance
    (e) Neurologic symptoms
        • Dysesthesias/paresthesias in ulnar nerve distribution
        • Hand intrinsic weakness
    (f) Aggravating and relieving factors
    (g) Prior treatments attempted
2. Physical exam
    (a) Inspection
        • Carrying angle of elbow—compare to contralateral arm
            – Throwing athletes may have nonpathologic increase in this angle in the dominant arm [6, 7]
        • Ecchymosis over medial elbow
        • Medial soft tissue swelling
        • Previous surgical incisions
        • Presence/absence of palmaris longus tendon at wrist
            – Used in reconstruction scenarios
    (b) Palpation
        • Entire course of UCL—medial epicondyle of humerus to sublime tubercle of ulna
        • Flexor-pronator mass
            – Displaces anterior to UCL with 50 to 90° elbow flexion [8]
        • Olecranon
            – Tenderness may suggest other diagnosis, i.e., stress fracture or valgus extension overload
        • Ulnar nerve
            – Tenderness
            – Subluxation out of cubital tunnel with elbow motion [9]
        • Lateral epicondyle of humerus
        • Radiocapitellar joint
    (c) Range of motion—compare to contralateral extremity
        • Flexion
        • Extension
            – Slight asymptomatic flexion contractures may be nonpathologic in thrower's dominant arm [10]
        • Pronosupination

(d) Strength
- Forearm pronation
- Digit/wrist flexion

(e) Provocative maneuvers
- Manual valgus stress test—performed in 30° elbow flexion with forearm pronated [8]
  - Seated or supine
- Milking maneuver—abduct and externally rotate shoulder, supinate forearm and apply valgus stress by pulling on thumb
- Moving valgus stress test—apply valgus stress while ranging the elbow between 30 and 120° [10] (Fig. 21.2)
  - Best when patient supine with shoulder in abduction/external rotation
  - Pain at UCL site or apprehension are positive tests

(f) Neurovascular exam
- Ulnar nerve
  - Sensation in ulnar ring and small fingers
  - Tinel's sign at cubital tunnel
- Radial and ulnar arteries
  - Palpate pulses
  - Distal capillary refill

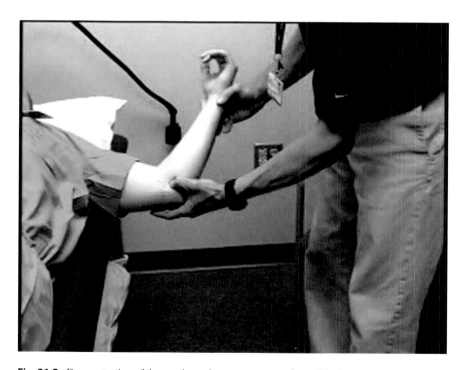

**Fig. 21.2** Demonstration of the moving valgus stress test performed in the supine position

(g) Kinetic chain
- Ipsilateral shoulder—glenohumeral internal rotation deficit (GIRD), scapular dyskinesias [11]
- Ipsilateral wrist
- Lower extremities/stance
- Core/balance [12]

3. Imaging
 (a) X-rays—AP, lateral, oblique
   - Useful for bony avulsions from medial epicondyle or sublime tubercle
   - HO or osteophytes in chronic injuries [13]
   - Valgus stress radiographs have limited utility and cause patient discomfort [14]
 (b) MRI—gold standard for diagnosis
   - Intraarticular gadolinium enhances sensitivity/specificity, better identification of partial tears [15–17] (Fig. 21.3)

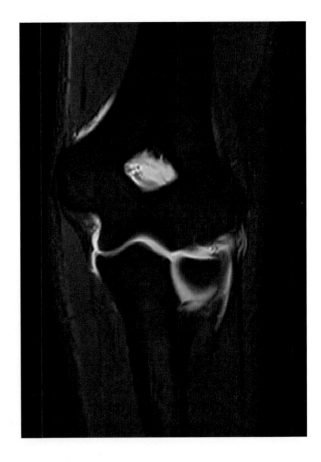

**Fig. 21.3** MR arthrogram of elbow demonstrating distal tear of the UCL. Patient went on to undergo UCL repair with internal brace augmentation

(c) Ultrasound
  - Advantages: low cost, noninvasive, allows dynamic evaluation of entire medial elbow [18]
  - Disadvantages: User-dependent
4. Treatment
  (a) Nonoperative treatment
    - Indicated in most non-athletes with partial or complete tears, some non-throwing athletes [19–21]
      - Rest, physical therapy targeting entire kinetic chain [22]
      - PRP—may have a role in the treatment of partial tears, athletes unwilling/unable to undergo surgery and participate in extended rehabilitation [23, 24]
  (b) Operative treatment
    - Indicated in throwing athletes with full-thickness UCL tears, partial thickness tears that failed nonoperative treatment
      - UCL repair
        Poor initial results, but new techniques/technologies demonstrate improving outcomes [25–28]
        Most likely to benefit patients with proximal or distal avulsion injuries (Fig. 21.4)
        Current technique—repair native ligament and reinforce with internal brace using suture tape material fixed with two suture anchors [27, 29, 30] (Figs. 21.5 and 21.6)
      - UCL reconstruction
        Gold standard for surgical treatment of overhead throwing athletes
        Reconstruct anterior band of MUCL, restoring valgus stability
        Original technique—medial approach to the elbow, flexor-pronator mass detachment, palmaris longus autograft passed in figure of eight fashion through V-shaped proximal ulna tunnel and Y-shaped tunnel in distal humerus [31] (Fig. 21.7)
        Routinely transferred ulnar nerve to avoid perineural scarring

**Fig. 21.4** Distal avulsion injury of the UCL as seen after a muscle-splitting approach and split of the native ligament. Patient went on to UCL repair with internal brace augmentation

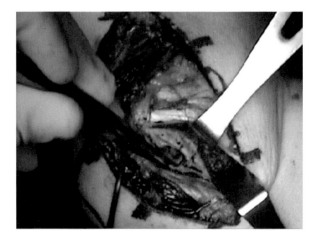

**Fig. 21.5** Distal avulsion
of the UCL after placement
of the first 3.5 mm
SwiveLock anchor
(Arthrex, Naples, FL,
USA) at the site of injury.
A vessel loop and retractor
protect the ulnar nerve

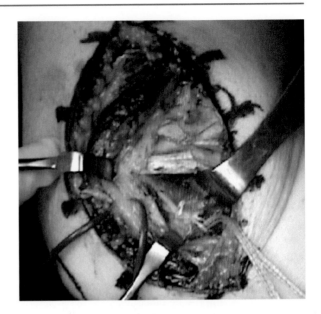

**Fig. 21.6** Final position
of the InternalBrace
(Arthrex, Naples, FL,
USA) augment of distal
UCL avulsion

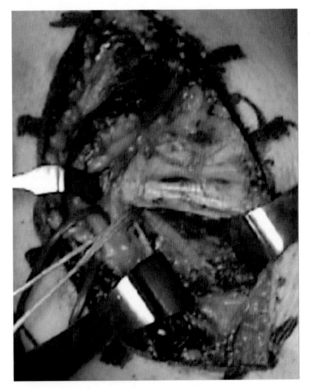

## Figure of 8 Constructs

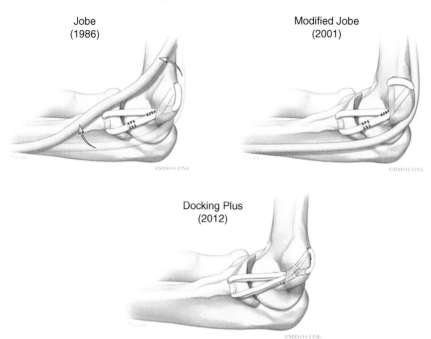

**Fig. 21.7** Figure of eight UCL reconstruction techniques. (Reprinted by permission from Springer Nature: The history and evolution of elbow medial ulnar collateral ligament reconstruction: from Tommy John to 2020 by Jensen AR et al. 2020)

Approach developments—muscle-splitting approach developed to decrease morbidity and rates of postoperative ulnar nerve issues

Split through the posterior 1/3 of the common flexor bundle from the medial epicondyle to 1 cm distal to the sublime tubercle [32]

Obviates need for routine ulnar nerve mobilization

Fixation developments

Modified Jobe technique—increase in size of humeral tunnels, change in configuration, whereby drill holes exit on anterior humeral surface to minimize postoperative ulnar neuropathy [33] (Fig. 21.7)

Docking technique—utilizes large dead-end humeral tunnel with two smaller connecting tunnels drilled to the proximal epicondyle, tension graft sutures through the connecting tunnels, and tie over a bone bridge on the proximal epicondyle [34] (Figs. 21.8, 21.9, 21.10, and 21.11)

## *Triangular Constructs*

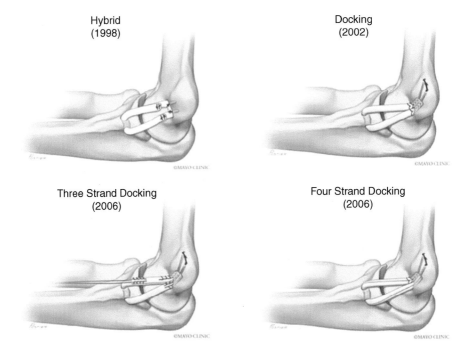

**Fig. 21.8** Triangular UCL reconstruction techniques. (Reprinted by permission from Springer Nature: The history and evolution of elbow medial ulnar collateral ligament reconstruction: from Tommy John to 2020 by Jensen AR et al. 2020)

**Fig. 21.9** UCL reconstruction using a muscle-splitting approach and the docking technique, the author's preferred method. Graft sutures are seen being tensioned over the medial epicondyle to the right. Vessel loops protect the ulnar nerve

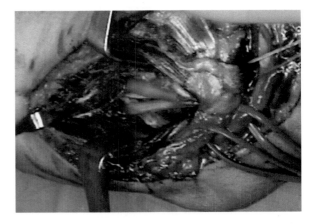

**Fig. 21.10** Close up of palmaris longus tendon graft used for reconstruction with the docking technique

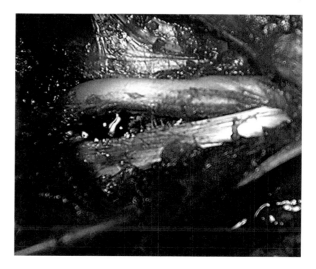

**Fig. 21.11** Final construct using the docking technique. Graft sutures tied over the humeral bone bridge can be seen in the top right

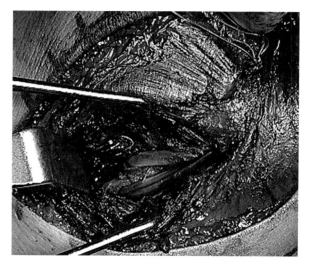

Three-strand docking/four-strand docking techniques—excess graft retained and folded back on itself to reinforce reconstructed limbs [35, 36] (Fig. 21.8)

DANE TJ technique—hybrid technique using docking tunnels in humerus with interference screw in the ulna [37] (Fig. 21.12)

Useful for patients whose sublime tubercle cannot accommodate a bone tunnel

Suture anchor fixation—less soft tissue dissection, avoid ulnar nerve transposition (Fig. 21.12)

### *Linear Constructs*

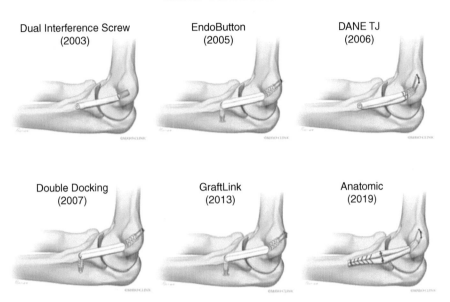

**Fig. 21.12** Linear UCL reconstruction techniques. (Reprinted by permission from Springer Nature: The history and evolution of elbow medial ulnar collateral ligament reconstruction: from Tommy John to 2020 by Jensen AR et al. 2020)

Initially used on ulna and humerus; new hybrid techniques use ulnar bone tunnels and a humeral anchor [38, 39]

Suspensory button fixation—utilizes cortical buttons developed for femoral ACL reconstruction fixation [40–42] (Fig. 21.12)

Avoids damaging grafts with interference screw threads [40]

Clinical outcomes still under investigation

- Surgical risks/complications
  - Ulnar nerve neuropraxia—most common complication [43]

    Usually presents as sensory paresthesias in ulnar ring and small fingers [44]

    Vast majority resolve within 6 weeks postoperatively [44]

    Decrease this risk with muscle-splitting approach [45]
  - Flexor-pronator rupture
  - Superficial wound infection
  - Hematoma formation
  - Heterotopic ossification [46]
  - Elbow stiffness

    Stress early gentle motion in rehabilitation [43, 45]

# References

1. Labott JR, Aibinder WR, Dines JS, Camp CL. Understanding the medial ulnar collateral ligament of the elbow: review of native ligament anatomy and function. World J Orthop. 2018;9(6):78–84. https://doi.org/10.5312/wjo.v9.i6.78.
2. Cinque ME, Schickendantz M, Frangiamore S. Review of anatomy of the medial ulnar collateral ligament complex of the elbow. Curr Rev Musculoskelet Med. 2020;13(1):96–102. https://doi.org/10.1007/s12178-020-09609-z.
3. Regan WD, Korinek SL, Morrey BF, An KN. Biomechanical study of ligaments around the elbow joint. Clin Orthop Relat Res. 1991;271:170–9.
4. Freehill MT, Safran MR. Diagnosis and management of ulnar collateral ligament injuries in throwers. Curr Sports Med Rep. 2011;10(5):271–8. https://doi.org/10.1249/JSR.0b013e31822d4000.
5. Nassab PF, Schickendantz MS. Evaluation and treatment of medial ulnar collateral ligament injuries in the throwing athlete. Sports Med Arthrosc Rev. 2006;14(4):221–31. https://doi.org/10.1097/01.jsa.0000212323.38807.fa.
6. Torg JS, Pollack H, Sweterlitsch P. The effect of competitive pitching on the shoulders and elbows of preadolescent baseball players. Pediatrics. 1972;49(2):267–72.
7. Gugenheim JJ Jr, Stanley RF, Woods GW, Tullos HS. Little league survey: the Houston study. Am J Sports Med. 1976;4(5):189–200. https://doi.org/10.1177/036354657600400501.
8. Patel RM, Lynch TS, Amin NH, Calabrese G, Gryzlo SM, Schickendantz MS. The thrower's elbow. Orthop Clin North Am. 2014;45(3):355–76. https://doi.org/10.1016/j.ocl.2014.03.007.
9. Eygendaal D, Safran MR. Postero-medial elbow problems in the adult athlete. Br J Sports Med. 2006;40(5):430–4; discussion 434. https://doi.org/10.1136/bjsm.2005.025437.
10. Ciccotti MC, Ciccotti MG. Ulnar collateral ligament evaluation and diagnostics. Clin Sports Med. 2020;39(3):503–22. https://doi.org/10.1016/j.csm.2020.02.002.
11. Ben Kibler W, Sciascia A. Kinetic chain contributions to elbow function and dysfunction in sports. Clin Sports Med. 2004;23(4):545–52, viii. https://doi.org/10.1016/j.csm.2004.04.010.
12. Garrison JC, Arnold A, Macko MJ, Conway JE. Baseball players diagnosed with ulnar collateral ligament tears demonstrate decreased balance compared to healthy controls. J Orthop Sports Phys Ther. 2013;43(10):752–8. https://doi.org/10.2519/jospt.2013.4680.
13. Gustas CN, Lee KS. Multimodality imaging of the painful elbow: current imaging concepts and image-guided treatments for the Injured Thrower's elbow. Radiol Clin N Am. 2016;54(5):817–39. https://doi.org/10.1016/j.rcl.2016.04.005.
14. Molenaars RJ, Medina GIS, Eygendaal D, Oh LS, Injured vs. Uninjured elbow opening on clinical stress radiographs and its relationship to ulnar collateral ligament injury severity in throwers. J Shoulder Elb Surg. 2020;29(5):982–8. https://doi.org/10.1016/j.jse.2020.01.068.
15. Magee T. Accuracy of 3-T MR arthrography versus conventional 3-T MRI of elbow tendons and ligaments compared with surgery. AJR Am J Roentgenol. 2015;204(1):W70–5. https://doi.org/10.2214/AJR.14.12553.
16. Carrino JA, Morrison WB, Zou KH, Steffen RT, Snearly WN, Murray PM. Noncontrast MR imaging and MR arthrography of the ulnar collateral ligament of the elbow: prospective evaluation of two-dimensional pulse sequences for detection of complete tears. Skelet Radiol. 2001;30(11):625–32. https://doi.org/10.1007/s002560100396.
17. Schwartz ML, al-Zahrani S, Morwessel RM, Andrews JR. Ulnar collateral ligament injury in the throwing athlete: evaluation with saline-enhanced MR arthrography. Radiology. 1995;197(1):297–9. https://doi.org/10.1148/radiology.197.1.7568841.
18. Hendawi TK, Rendos NK, Warrell CS, Hackel JG, Jordan SE, Andrews JR, Ostrander RV. Medial elbow stability assessment after ultrasound-guided ulnar collateral ligament transection in a cadaveric model: ultrasound versus stress radiography. J Shoulder Elb Surg. 2019;28(6):1154–8. https://doi.org/10.1016/j.jse.2018.11.060.

19. Nicolette GW, Gravlee JR. Ulnar collateral ligament injuries of the elbow in female division I collegiate gymnasts: a report of five cases. Open Access J Sports Med. 2018;9:183–9. https://doi.org/10.2147/OAJSM.S159624.

20. McCrum CL, Costello J, Onishi K, Stewart C, Vyas D. Return to play after PRP and rehabilitation of 3 elite ice hockey players with ulnar collateral ligament injuries of the elbow. Orthop J Sports Med. 2018;6(8):2325967118790760. https://doi.org/10.1177/2325967118790760.

21. Kenter K, Behr CT, Warren RF, O'Brien SJ, Barnes R. Acute elbow injuries in the National Football League. J Shoulder Elb Surg. 2000;9(1):1–5. https://doi.org/10.1016/s1058-2746(00)80023-3.

22. Langer P, Fadale P, Hulstyn M. Evolution of the treatment options of ulnar collateral ligament injuries of the elbow. Br J Sports Med. 2006;40(6):499–506. https://doi.org/10.1136/bjsm.2005.025072.

23. Podesta L, Crow SA, Volkmer D, Bert T, Yocum LA. Treatment of partial ulnar collateral ligament tears in the elbow with platelet-rich plasma. Am J Sports Med. 2013;41(7):1689–94. https://doi.org/10.1177/0363546513487979.

24. Dines JS, Williams PN, ElAttrache N, Conte S, Tomczyk T, Osbahr DC, Dines DM, Bradley J, Ahmad CS. Platelet-rich plasma can be used to successfully treat elbow ulnar collateral ligament insufficiency in high-level throwers. Am J Orthop (Belle Mead NJ). 2016;45(5):296–300.

25. Savoie FH 3rd, Trenhaile SW, Roberts J, Field LD, Ramsey JR. Primary repair of ulnar collateral ligament injuries of the elbow in young athletes: a case series of injuries to the proximal and distal ends of the ligament. Am J Sports Med. 2008;36(6):1066–72. https://doi.org/10.1177/0363546508315201.

26. Dugas JR, Looze CA, Jones CM, Walters BL, Rothermich MA, Emblom BA, Fleisig GS, Aune K, Cain EL. Ulnar collateral ligament repair with internal brace augmentation in amateur overhead throwing athletes. Orthop J Sports Med. 2018;6(7):1096–102.

27. Dugas JR, Looze CA, Capogna B, Walters BL, Jones CM, Rothermich MA, Fleisig GS, Aune KT, Drogosz M, Wilk KE, Emblom BA, Cain EL Jr. Ulnar collateral ligament repair with collagen-dipped fibertape augmentation in overhead-throwing athletes. Am J Sports Med. 2019;47(5):1096–102. https://doi.org/10.1177/0363546519833684.

28. Paletta GA Jr, Milner J. Repair and InternalBrace augmentation of the medial ulnar collateral ligament. Clin Sports Med. 2020;39(3):537–48. https://doi.org/10.1016/j.csm.2020.04.001.

29. Dugas JR, Walters BL, Beason DP, Fleisig GS, Chronister JE. Biomechanical comparison of ulnar collateral ligament repair with internal bracing versus modified Jobe reconstruction. Am J Sports Med. 2016;44(3):735–41. https://doi.org/10.1177/0363546515620390.

30. Bodendorfer BM, Looney AM, Lipkin SL, Nolton EC, Li J, Najarian RG, Chang ES. Biomechanical comparison of ulnar collateral ligament reconstruction with the docking technique versus repair with internal bracing. Am J Sports Med. 2018;46(14):3495–501. https://doi.org/10.1177/0363546518803771.

31. Jobe FW, Stark H, Lombardo SJ. Reconstruction of the ulnar collateral ligament in athletes. J Bone Joint Surg. 1986;68(8):1158–63.

32. Smith GR, Altchek DW, Pagnani MJ, Keeley JR. A muscle-splitting approach to the ulnar collateral ligament of the elbow. Neuroanatomy and operative technique. Am J Sports Med. 1996;24(5):575–80. https://doi.org/10.1177/036354659602400503.

33. Thompson WH, Jobe FW, Yocum LA, Pink MM. Ulnar collateral ligament reconstruction in athletes: muscle-splitting approach without transposition of the ulnar nerve. J Shoulder Elb Surg. 2001;10(2):152–7. https://doi.org/10.1067/mse.2001.112881.

34. Rohrbough JT, Altchek DW, Hyman J, Williams RJ 3rd, Botts JD. Medial collateral ligament reconstruction of the elbow using the docking technique. Am J Sports Med. 2002;30(4):541–8. https://doi.org/10.1177/03635465020300041401.

35. Koh JL, Schafer MF, Keuter G, Hsu JE. Ulnar collateral ligament reconstruction in elite throwing athletes. Arthroscopy. 2006;22(11):1187–91. https://doi.org/10.1016/j.arthro.2006.07.024.

36. Paletta GA Jr, Klepps SJ, Difelice GS, Allen T, Brodt MD, Burns ME, Silva MJ, Wright RW. Biomechanical evaluation of 2 techniques for ulnar collateral ligament reconstruction of the elbow. Am J Sports Med. 2006;34(10):1599–603. https://doi.org/10.1177/0363546506289340.

37. Conway JE. The DANE TJ procedure for elbow medial ulnar collateral ligament insufficiency. Tech Shoulder Elb Surg. 2006;7(1):6–43.

38. Hechtman KS, Tjin-A-Tsoi EW, Zvijac JE, Uribe JW, Latta LL. Biomechanics of a less invasive procedure for reconstruction of the ulnar collateral ligament of the elbow. Am J Sports Med. 1998;26(5):620–4. https://doi.org/10.1177/03635465980260050401.

39. Hechtman KS, Zvijac JE, Wells ME, Botto-van Bemden A. Long-term results of ulnar collateral ligament reconstruction in throwing athletes based on a hybrid technique. Am J Sports Med. 2011;39(2):342–7. https://doi.org/10.1177/0363546510385401.

40. Armstrong AD, Dunning CE, Ferreira LM, Faber KJ, Johnson JA, King GJ. A biomechanical comparison of four reconstruction techniques for the medial collateral ligament-deficient elbow. J Shoulder Elb Surg. 2005;14(2):207–15. https://doi.org/10.1016/j.jse.2004.06.006.

41. Lynch JL, Maerz T, Kurdziel MD, Davidson AA, Baker KC, Anderson K. Biomechanical evaluation of the TightRope versus traditional docking ulnar collateral ligament reconstruction technique: kinematic and failure testing. Am J Sports Med. 2013;41(5):1165–73. https://doi.org/10.1177/0363546513482567.

42. Lynch JL, Pifer MA, Maerz T, Kurdziel MD, Davidson AA, Baker KC, Anderson K. The GraftLink ulnar collateral ligament reconstruction: biomechanical comparison with the docking technique in both kinematics and failure tests. Am J Sports Med. 2013;41(10):2278–87. https://doi.org/10.1177/0363546513498999.

43. Watson JN, McQueen P, Hutchinson MR. A systematic review of ulnar collateral ligament reconstruction techniques. Am J Sports Med. 2014;42(10):2510–6. https://doi.org/10.1177/0363546513509051.

44. Cain EL Jr, Andrews JR, Dugas JR, Wilk KE, McMichael CS, Walter JC 2nd, Riley RS, Arthur ST. Outcome of ulnar collateral ligament reconstruction of the elbow in 1281 athletes: results in 743 athletes with minimum 2-year follow-up. Am J Sports Med. 2010;38(12):2426–34. https://doi.org/10.1177/0363546510378100.

45. Vitale MA, Ahmad CS. The outcome of elbow ulnar collateral ligament reconstruction in overhead athletes: a systematic review. Am J Sports Med. 2008;36(6):1193–205. https://doi.org/10.1177/0363546508319053.

46. Andrachuk JS, Scillia AJ, Aune KT, Andrews JR, Dugas JR, Cain EL. Symptomatic heterotopic ossification after ulnar collateral ligament reconstruction: clinical significance and treatment outcome. Am J Sports Med. 2016;44(5):1324–8. https://doi.org/10.1177/0363546515626185.

# Arthritis of the Elbow

# 22

Emilie Cheung and Stephanie Tieu Kha

## Introduction

Primary osteoarthritis (OA) of the elbow is characterized by progressive loss of motion with mechanical symptoms most commonly seen in the active, male laborer population. Rheumatoid arthritis (RA) of the elbow is an inflammatory type of arthritis, characterized by diffuse pain and stiffness, often amid a clinical picture of polyarticular disease. Advanced RA is less frequently seen in the elbow due to the advancement and efficacy of disease-modifying medication. Post-traumatic arthritis occurs in patients with a history of prior elbow fracture or dislocation with damage to the articular surface. Medical treatment and physical therapy may be initiated in the early stages of arthritic disease. Surgical treatment options include arthroscopic debridement, open debridement, and total elbow arthroplasty.

1. History—three main types of elbow arthritis (primary, inflammatory, and post-traumatic):
   (a) Primary osteoarthritis (OA) of the elbow.
   - Most commonly seen in the dominant upper extremity of middle-aged men, manual laborers, weight-lifters, and throwing athletes.
   - Symptoms: impingement-type pain with carrying heavy objects next to body with the elbow extended, or pain at end range of motion.
     - Periarticular hypertrophic osteophytes can fracture after a traumatic event, form loose bodies, and lead to mechanical symptoms (i.e., locking and catching).
   - Often involves radiocapitellar joint and spares the ulnohumeral joint.

E. Cheung · S. T. Kha (✉)
Department of Orthopaedic Surgery, Stanford University, Redwood City, CA, USA
e-mail: evcheung@stanford.edu; skha@stanford.edu

© The Author(s), under exclusive license to Springer Nature Switzerland AG 2022
C. M. Chebli, A. M. Murthi (eds.), *The Resident's Guide to Shoulder and Elbow Surgery*, https://doi.org/10.1007/978-3-031-12255-2_22

(b) Rheumatoid arthritis (RA) of the elbow:
  - Inflammatory arthropathy more commonly affects females than males.
  - Elbow involvement seen in 20–60% of patients diagnosed with RA.
    - Often seen in the setting of polyarticular disease and extra-articular rheumatoid manifestations.
  - Symptoms: Diffuse pain and stiffness from episodes of inflammation of the synovium leading to capsular distension and fixed flexion contracture [1].
  - Some patients may report numbness/tingling in ulnar nerve distribution (from ulnar nerve compression at the cubital tunnel or during terminal flexion of the elbow).
  - As RA progresses to advanced stages, proliferative granulation tissue or inflammatory pannus extends into the joint causing erosive destruction of the bone and cartilage and nearby tendons and ligaments [2].
    - Leads to deformity, subluxation or dislocation of the elbow joint, fracture, bone loss, or ankylosis.
    - Advanced-stage RA is less frequently seen in the elbow due to the advancement and efficacy of disease-modifying treatments (DMARDs) over the past two decades [3].
(c) Post-traumatic arthritis.
  - Commonly seen in patients with a prior elbow fracture (i.e., distal humerus, radial head, and olecranon) or elbow dislocation, with damage to the articular cartilage.
  - Early onset degenerative changes and arthritis result from altered load distribution across the damaged articular surface.
  - Symptoms: patients can report pain at end range of motion (from osteophyte impingement) and pain throughout range of motion (from advanced OA) and may also have chronic instability or stiffness.
2. Physical Exam.
  (a) Inspection/palpation:
    - Assess for elbow deformity, prior incisions or scars, and elbow joint effusion.
    - Assess for location of pain on palpation or pain with range of motion.
    - In patients with RA, examine the bilateral hand, wrist, and shoulder joints as well as the cervical spine, since rheumatoid disease rarely occurs in isolation in the elbow [4].
  (b) Range of motion.
    - Loss of terminal elbow extension can be seen in all types of elbow arthritis.
    - Limited midrange of motion—can be seen in rheumatoid arthritis or non-union/malunion cases of post-traumatic arthritis of the elbow.
    - Assess for instability or subluxation—often seen in end-stage inflammatory arthritis or post-traumatic arthritis.

(c) Neurologic and vascular.
  • Assess motor and sensory function of the ulnar, radial, and median nerves in both upper extremities:
    – Ulnar neuropathy is frequently associated with elbow arthritis; examine for ulnar nerve symptoms (paresthesia) from compression at the cubital tunnel or with terminal flexion of the elbow.
  • Palpate the radial pulse or evaluate distal capillary refill in the digits to assess distal perfusion.
3. Imaging.
  (a) X-rays—obtain standard elbow radiographs (AP, lateral, and oblique projections):
    • X-ray findings in primary elbow OA.
      – Hypertrophic osteophyte and loose body formation at the ulnohumeral articulation.
      – Can visualize osteophyte on the olecranon and coronoid processes, extending into their fossae at the distal humerus.
      – Minor osteophytes and squaring around the radial head may be seen relatively early in the disease process (Fig. 22.1).
      – Relative preservation of the ulnohumeral joint space.
    • X-ray findings in RA of the elbow:
      – Concentric joint space narrowing.
      – Typically no osteophyte formation.
      – In advanced RA, can see periarticular cyst formation and architectural bony changes due to progressive bony erosion.

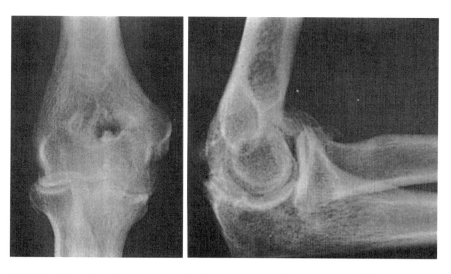

**Fig. 22.1** AP and lateral radiographs of typical appearance of primary osteoarthritis of the elbow. There is radiocapitellar joint space narrowing, relative preservation of the ulnohumeral joint space, and hypertrophic osteophyte formation

- X-ray findings in post-traumatic arthritis of the elbow.
  - Assess articular congruence along ulnohumeral joint and radiocapitellar joint.
  - In the setting of prior fracture or fixation, assess for implant failure, nonunion, or malunion at the fracture site.
  (b) Computerized tomography (CT) scan with 3-D reconstructions—useful for surgical planning.
  - Primary elbow OA.
    - Routinely performed to visualize the location and size of osteophytes.
    - Identify horizontally shaped "shelf osteophytes" in the olecranon fossa, radial fossa, and coronoid fossa, which are less easily seen on plain films.
    - Location, size, and geometry of osteophytes are especially helpful to visualize when planning open or arthroscopic bony debridement.
  - RA of the elbow.
    - CT scan is typically not needed in RA because the surgical intervention for end-stage RA of the elbow is total elbow arthroplasty.
  - Post-traumatic arthritis of the elbow.
    - Routinely performed to assess articular surfaces and congruence and severity of arthritis and to evaluate for nonunion or malunion in patients with history of a fracture.
  (c) MRI.
  - MRI is not as helpful in primary elbow OA and is not usually performed in.
  - MRI may be helpful to visualize synovitis in early stages of RA and confirm diagnosis.
  (d) Ultrasound.
  - Limited utility in evaluating elbow arthritis, although can help visualize soft tissue changes, joint erosion, or synovitis in the early stages of RA.
4. Treatment algorithm.
  (a) Nonoperative treatment.
  - Medical treatment and physical therapy may be initiated in the early stages of arthritis (Fig. 22.2).
  - Physical therapy may include pain-control measures, such as avoidance of activities, which place high stresses on the elbow, and gentle range-of-motion exercises to maintain mobility and strength about the muscles.
  - A trial of nonsteroidal anti-inflammatory medication and intra-articular injection of corticosteroid can be helpful to alleviate symptoms from inflammation.
  - For patients with RA, initiating disease-modifying medications (DMARDs) can help slow the progression of disease.
  (b) Operative treatment indicated following failure of conservative treatment:
  - Surgical options:
    - Arthroscopic elbow debridement with resection of osteophytes and loose body removal.

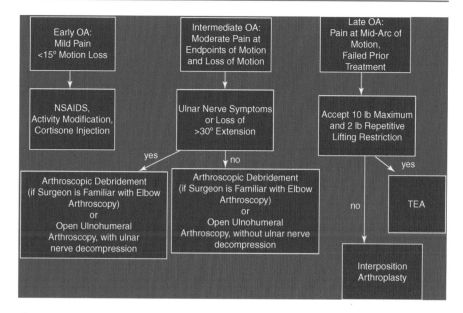

**Fig. 22.2** Treatment algorithm for primary osteoarthritis of the elbow

Also called arthroscopic ulnohumeral arthroplasty or osteocapsular arthroplasty.

Indicated in the young, active patient with OA who has impingement pain at the extremes of motion.

The principle of treatment involves resecting the impinging osteophytes, capsulectomy, and removal of loose bodies.

Advantages to arthroscopic versus open treatment include less postoperative pain and decreased intracapsular bleeding, leading to less capsular scar formation, facilitating early gains in motion and recovery [5].

Surgical approach and operative technique.

> The patient is placed in the lateral decubitus position for elbow arthroscopy [6, 7]. The forearm and hand are allowed to hang free with the elbow flexed 90 deg (Fig. 22.3a, b).
>
> The ulnar nerve and bony landmarks are marked by a pen: lateral epicondyle, medial epicondyle, radial head, capitellum, and olecranon.
>
>> The ulnar nerve is also palpated to be sure of its location and to check that it does not subluxate with elbow flexion (Fig. 22.4).
>
> The elbow is injected through the lateral soft spot, bound by the radial head, lateral epicondyle, and olecranon, with 20–30 cc of saline solution.

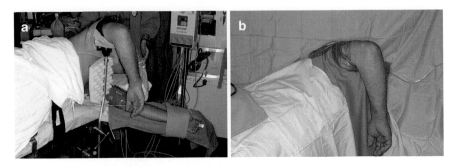

**Fig. 22.3** (**a, b**) Elbow arthroscopy setup before and after draping. The patient is positioned in the lateral decubitus position with the forearm allowed to hang free with the elbow at 90 deg

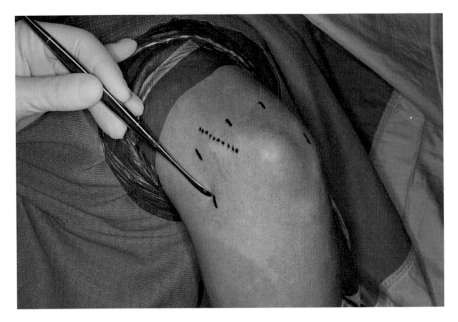

**Fig. 22.4** Portals for elbow arthroscopy, with the pointer indicating the anteromedial portal. The dotted line represents the location of the ulnar nerve

When the elbow is distended, the major neurovascular structures are positioned farther away from the portal sites, and entry is theoretically safer.

The elbow is initially entered through an anteromedial portal by the arthroscope. An anterolateral portal, used as an instrument portal, is created by direct visualization. A retractor can be placed into the elbow joint through an accessory portal, which is typically 2–3 cm proximal to the working portals, and requires an assistant to maintain its position.

**Fig. 22.5** Arthroscopic view of anterior elbow capsule from anteromedial viewing portal. Distal humerus is on the left in this photograph. Arthroscopic shaver is used to complete the anterior capsulectomy

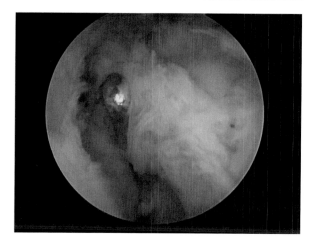

Loose bodies are removed, osteoarthritic spurs are debrided from the coronoid, coronoid fossa, and radial fossa, and anterior capsulectomy is performed (Fig. 22.5).

The posterior compartment is then entered via a posterolateral portal for visualization and one central portal for instruments.

After complete capsulectomy, loose bodies and impinging osteophytes on the tip and sides of the olecranon and posterior capitellum are removed.

Risks and complications.

Elbow arthroscopy is technically demanding and associated with a risk of injury to neurovascular structures. Surgeon experience and familiarity with this technique is perhaps the most important factor in preventing neurovascular injury.

Radial, median, and ulnar nerve injuries following elbow arthroscopy have been reported [8–11]. The use of retractors is an important strategy in preventing nerve injury because this protects the neurovascular structures anterior to the anterior capsule [12].

Clinical outcomes.

Reports on arthroscopic debridement for treatment of osteoarthritis of the elbow have shown satisfactory results.

Phillips and Strasburger [13] reported satisfactory results in all 25 patients in their series, with an average improvement in arc of motion of 41 deg, at a mean of 1.5 years follow-up. There were no complications, but one patient required reoperation for recalcitrant symptoms.

Kim and Shin [14] reported on 63 elbows, mean follow-up of 3.5 years, with 92% having significant improvement in their arc of motion (mean 81 deg preoperatively to 121 deg postoperatively). They found that there was no difference between patients with post-traumatic and those with degenerative etiology. Motion achieved at the time of surgery was predictive of gains in postoperative motion. Patients with symptoms of less than one year duration were able to achieve better postoperative motion than those with longer duration of symptoms.

Krishnan et al. [15] reported on 11 patients, all under the age of 50, who underwent arthroscopic ulnohumeral arthroplasty for degenerative arthritis. All patients had a good to excellent result at mean 26 months follow-up, and mean MEPS scores improved from 58 points preoperatively to 89 points postoperatively.

Adams et al. [16] reported on the largest cohort of patients who have had arthroscopic osteocapsular debridement of the elbow for the indication of osteoarthritis. At an average follow-up of 3.4 years, there were statistically significant improvements in pain and motion. Elbow scores were significantly improved at follow-up (postoperative scores averaged 84.4 points, from 67.5 points preoperatively), with 81% good to excellent results. Two complications occurred: one case of heterotopic ossification, and one case of ulnar dysthesias. In experienced hands, arthroscopic osteocapsular debridement can be a safe and effective treatment option.

– Open elbow debridement ± ulnar nerve decompression.

Indications (similar to that for arthroscopic osteocapsular arthroplasty)—the younger patient who has impingement pain at the extremes of motion.

Surgeons who perform arthroscopy should be familiar with open technique if technical difficulties emerge during arthroscopy.

Surgical approach and operative technique.

Ulnohumeral arthroplasty is a variation of the Outerbridge-Kashiwagi procedure [17], which involves a core excision of the distal humerus, and resection of the tips of the olecranon and coronoid (Fig. 22.6a–d).

The patient is supine with a sandbag under the scapula. A tourniquet is applied, and the arm is prepared and brought across the chest. A posterior skin incision is utilized, and the triceps split in the midline, and up to 25% of the attachment of the triceps is elevated from the distal humerus in order to achieve visualization into the posterior compartment. The hypertrophic olecranon tip is then excised, and the shelf osteophyte within the olecranon fossa is also resected under direct visualization.

Access to the anterior compartment through an anterior "column procedure" is performed next (Fig. 22.7). The common extensor group is split longitudinally through Kaplan's interval. The anterior musculature is then bluntly reflected off of the

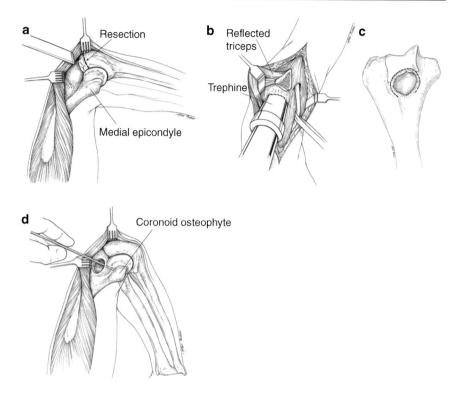

**Fig. 22.6** Operative technique of ulnohumeral arthroplasty. (**a**) The tip of the olecranon is osteotomized, and loose bodies are removed from the olecranon fossa. (**b, c**) A trephine is used to fenestrate the humerus at the level of the olecranon fossa. (**d**) The elbow is then flexed, which brings the coronoid process into view through the trephine hole. The anterior osteophyte is removed using an osteotome, and anterior loose bodies are identified by palpation and are excised. (Adapted with permission from: Morrey BF, editor. *The elbow.* Lippincott Williams & Wilkins; 2002)

**Fig. 22.7** Anterior capsulectomy through a lateral "column procedure" is performed if residual flexion contracture persists. Olecranon and coronoid osteophytes are removed, and anterior and posterior capsulectomies are performed. (Adapted with permission from: Morrey BF, editor. *The elbow.* Lippincott Williams & Wilkins; 2002)

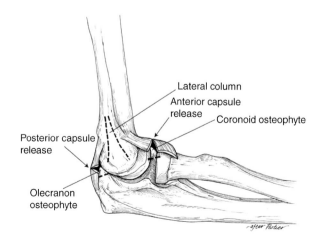

anterior capsule. The anterior capsule is completely isolated, then carefully excised. An anterior elbow retractor is placed, and osteophyte resection is completed with osteotomes and pituitary rongeurs.

Risks and complications.

The ulnar nerve is commonly irritated, and decompression may be indicated if there are symptoms of ulnar neuritis or the elbow lacks flexion greater than 100 deg. This is because postoperative increases in flexion may result in traction-induced ulnar neuritis, which has been the limiting factor in the clinical success of open debridement.

Positive outcomes may not be maintained over long periods of time.

Minami et al. [18] reviewed the results of ulnohumeral arthroplasty in 44 elbows with follow-up of 8–16 years. Sixty-one percent reported no or slight pain, and range of motion was from 32 to 122 deg. This represented a 10% deterioration in subjective outcome and a 17 deg of loss of motion when compared with their initial report [17], in which the mean duration of follow-up was 4.5 years.

Clinical outcomes.

Cohen et al. [19] compared the effectiveness of open and arthroscopic debridement of the elbow at mean 2.9 years follow-up and found that both procedures were effective, with no difference in patients' perceived effectiveness, and no major complications.

However, synovectomy and capsulectomy was not performed in this study. Patients who had arthroscopy had a trend toward better pain relief, but patients who had the open procedure had greater improvement in elbow flexion.

This was thought to be due to the fact that the arthroscopic procedure involves less intraoperative trauma and less scar formation, resulting in less pain, whereas the open procedure enables a more generous debridement of the posterior compartment, allowing for more flexion.

Antuna et al. [20] reported the long-term outcome of this procedure in 46 elbows, with the average arc of motion significantly improved from 79 deg preoperatively to 101 deg at a mean of 6.7 years postoperatively. Seventy-six percent were only mildly painful to not painful. According to the Mayo Elbow Performance Score (MEPS), the results were good to excellent in 74% elbows.

Complications related to the ulnar nerve limited the success of this operation. Twenty-nine percent of patients reported ulnar nerve symptoms postoperatively, and 13% required another operation to decompress or translocate the nerve.

Ulnar nerve decompression or mobilization was recommended in circumstances where patients have limitation of elbow extension of >60 deg and flexion <100 deg, or if the patient has preoperative nerve symptoms.

- Interposition arthroplasty.

Currently has extremely limited indications.

Involves disarticulating the elbow joint, removing and reshaping articular surfaces of the ulna and distal humerus with a burr, removing osteophytes, and then resurfacing the distal humeral surface with fascia lata, dermal matrix, or Achilles tendon allograft, which is trimmed to fit the distal humerus and secured in place with transosseous fixation [21, 22].

- Total elbow arthroplasty (TEA).

Indicated for patients with RA who are willing to accept low activity levels.

Less common indications for TEA: complex or comminuted distal humerus fractures in low-demand elderly patients, post-traumatic arthritis, and primary osteoarthritis.

Complication rates are relatively high, and durability of the implant for these indications is guarded.

Over the past decade, the annual frequency of TEA for treating distal humerus fractures has increased [23].

Complication rates range from 10% to 35% across studies, with periprosthetic fracture, component loosening, component fracture, and infection cited as the most frequent complications requiring implant revision or reoperation [24–26].

Meanwhile, TEA for post-traumatic arthritis has a different complication profile secondary to soft tissue management, as most patients typically have already underwent more than one surgery and have residual scar or soft-tissue contracture [27].

Functional outcomes are also less satisfactory. Hildebrand et al. [28] reported patient undergoing TEA for post-traumatic indication has a significantly lower mean MEPS compared with patient undergoing TEA for inflammatory arthritis.

For patients with primary OA, the use of TEA is a reliable option for achieving pain relief, but not for restoring elbow extension. The typical patient with primary OA tends to have a higher baseline activity level than patients with inflammatory arthritis. Mechanical failure and aseptic loosening are more frequently encountered complications in this population [29].

Implant design: most designs mechanically link ulnar and humeral components, but the linkage allows 6–8 deg of laxity that permits the soft tissues to absorb some of the stresses that would normally be applied to the prosthesis–cement–bone interface (Fig. 22.8a, b).

Surgical approach and operative technique.

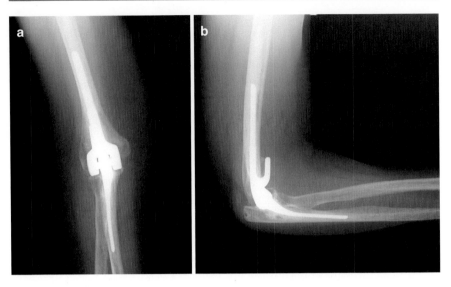

**Fig. 22.8** (**a, b**) AP and lateral radiographs of a 60 year old patient with primary osteoarthritis, demonstrating the Coonrad-Morrey (Zimmer, Warsaw, IN) linked total elbow prosthesis at 5 years postoperative

Patient is positioned supine on the operative table with a tourniquet placed on the proximal arm, and the arm draped over the patient's chest.

The skin incision is posterior and full-thickness skin flaps are created medially and laterally. The ulnar nerve is routinely transposed subcutaneously.

Management of the triceps tendon varies:

The Bryan-Morrey approach [30] reflects the triceps attachment along the olecranon tip in continuity with the forearm fascia.

Alternatively, the Gschwend paratricipital triceps-on approach [31] preserves the triceps insertion, which may be technically more difficult.

Olecranon and coronoid osteophytes are excised, as well as complete release of the collateral ligaments and anterior capsule to gain extension.

The humeral component may need to be seated more proximally than usual to help relax the anterior soft tissue envelope in extension.

The triceps is repaired back to the olecranon through drill holes if it has been released. The tourniquet is deflated, meticulous hemostasis is achieved, and a drain is often placed for a few days postoperatively.

Postoperative protocol:

> The elbow is immobilized in extension and elevated for the first 48 h postoperatively for edema control.
>
> Active range of motion has begun on the second postoperative day, and the patient is usually dismissed the third day after surgery.
>
> The patient is cautioned against active extension against resistance for the first 6 weeks in order to protect the triceps repair if the triceps has been detached.

Risks and complications.

> The overall complication rate for TEA in the management of RA of the elbow varies, with complication rates cited as high as 26% [32, 33].
>
> Most commonly cited complications and modes of failure requiring revision surgery include periprosthetic joint infection, aseptic loosening, periprosthetic fracture, triceps insufficiency, bushing wear, wound breakdown near the olecranon, and postoperative ulnar nerve symptoms.

Clinical outcomes.

> Recent studies on the overall clinical outcomes of total elbow arthroplasty report improvements in pain, function, and range of motion [34].
>
> In the systematic review of over 9000 TEA's performed between 2003 and 2015, Welsink et al. reported pain was improved in 60% of cases at final time of follow-up (mean 6.3 years). Functional outcome, most frequently measured by MEPS, was good to excellent after TEA, with the mean weighted MEPS ranging from 80.5 to 94.1 (good functional outcome = 75–89, Excellent >90) [34].
>
> Biomechanical studies on normal elbow range of motion for activities of daily living demonstrate that most activities can be accomplished with a 30–130 deg flexion arc and 100 deg of forearm rotation (50 deg pronation to 50 deg supination) [35], although more recent studies suggest greater pronation and flexion is needed for contemporary tasks such as typing on a keyboard or using a cellular phone, respectively [36]. In comparison with these biomechanical studies, the overall range of motion after TEA is acceptable, with mean elbow flexion angle of 129 deg, mean extension lag of 30 deg, and mean pronation and supination of 71 and 66 deg, respectively [34].
>
> Welsink et al. also calculated the overall survival rate of TEA implants for all indications to be 79% after 11 years (range 70.6–90.1%) [34]. Similarly, the Norwegian Arthroplasty

Registry demonstrated overall 5-year and 10-year survival rates of TEA implants to be 92% and 81%, respectively [37].

The overall TEA survival rates are less than the survival rates of implants used in knee and hip arthroplasty; however, this highlights the need and opportunity for further research and improvement.

Specifically in TEA for the treatment of advanced RA of the elbow, studies have demonstrated favorable clinical outcomes in terms of survivorship, pain improvement, functional outcome scores, and range of motion. Multiple studies have demonstrated five-year survival rates (with revision surgery as the endpoint) ranging from 80% (little, 2005) to 97% (Thomas 2009, Pham 2018) [32, 33, 38], with ten-year survival rates as high as 92% [39], and 20-year revision-free survivorship of 88% in one study of 461 TEAs [40]. In these studies, the vast majority (over 90%) of patients at last follow-up report minimal to no pain. Furthermore, functional outcome scores are also encouraging, with an average MEPS of 86–91 points at latest follow-up [32, 33, 40].

In a retrospective review of 54 TEA's performed for RA, Pham et al. [32] also reported statistically significant improvement in MEPS ($37 \pm 11$ to $91 \pm 12$; $p < 0.0001$) and in range of motion when comparing latest follow-up to preoperative values. Similarly, Sanchez-Sotelo et al. [40] found promising flexion-extension arcs at latest follow-up, with >100 deg arc noted in 72% of patients.

## Summary

Surgical treatment options for OA of the elbow include arthroscopic or open debridement, interpositional arthroplasty, or TEA. Advancements in the treatment of arthritis of the elbow are the recognition of the concurrent involvement of the ulnar nerve and the evolution of arthroscopic techniques. Total elbow arthroplasty is reserved for sedentary patients with end-stage RA. Future directions for the treatment of may include advances in elbow prosthetic design.

## References

1. Studer A, Athwal GS. Rheumatoid arthritis of the elbow. Hand Clin. 2011;27(2):139–50. https://doi.org/10.1016/j.hcl.2011.01.001.
2. Sanchez-Sotelo J. Elbow rheumatoid elbow: surgical treatment options. Curr Rev Musculoskelet Med. 2016;9(2):224–31. https://doi.org/10.1007/s12178-016-9328-9.
3. Jämsen E, Virta LJ, Hakala M, Kauppi MJ, Malmivaara A, Lehto MUK. The decline in joint replacement surgery in rheumatoid arthritis is associated with a concomitant increase in the intensity of anti-rheumatic therapy. Acta Orthop. 2013;84(4):331–7. https://doi.org/10.310 9/17453674.2013.810519.

4. Dyer GSM, Blazar PE. Rheumatoid elbow. Hand Clin. 2011;27(1):43–8. https://doi. org/10.1016/j.hcl.2010.10.003.

5. O'Driscoll SW. Arthroscopic treatment for osteoarthritis of the elbow. Orthop Clin North Am. 1995;26(4):691–706. https://doi.org/10.1016/s0030-5898(20)32030-7.

6. Morrey B. Arthroscopy of the elbow . Instr Course Lect 1986;35:102–107. https://pubmed. ncbi.nlm.nih.gov/3819396/. Accessed 23 Feb 2021.

7. Steinmann SP, King GJW, Savoie FH. Arthroscopic treatment of the arthritic elbow. J Bone Joint Surg Am. 2005;87:2114–21. https://doi.org/10.2106/00004623-200509000-00026.

8. Haapaniemi T, Berggren M, Adolfsson L. Complete transection of the median and radial nerves during arthroscopic release of post-traumatic elbow contracture. Arthroscopy. 1999;15(7):784–7. https://doi.org/10.1016/S0749-8063(99)70015-0.

9. Hahn M, Grossman JAI. Ulnar nerve laceration as a result of elbow arthroscopy. J Hand Surg Eur Vol. 1998;23(1):109. https://doi.org/10.1016/S0266-7681(98)80236-2.

10. Papilion JD, Neff RS, Shall LM. Compression neuropathy of the radial nerve as a complication of elbow arthroscopy: a case report and review of the literature. Arthroscopy. 1988;4(4):284–6. https://doi.org/10.1016/S0749-8063(88)80046-X.

11. Ruch DS, Poehling GG. Anterior interosseus nerve injury following elbow arthroscopy. Arthroscopy. 1997;13(6):756–8. https://doi.org/10.1016/S0749-8063(97)90014-1.

12. Kelly EW, Morrey BF, O'Driscoll SW. Complications of elbow arthroscopy. J Bone Joint Surg Am. 2001;83(1):25–34. https://doi.org/10.2106/00004623-200101000-00004.

13. Phillips BB, Strasburger S. Arthroscopic treatment of arthrofibrosis of the elbow joint. Arthroscopy. 1998;14(1):38–44. https://doi.org/10.1016/S0749-8063(98)70118-5.

14. Kim SJ, Shin SJ. Arthroscopic treatment for limitation of motion of the elbow. Clin Orthop Relat Res. 2000;375:140–8. https://doi.org/10.1097/00003086-200006000-00017.

15. Krishnan SG, Harkins DC, Pennington SD, Harrison DK, Burkhead WZ. Arthroscopic ulno-humeral arthroplasty for degenerative arthritis of the elbow in patients under fifty years of age. J Shoulder Elb Surg. 2007;16(4):443–8. https://doi.org/10.1016/j.jse.2006.09.001.

16. Adams JE, Wolff LH, Merten SM, Steinmann SP. Osteoarthritis of the elbow: results of arthroscopic osteophyte resection and capsulectomy. J Shoulder Elb Surg. 2008;17(1):126–31. https://doi.org/10.1016/j.jse.2007.04.005.

17. Minami M, Ishii S. Outerbridge-Kashiwagi arthroplasty for osteoarthritis of the elbow joint. Elb Jt 1985:189–196. https://ci.nii.ac.jp/naid/10011129169. Accessed 23 Feb 2021.

18. Minami M, Kato S, Kashiwagi D. Outerbridge-Kashiwagi's method for arthroplasty of osteo-arthritis of the elbow — 44 elbows followed for 8–16 years. J Orthop Sci. 1996;1(1):11–5. https://doi.org/10.1007/bf01234111.

19. Cohen AP, Redden JF, Stanley D. Treatment of osteoarthritis of the elbow: a comparison of open and arthroscopic debridement. Arthroscopy. 2000;16(7):701–6. https://doi.org/10.1053/jars.2000.8952.

20. Antuña SA, Morrey BF, Adams RA, O'Driscoll SW. Ulnohumeral arthroplasty for primary degenerative arthritis of the elbow: long-term outcome and complications. J Bone Joint Surg Am. 2002;84(12):2168–73. https://doi.org/10.2106/00004623-200212000-00007.

21. Morrey BF. Post-traumatic contracture of the elbow. Operative treatment, includ-ing distraction arthroplasty. J Bone Joint Surg Am. 1990;72(4):601–18. https://doi. org/10.2106/00004623-199072040-00019.

22. Walker JW, Merrell GA, Reiter BD, Hastings H. Interposition arthroplasty of the elbow utiliz-ing a lateral epicondyle osteotomy. Tech Hand Up Extrem Surg. 2019;23(2):54–8. https://doi. org/10.1097/BTH.0000000000000235.

23. Rajaee SS, Lin CA, Moon CN. Primary total elbow arthroplasty for distal humeral fractures in elderly patients: a nationwide analysis. J Shoulder Elb Surg. 2016;25(11):1854–60. https:// doi.org/10.1016/j.jse.2016.05.030.

24. Barco R, Streubel PN, Morrey BF, Sanchez-Sotelo J. Total elbow arthroplasty for distal humeral fractures: a ten-year-minimum follow-up study. J Bone Joint Surg Am. 2017;99(18):1524–31. https://doi.org/10.2106/JBJS.16.01222.

25. Lami D, Chivot M, Caubere A, Galland A, Argenson JN. First-line management of distal humerus fracture by total elbow arthroplasty in geriatric traumatology: results in a 21-patient

series at a minimum 2 years' follow-up. Orthop Traumatol Surg Res. 2017;103(6):891–7. https://doi.org/10.1016/j.otsr.2017.06.009.

26. Pogliacomi F, Aliani D, Cavaciocchi M, Corradi M, Ceccarelli F, Rotini R. Total elbow arthroplasty in distal humeral nonunion: clinical and radiographic evaluation after a minimum follow-up of three years. J Shoulder Elb Surg. 2015;24(12):1998–2007. https://doi.org/10.1016/j.jse.2015.08.010.

27. Kwak JM, Koh KH, Jeon IH. Total elbow arthroplasty: clinical outcomes, complications, and revision surgery. Clin Orthop Surg. 2019;11(4):369–79. https://doi.org/10.4055/cios.2019.11.4.369.

28. Hildebrand KA, Patterson SD, Regan WD, MacDermid JC, King GJW. Functional outcome of semiconstrained total elbow arthroplasty. J Bone Joint Surg Am. 2000;82(10):1379–86. https://doi.org/10.2106/00004623-200010000-00003.

29. Schoch BS, Werthel JD, Sánchez-Sotelo J, Morrey BF, Morrey M. Total elbow arthroplasty for primary osteoarthritis. J Shoulder Elb Surg. 2017;26(8):1355–9. https://doi.org/10.1016/j.jse.2017.04.003.

30. Bryan RS, Morrey BF. Extensive posterior exposure of the elbow. A triceps-sparing approach. Clin Orthop Relat Res. 1982;(166):188–92. https://doi.org/10.1097/00003086-198206000-00033.

31. Gschwend N. Our operative approach to the elbow joint. Arch Orthop Trauma Surg. 1981;98(2):143–6. https://doi.org/10.1007/BF00460803.

32. Pham TT, Delclaux S, Huguet S, Wargny M, Bonnevialle N, Mansat P. Coonrad-Morrey total elbow arthroplasty for patients with rheumatoid arthritis: 54 prostheses reviewed at 7 years' average follow-up (maximum, 16 years). J Shoulder Elb Surg. 2018;27(3):398–403. https://doi.org/10.1016/j.jse.2017.11.007.

33. Thomas M, Adeeb M, Mersich I, Neumann L. Kudo 5 total elbow replacement in patients with rheumatoid arthritis. A two centre 2 year to 11 year follow-up study. Shoulder Elb. 2009;1(1):43–50. https://doi.org/10.1111/j.1758-5740.2009.00011.x.

34. Welsink CL, Lambers KTA, van Deurzen DFP, Eygendaal D, van den Bekerom MPJ. Total elbow arthroplasty. JBJS Rev. 2017;5(7):e4. https://doi.org/10.2106/JBJS.RVW.16.00089.

35. Morrey BF, Askew LJ, An KN, Chao EY. A biomechanical study of normal functional elbow motion. J Bone Joint Surg Am. 1981;63(6):872–7. https://doi.org/10.2106/00004623-198163060-00002.

36. Sardelli M, Tashjian RZ, MacWilliams BA. Functional elbow range of motion for contemporary tasks. J Bone Joint Surg Am. 2011;93(5):471–7. https://doi.org/10.2106/JBJS.I.01633.

37. Krukhaug Y, Hallan G, Dybvik E, Lie SA, Furnes ON. A survivorship study of 838 total elbow replacements: a report from the Norwegian Arthroplasty Register 1994-2016. J Shoulder Elb Surg. 2018;27(2):260–9. https://doi.org/10.1016/j.jse.2017.10.018.

38. Little CP. Outcomes of total elbow arthroplasty for rheumatoid arthritis: comparative study of three implants. J Bone Joint Surg Am. 2005;87(11):2439. https://doi.org/10.2106/JBJS.D.02927.

39. Gill DRJ, Morrey BF. The Coonrad-Morrey total elbow arthroplasty in patients who have rheumatoid arthritis: a ten to fifteen-year follow-up study. J Bone Joint Surg Am. 1998;80(9):1327–35. https://doi.org/10.2106/00004623-199809000-00012.

40. Sanchez-Sotelo J, Baghdadi YMK, Morrey BF. Primary linked semiconstrained total elbow arthroplasty for rheumatoid arthritis. J Bone Joint Surg Am. 2016;98(20):1741–8. https://doi.org/10.2106/JBJS.15.00649.

# Distal Humerus Fractures

# 23

Spencer Albertson and Christopher Chuinard

## Introduction

Distal humerus fractures are relatively uncommon injury involving low energy mechanisms in the geriatric population or those with poor bone quality and high energy mechanisms in the young to middle aged population [1–5]. Frequently, interarticular involvement is seen with these injuries requiring anatomic reduction along with the fixation of multiple fracture fragments [2, 4, 6]. Several approaches can be performed based upon the anatomy, fracture pattern, and surgeon experience/ training [7–12]. Fixation can be obtained through percutaneous approaches, open approaches with plates and screws, or even total elbow arthroplasty in the select patient population with a goal of early motion in order to prevent stiffness at the elbow joint [2, 3, 13–15].

1. History:
   (a) What is the Mechanism? High energy vs low energy:
      - Young patient = High energy.
        - Ex: MVC, fall from height, sport
      - Elderly patient = Low energy.
        - Ex: Ground level fall onto outstretched arm.
          Cause of the patient's fall
      - Hand dominance.
      - Medical comorbidities and social factors: cardiac hx, polypharmacy, diabetes, seizure disorder, and EtOH use.

S. Albertson
University of South Florida/Florida Orthopedic Institute, Tampa, FL, USA
e-mail: salberts@usf.edu

C. Chuinard (✉)
Great Lakes Orthopedic Center, Traverse City, MI, USA

© The Author(s), under exclusive license to Springer Nature Switzerland AG 2022
C. M. Chebli, A. M. Murthi (eds.), *The Resident's Guide to Shoulder and Elbow Surgery*, https://doi.org/10.1007/978-3-031-12255-2_23

2. Pathoanatomy:
   (a) What position was the elbow in at the time of injury?
   - Axial load to elbow at less than 90° = transcolumnar fracture.
   - Axial load to elbow at greater than 90° = intercondylar fracture.
3. Physical exam:
   (a) The young patient may be a polytrauma.
   - Evaluate all extremities, and follow ALS guidelines.
   - Examine ipsilateral wrist and shoulder.
   (b) Inspection and palpation of the distal humerus.
   - Skin exam: swelling, bruising, and lacerations/abrasions.
   - Is this open or closed?
     - Particularly important in the elderly patient who may be treated with a TEA.
4. Neurological exam:
   (a) Ulnar nerve: most commonly injured.
   - FCU, finger adductors, interossei, and small/ring finger sensibility.
   (b) Radial nerve: posterior/lateral lacerations or lateral column injuries.
   - Wrist and finger dorsiflexion; first webspace sensibility.
   (c) Median nerve: deep anterior lacerations.
   - Opponens pollicis function and palmar sensibility.
5. Vascular exam.
   (a) Concern for brachial artery injury; palpate radial pulse at minimum.
   - Low likelihood, but concern with an anterior open fracture and/or loss of median nerve function.
   - May perform brachial-brachial index: Normal approximately 0.95.
     - Vascular consultation if abnormal.
   (b) Concern for compartment syndrome particularly in the young patient with a high energy mechanism.
   - May require serial examinations; have low threshold for fasciotomies to avoid Volkmann's ischemic contracture.
6. Imaging.
   (a) X-rays (views): AP, lateral, oblique [16].
   - Preferably without a splint in place.
   - Consider traction views to further delineate intra-articular fragments.
     - May be performed under sedation or at time of operative management.
     - Make sure to image entire humerus and forearm.
     - If significant shortening, rotation, or angulation is present, can perform traction views under conscious or at the time of fixation.
     - Traction views are helpful to evaluate reduction and ligamentous integrity.
   (b) Classification.
   - Milch classification (Fig. 23.1)
     - Single column fracture.
   - Jupiter classification (Figs. 23.2 and 23.3).
     - Two column fractures.
   - AO/OTA (Fig. 23.4).

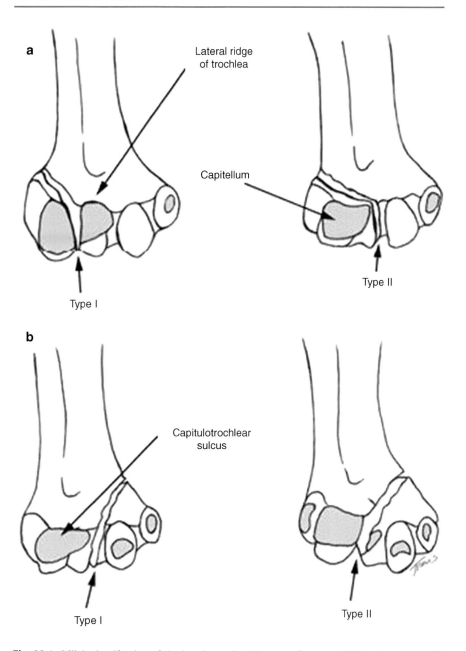

**Fig. 23.1** Milch classification of single column distal humerus fractures: (**a**) lateral condyle; (**b**) Medial condyle. Type 1 lateral condyle fractures involve the capitellum only and are stable. Type 2 involves the capitellum and a portion of the trochlea and is unstable. Type 1 medial condyle fractures involve a split within the trochlear grove; type 2 medial fracture involves the entire trochlear portion (Milch et al. [17])

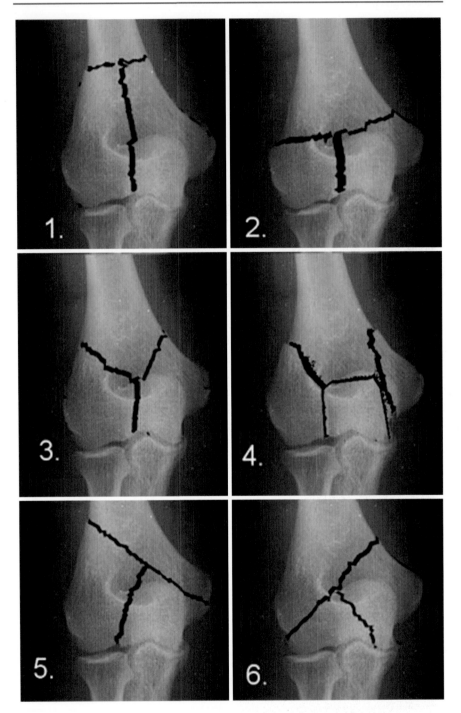

**Fig. 23.2** Jupiter classification of bicolumnar distal humerus fractures: (1) a t-split fracture at or above the tip of the olecranon, (2) a low t-split at the apex of the trochlea, (3) a "Y"-shaped split, (4) an "H"-shaped fracture that carries a high risk of AVN for the free-floating trochlea, (5) medial lambda pattern, and (6) lateral lambda pattern (Jupiter et al. [4])

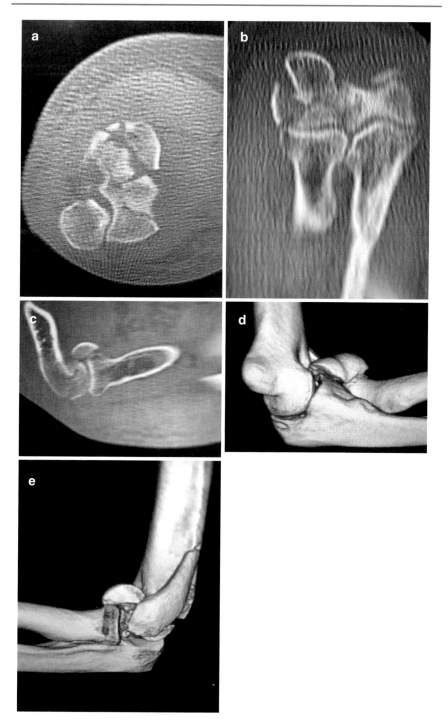

**Fig. 23.3** CT scan of multiplane Jupiter T-Type with coronal fracture—(**a**) axial, (**b**) coronal, and (**c**, **d**, and **e**) sagittal images

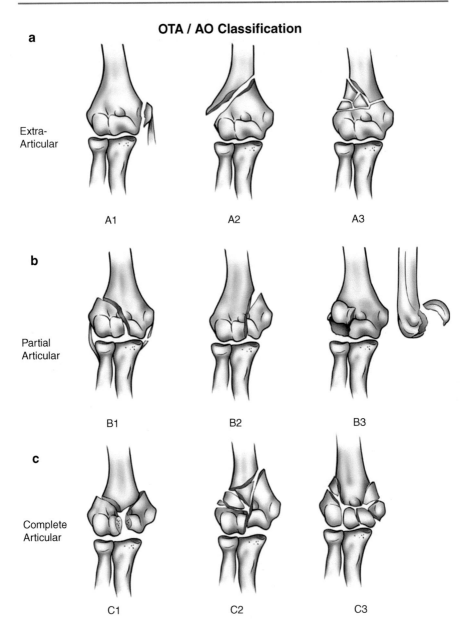

**Fig. 23.4** OTA classification: (**a**) extra-articular, (**b**) partial articular, and (**c**) complete articular fracture (Mckee et al. Distal humerus fractures in adults [14])

(c) CT.
- Assists in operative approach and planning.
- Helpful when there is severe comminution in elderly.
  - Assist in operative planning between ORIF and TEA.
  - Three dimensional reconstructions may be most beneficial with severe comminution.

7. Treatment

Open fractures should receive first generation cephalosporin with addition of aminoglycoside in the instance of a Gustilo-Anderson type III open fracture

- Make sure tetanus is up to date.
- Irrigate at bedside.
- Plan for formal irrigation and debridement.
- Splint in a position of comfort using long arm posterior splint with or without medial and lateral struts prior to definitive fixation.

(a) Nonoperative indications.

- Rare in young patients: only if they are unfit for surgery: hemodynamic instability, severe TBI, etc.
- "Bag of bones" treatment
  - Geriatric, low demand patients for whom surgery is contraindicated.
  - Well-padded splinting then gradual bracing and therapy for range of motion.
- Nondisplaced fractures.
  - Serial radiographs weekly for 4 weeks.
  - Cast and brace immobilization.
  - Gradual range of motion therapy upon consolidation.
- AO B3: Partial articular fracture.
  - Reduction technique.
    Elbow in full extension, forearm in supination.
    Immobilized in above elbow plaster for 3 weeks with weekly radiographs.
    Postreduction CT.
- Definitive casting.
  - Lateral condylar fractures = supination.
  - Medial condylar fractures = pronation.
- Outcomes: Higher pain scores, decreased function compared with operative cohort [1, 14].

(b) Operative treatment.

- Open reduction and internal fixation.
  - No consensus regarding orthogonal plating versus parallel plating.
  - Precontoured anatomic plates make either orthogonal plating or parallel plating easier by assisting with the reduction.
  - Goal is to obtain rigid fixation with anatomic articular reduction to allow early joint mobilization.
  - Technical objectives:
    Rigid articular surface reconstruction.
    Cannulated or solid lag screws.
    Align columns to distal portion then to each other.
    May shorten and bone graft metaphyseal zone.
    Crossed columnar screws may be used for low demand elderly patients.
  - O'Driscoll Mayo Technique: [2]
    All screws through plate.
    Each screw captures distal fragment that is fixed by a plate as well.

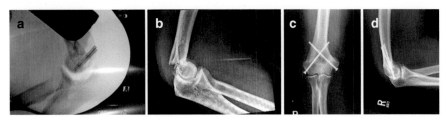

**Fig. 23.5** (**a**) Intraoperative lateral X-ray of an arthroscopic-assisted capitellar shear fixation and (**b**) lateral X-ray of low supracondylar humerus fracture in an adult treated with percutaneous screws (**c** and **d**)

> As many screws in distal fragments.
> Longest screw possible.
> Capture the most possible articular fragments with each screw.
> Interdigitate screws in distal fragment.
> Plate compression achieved at supracondylar level.
> Plates need to be stiff and strong enough.

- Arthroscopy and percutaneous fixation.
  - Very uncommon, narrow indications.
    Isolated capitellar fractures.
    Low transverse extra-articular fractures in adults (Fig. 23.5).
- Total elbow arthroplasty.
  - Indications.
    Geriatric patient.
    Poor bone density.
    Comminuted, bicolumnar fractures.
    Allows for early mobilization and activities of daily living (ADLs), especially when performed with a "triceps on" approach [12–14].
  - Disadvantages.
    Lifetime lifting restriction.
    Concern for prosthesis failure.
      Survivability is improved with preservation of the condyles.

- Postoperative management.
  - Relies heavily on approach (Table 23.1).
    If olecranon osteotomy is used, longer period of immobilization is necessary.
    Extensor mechanism sparing approaches may begin passive ROM of the elbow within the first 7 days.
    If triceps splitting approach is used, consider prolonged avoidance of resisted elbow extension maneuvers.
  - It is imperative to begin early ROM in order to avoid a stiff elbow.

**Table 23.1** Approaches: largely determined by fracture location [12]

| Posterior | Lateral | Medial | Anterior |
|---|---|---|---|
| • Olecranon osteotomy<br>– Indications:<br>  Articular surface involvement<br>– Advantages:<br>  Best to see articular surface.<br>  Useful for AO/OTA type 3.<br>  Develop plane medially along the intermuscular septum and cubital tunnel, laterally along Kocher's interval<br>– Disadvantages:<br>  Osteotomy nonunion<br>  Prominent hardware with osteotomy reduction.<br>*Not ideal if considering TEA* | • Kocher<br>– Indications, lateral column type fracture<br>  Milch type 1, Milch type 2<br>  If ipsilateral radial head/neck fracture requires intervention<br>  Interval is between the extensor carpi ulnaris and the anconeus<br>  Pronation helps to move the PIN out of the operative field<br>  Brachioradialis can be released off of lateral supracondylar ridge for better exposure of capitellum and radial head | • Taylor and Schamm<br>– Indication<br>  Medial column fractures<br>  Elevate entire FCU and flexor pronator mass from posterior to anterior<br>  If MCL involvement; dissect from distal to proximal to avoid injury<br>  Split between FCU heads after transposing ulnar nerve can be used to access medial facet<br>– Advantages:<br>  Good visualization of coronoid and trochlea<br>– Disadvantages<br>  Poor lateral column exposure | • Henry<br>– Indication<br>  Rare instance involving neurovascular injury (brachial a.; median n.)<br>– Advantage<br>  Articular surface exposure<br>  Visualization of NV structures<br>  The interval is between the biceps tendon and pronator teres. The lateral dissection is between the radial nerve and the brachialis<br>  The lateral antebrachial cutaneous and radial nerves are at risk on the lateral side while the median nerve and brachial artery are at risk medially<br>– Disadvantage<br>  Poor column access |

(continued)

**Table 23.1** (continued)

| Posterior | Lateral | Medial | Anterior |
|---|---|---|---|
| • Triceps splitting<br>  – Indications<br>    Tea<br>    Intra-articular or extra-articular fractures<br>    Split midline between triceps tendon and medial head of triceps<br>    Proximal extent is radial nerve<br>    Distal exposure can be extended by elevating the triceps off of the olecranon through Sharpey's fibers<br>  – Advantages<br>    Unlike olecranon osteotomy, no concern for nonunion at osteotomy site<br>  – Disadvantages<br>    Less articular exposure<br>    Triceps insufficiency<br>• Triceps sparing<br>  – Indications<br>    Tea<br>    Distal periarticular and articular fractures<br>    Lateral extension is taken through Kocher's interval; medial extension is taken into the flexor/pronator split<br>  – Advantages: Early mobilization as the triceps is intact, no risk of hardware complications or nonunion; easy to convert to a total elbow<br>  – Disadvantages: Mirror triceps splitting with potentially limited articular exposure | • Kaplan<br>  – Indications<br>    Similar to Kocher<br>    Radial head fracture requiring intervention<br>    The interval is between the extensor carpi radialis brevis and extensor digitorum communis<br>    PIN and LABC nerves are at risk | | |

Risk and complications

1. Stiffness.
2. Neurovascular injury.
   (a) Ulnar nerve can be subject to delayed onset ulnar neuropathy (DOUN); therefore, a simple in situ decompression may be warranted at the time of surgery.
   (b) Radial nerve injury can occur with prolonged tourniquet time but is often transitory.
3. Heterotopic ossification prophylaxis is recommended in cases of associated head injury or poly trauma.

# References

1. Srinivasan K, Agarwal M, Matthews SJ, Giannoudis PV. Fractures of the distal humerus in the elderly: is internal fixation the treatment of choice? Clin Orthop Relat Res. 2005;434:222–30.
2. O'Driscoll SW. Optimizing stability in distal humeral fracture fixation. J Shoulder Elb Surg. 2005;14(1 Suppl S):186S–94S.
3. Barco R, Streubel PN, Morrey BF, Sanchez-Sotelo J. Total elbow arthroplasty for distal humeral fractures: a ten-year-minimum follow-up study. J Bone Joint Surg Am. 2017;99(18):1524–31. https://doi.org/10.2106/JBJS.16.01222.
4. Jupiter JB, Mehne DK. Fractures of the distal humerus. Orthopedics. 1992;15(7):825–33.
5. Nauth A, McKee MD, Ristevski B, Hall J, Schemitsch EH. Distal humeral fractures in adults. J Bone Joint Surg Am. 2011;93(7):686–700. https://doi.org/10.2106/JBJS.J.00845.
6. Helfet DL, Hotchkiss RN. Internal fixation of the distal humerus: a biomechanical comparison of methods. J Orthop Trauma. 1990;4(3):260–4.
7. Bryan RS, Morrey BF. Extensive posterior exposure of the elbow. A triceps-sparing approach. Clin Orthop Relat Res. 1982;166:188–92.
8. Campbell WC. Incision for exposure of the elbow joint. Am J Surg. 1932;15:65–7.
9. Coles CP, Barei DP, Nork SE, et al. The olecranon osteotomy: a six-year experience in the treatment of intraarticular fractures of the distal humerus. J Orthop Trauma. 2006;20(3):164–71.
10. Taylor TK, Scham SM. A posteromedial approach to the proximal end of the ulna for the internal fixation of olecranon fractures. J Trauma. 1969;9(7):594–602.
11. Henry AK. Extensile exposure applied to limb surgery. Baltimore: Williams & Wilkins; 1945.
12. Pollock JW, Athwal GS, Steinmann SP. Surgical exposures for distal humerus fractures: a review. Clin Anat. 2008;21(8):757–68. https://doi.org/10.1002/ca.20720.
13. Barco R, Streubel PN, Morrey BF, et al. Total elbow arthroplasty for distal humeral fractures: a ten-year-minimum follow-up study. J Bone Joint Surg Am. 2017;99(18):1524–31.
14. McKee MD, Veillette CJ, Hall JA, Schemitsch EH, Wild LM, McCormack R, Perey B, Goetz T, Zomar M, Moon K, Mandel S, Petit S, Guy P, Leung I. A multicenter, prospective, randomized, controlled trial of open reduction--internal fixation versus total elbow arthroplasty for displaced intra-articular distal humeral fractures in elderly patients. J Shoulder Elb Surg. 2009;18(1):3–12. https://doi.org/10.1016/j.jse.2008.06.005; Epub 2008 Sep 26.
15. MacAusland WR. Ankylosis of the elbow: with report of four cases treated by arthroplasty. JAMA. 1915;64(4):312–8.
16. Williams JR, Wainwright AM, Carr AJ. Interobserver and intraobserver variation in classification systems for fractures of the distal humerus. J Bone Joint Surg Br. 2000;82(5):636.
17. Milch H. Fractures and fracture dislocations of the humeral condyles. J Trauma. 1964;4:592–607.

# Monteggia Fractures

# 24

Carl M. Cirino and Brad O. Parsons

## Introduction

- Classically involves a proximal ulna fracture with an associated radial head dislocation.
- Affect children and adults alike, with specific management options in each subset.
- Presence of radial head or neck fractures, coronoid fractures, and/or proximal ulna comminution elevates the complexity of surgical reconstruction.
- Historically, the outcomes seen in Monteggia injuries have been suboptimal and improved clinical results more recently.

## History

1. Accounts for approximately 5–7% of forearm fractures [1].
2. First described by Giovanni Battista Monteggia in 1814.
3. Typically result of low-energy fall in elderly or high-energy blunt trauma in younger patients [2].
4. Involves not only proximal ulna fracture but also important soft-tissue disruptions including annular ligament, quadrate ligament, and interosseous membrane as result of radial head dislocation [3].
5. Classified by Jose Luis Bado in 1958 (Table 24.1 and Fig. 24.1), which also describes mechanism of injury:
   (a) The Bado type II fractures further subclassified by Jupiter in 1991 [4] (Table 24.2, Figs. 24.2 and 24.5).

C. M. Cirino (✉) · B. O. Parsons
Department of Orthopedics, Mount Sinai Health System, New York, NY, USA
e-mail: carl.cirino@mountsinai.org; Bradford.Parsons@mountsinai.org

**Table 24.1** Bado classification

| Bado classification | | |
| --- | --- | --- |
| Type | Description | Mechanism |
| I | Anterior dislocation of radial head with apex anterior angulation of ulnar shaft fracture (most common in pediatric population) | Forced pronation of the forearm |
| II | Posterior or posterolateral dislocation with apex posterior angular of ulnar shaft | Axial loading of the forearm with flexed elbow |
| III | Lateral/anterolateral dislocation with fracture of ulnar metaphysis (more common in children) | Forced abduction of the arm |
| IV | Anterior dislocation with fractures of both ulna and radius | Similar to type I |

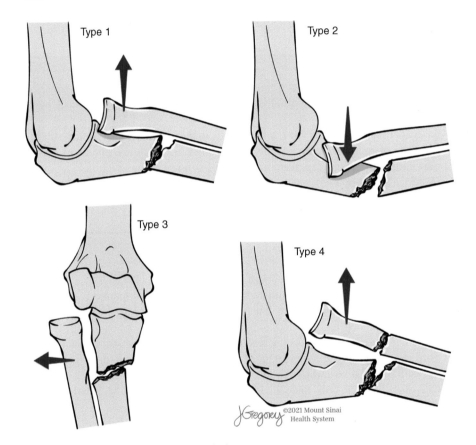

**Fig. 24.1** Bado classification of Monteggia fractures

6. Ask about prior elbow function, history of trauma or other potential injuries (shoulder, wrist, and head trauma).
7. High incidence of missed fractures in children due to potential for plastic deformation over complete fracture [5].

**Table 24.2**   Jupiter modification of Bado type II fracture-dislocations

| Jupiter classification of Bado II fracture-dislocations | |
| --- | --- |
| Type | Description |
| IIa | Ulna fracture at level of coronoid |
| IIb | Ulna fracture at metaphyseal-diaphyseal junction (distal to coronoid) |
| IIc | Ulna fracture at diaphysis |
| IId | Ulna fracture at trochlear notch with extension to metaphysis and separate coronoid fragment |

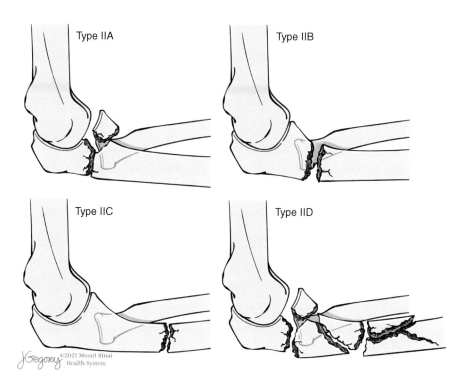

**Fig. 24.2**   Jupiter subclassification of Bado type II Monteggia fractures

## Physical Exam

1. *Inspection.*
   (a) Assess for ecchymosis, swelling, skin tenting, lacerations, and deformity.
      - High incidence of open fractures due to lack of soft tissue along length of ulna.
   (b) Assess shoulder, humerus, wrist and hand, and forearm/elbow for associated injuries.

2. *Palpation.*
    (a) Tenderness along the ulna due to fracture and the elbow due to the radial head dislocation.
3. *Range of motion.*
    (a) Both active and passive range of motion will be severely limited due to pain and in general should be avoided.
    (b) The ability to perform elbow flexion/extension will be dependent upon the morphology of the proximal ulna fracture (i.e., involvement of the coronoid).
    (c) Pronosupination will also be limited, especially in the setting of associated radial head or neck fractures.
4. *Strength/neurovascular exam.*
    (a) High incidence of nerve injury, especially PIN due to its proximity to the radial head [6].
    (b) Motor and sensory exam.
        • Radial/PIN function via thumb interphalangeal (IP) joint extension.
            – If absent, check wrist extension.
            – If radial nerve is functioning, there will be radial deviation of the wrist.
        • Medial/AIN function via thumb IP flexion.
            – If absent, it can be difficult to differentiate high versus low median nerve injury with motor exam alone.
            – AIN is primarily motor; therefore, the loss of sensation would suggest high median nerve injury but may warrant additional studies (EMG).

## Imaging

1. *XR.*
    (a) Standard anterior-posterior and lateral radiographs of elbow, forearm, and wrist.
        • Internal and external obliques of the elbow can be considered.
    (b) Assess radiocapitellar line on all views (Fig. 24.3) [7–9].
        • Line along the intramedullary canal of the ulna should intersect the middle of the capitellum.
    (c) Children may present with plastic deformation to the ulna (Fig. 24.4).
        • Dorsal surface of the ulna should be straight, and just 0.1 mm of displacement is associated radial head subluxation [10].
    (d) Assess the proximal radioulnar joint (PRUJ) to differentiate Monteggia fracture-dislocations from trans-olecranon fracture-dislocations.
        • PRUJ will be intact in trans-olecranon injuries but disrupted in Monteggias.
    (e) Assess ulno-humeral for incongruity, which may suggest additional injuries to the medial or lateral ulnar collateral ligaments.

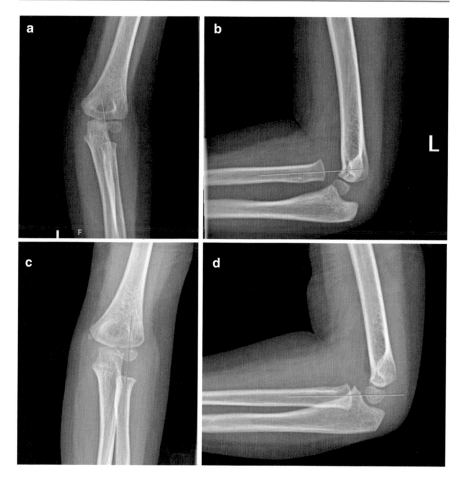

**Fig. 24.3** Radiocapitellar line. Figure **a** and **b** demonstrates disruption of the radiocapitellar line as seen on the AP and lateral views, respectively. In figures **c** and **d**, the line is intact

2. *CT.*
   (a) Low threshold to obtain CT.
       • Three-dimensional reconstruction can be essential to surgical planning.
       • Assessment of the presence and/or morphology of coronoid fractures, radial head/neck fractures, and ulnar comminution.
   (b) Children typically present with simple ulna fractures and therefore advanced imaging is not essential.
3. *MRI.*
   (a) Helpful in assessment of ulnar collateral ligaments if concomitant ulno-humeral instability is suspected.

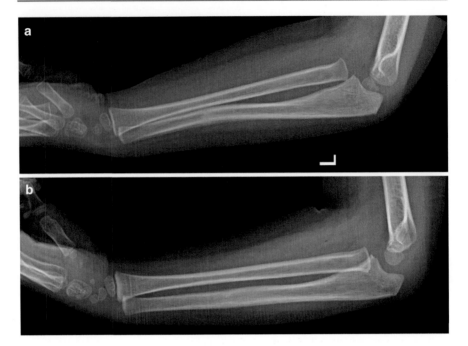

**Fig. 24.4** Figure **a** is an example of plastic deformation of the ulna with an associated radial head dislocation. This can be a subtle finding and radiographs in children with elbow pain require extra-scrutiny. Figure **b** is a postreduction radiograph in which the alignment of the ulna has been restored and the radiocapitellar joint is reduced

## Treatment

1. *Principles.*
   (a) Restoration of ulnar length and alignment should reduce radial head via ligamentotaxis.
   (b) If radial head does not spontaneously reduce, principal cause is ulnar malre-duction, not interposition of soft tissues within radiocapitellar joint [11, 12]:
      • Only after careful assessment of ulnar reduction should opening of radio-capitellar joint be considered.
   (c) Nonoperative management has a role in selecting pediatric fractures, but little to no role in adult fractures.
2. *Pediatric Injuries.*
   (a) Acute incomplete fractures (Fig. 24.4).
      • Generally stable and amenable to closed reduction and long-arm cast-ing [13].
         – Should be performed under conscious sedation or general anesthesia.
      • Fluoroscopy should be utilized to ensure restoration of the radiocapitellar and alignment of the ulnar shaft line prior to casting.

- Requires frequent (weekly) monitoring for displacement.
    - Loss of reduction can be related to residual malalignment, interposition of soft-tissues, or lack of compliance.
- Long-arm cast immobilization for 4–6 weeks depending on age and morphology.
(b) Acute complete fractures (and recurrent incomplete fractures).
- Short-oblique or transverse ulnar shaft fractures treated with intramedullary fixation [14].
    - Typically, with flexible titanium nails via anterograde triceps splitting approach.
    - Open reduction at ulnar fracture site may be required to remove periosteum or other soft-tissues.
    - While anatomic reduction is essential in adults, children can tolerate some residual deformity due to remodeling potential.
- Long-oblique or comminuted ulnar shaft fractures treated with plate-screw constructs.
    - Approach via longitudinal incision along the dorsal subcutaneous border of ulna.
    - While adults require 3.5 mm LCP plating, one-third tubular may suffice in smaller children as long as fixation in 4–6 cortices is obtained in proximal and distal segments [14]:
    - Multiple plates in orthogonal planes may be warranted in severely comminuted fractures.
    - Plates are often symptomatic and removed after fracture healing has occurred.
- May require open debridement of radiocapitellar joint via Kaplan or Kocher approach due to interposition of annular ligament or other soft tissues.
- Long-arm casting until radiographic union of the ulna is present.
(c) Chronic or missed fractures.
- Unfortunately missed in up to 1/3 of injuries [5].
    - Considered chronic after >4 weeks due to rapid healing in children.
- Requires ulnar osteotomy via dorsal approach.
    - Some advocate for overcorrection to maintain radiocapitellar stability.
    - Plating similar to acute, complete fractures.
- May require open debridement of radiocapitellar joint via Kaplan or Kocher approach due to fibrous scar tissue or interposition of annular ligament or other soft tissues.
- Role of annular ligament reconstruction is controversial.
- Long-arm casting for 6 weeks.
3. *Adult Injuries.*
(a) Ulnar shaft fracture (Fig. 24.5):
- Approached via dorsal incision along subcutaneous border of ulna.
    - Can extend proximally over olecranon with either curved or straight incision.

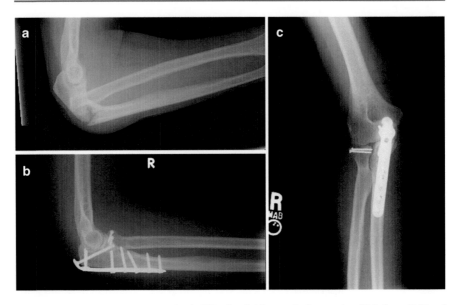

**Fig. 24.5** Figure **a** demonstrates an Bado II/Jupiter B Monteggia fracture in which the radial head is dislocated posteriorly and the ulna fracture is at the diaphyseal-metaphyseal junction distal to the coronoid. There is an associated radial head fracture. Figures **b** and **c** represents open reduction internal fixation of the fracture-dislocation using modern instrumentation with headless compression screws in the radial head and a pre-contoured proximal ulna locking plate

– Develop interval between flexor and extensor musculature and elevate subperiosteally.
– Must identify and consider transposition of ulnar nerve as necessary.
• Fixation with standard or proximal ulna-specific 3.5 mm LCP plate along dorsal surface [15–17].
– Proximal contour around olecranon allows for longer screws in multiple planes.
• Additional small fragment plates can be used in severely comminuted fractures.
(b) Coronoid fractures.
• Can range from small, capsular avulsions to large, basal fractures.
– Failure to address coronoid associated with fixation failure and inferior outcomes [17].
• Visualization and reduction either through mobilization of olecranon fracture or by elevating flexor muscle mass.
• Small, capsular avulsions can be fixed with a suture lasso technique.
• Larger fragments can be temporarily stabilized with K-wires and fixed with a separate coronoid plate, screw fixation, or integration into the dorsal plate construct.
– In the setting of severely comminuted coronoid fractures, iliac crest autograft or allografts may be considered.

(c) Radial head and neck fractures (Fig. 24.5).
   • Should be addressed after fixation of ulnar fracture.
   • Addressed via Kaplan or Kocher approach.
       – Modified Boyd approach can be utilized but is associated with high incidence of synostosis.
   • Fixation depends upon fracture morphology.
       – Mason 1 fractures can be treated nonoperatively.
       – Mason 2 and 3 fractures should be fixed via internal fixation (headless compression screws, small or mini-fragment instrumentation) [18–20].
       – Must be cognizant of 110° nonarticulating "safe-zone" for implants.
   • Radial head arthroplasty may be required for fractures that are unable to be constructed.
(d) Ulnohumeral instability.
   • Most common in Bado 2 fractures [21].
   • With LCL injury, primary repair is usually possible.
   • MUCL injuries benefit from the use of an internal joint stabilizer, external fixator, or trans-articular pins over acute MUCL repair/reconstruction.
(e) Postoperative management.
   • Splint immobilization for ~2 weeks followed by initiation of physical therapy:
       – In cases of ulnohumeral instability or significant comminution, prolonged immobilization may be warranted but should be weighed against the risk of post-operative stiffness.
   • Hardware removal is common as the ulnar plate can be symptomatic.
4. *Risks and Complications.*
   (a) High complication rate regardless of operative or nonoperative intervention [15, 16, 22].
       • Upward of 50% in some series of experienced surgeons.
       • Higher complication rates with Jupiter 2A and 2D morphologies.
   (b) Most common: post-traumatic stiffness, nonunion, malunion, early fixation failure, persistent radiocapitellar or ulnohumeral instability, nerve palsy, heterotopic ossification, radioulnar synostosis, painful or symptomatic hardware, and infection [4, 14, 16].

## References

1. Reckling FW, Cordell LD. Unstable fracture-dislocations of the forearm. The Monteggia and Galeazzi lesions. Arch Surg. 1968;96(6):999–1007.
2. Rehim SA, Maynard MA, Sebastin SJ, Chung KC. Monteggia fracture dislocations: a historical review. J Hand Surg Am. 2014;39(7):1384–94.
3. Givon U, Pritsch M, Levy O, Yosepovich A, Amit Y, Horoszowski H. Monteggia and equivalent lesions. A study of 41 cases. Clin Orthop Relat Res. 1997;337:208–15.
4. Jupiter JB, Leibovic SJ, Ribbans W, Wilk RM. The posterior Monteggia lesion. J Orthop Trauma. 1991;5(4):395–402.

5. Goyal T, Arora SS, Banerjee S, Kandwal P. Neglected Monteggia fracture dislocations in children: a systematic review. J Pediatr Orthop B. 2015;24(3):191–9.
6. Stein F, Grabias SL, Deffer PA. Nerve injuries complicating Monteggia lesions. J Bone Joint Surg Am. 1971;53(7):1432–6.
7. Miles KA, Finlay DB. Disruption of the radiocapitellar line in the normal elbow. Injury. 1989;20(6):365–7.
8. Ramirez RN, Ryan DD, Williams J, et al. A line drawn along the radial shaft misses the capitellum in 16% of radiographs of normal elbows. J Pediatr Orthop. 2014;34(8):763–7.
9. Kunkel S, Cornwall R, Little K, Jain V, Mehlman C, Tamai J. Limitations of the radiocapitellar line for assessment of pediatric elbow radiographs. J Pediatr Orthop. 2011;31(6):628–32.
10. Lincoln TL, Mubarak SJ. "Isolated" traumatic radial-head dislocation. J Pediatr Orthop. 1994;14(4):454–7.
11. Jennings JD, Hahn A, Rehman S, Haydel C. Management of adult elbow fracture dislocations. Orthop Clin North Am. 2016;47(1):97–113.
12. Eglseder WA, Zadnik M. Monteggia fractures and variants: review of distribution and nine irreducible radial head dislocations. South Med J. 2006;99(7):723–7.
13. Ramski DE, Hennrikus WP, Bae DS, et al. Pediatric monteggia fractures: a multicenter examination of treatment strategy and early clinical and radiographic results. J Pediatr Orthop. 2015;35(2):115–20.
14. Ring D, Jupiter JB, Waters PM. Monteggia fractures in children and adults. J Am Acad Orthop Surg. 1998;6(4):215–24.
15. Ring D. Monteggia fractures. Orthop Clin North Am. 2013;44(1):59–66.
16. Konrad GG, Kundel K, Kreuz PC, Oberst M, Sudkamp NP. Monteggia fractures in adults: long-term results and prognostic factors. J Bone Joint Surg Br. 2007;89(3):354–60.
17. Ring D, Jupiter JB, Simpson NS. Monteggia fractures in adults. J Bone Joint Surg Am. 1998;80(12):1733–44.
18. Klug A, Konrad F, Gramlich Y, Hoffmann R, Schmidt-Horlohe K. Surgical treatment of the radial head is critical to the outcome of Monteggia-like lesions. Bone Joint J. 2019;101-B(12):1512–9.
19. Sun H, Duan J, Li F. Comparison between radial head arthroplasty and open reduction and internal fixation in patients with radial head fractures (modified Mason type III and IV): a meta-analysis. Eur J Orthop Surg Traumatol. 2016;26(3):283–91.
20. Zarattini G, Galli S, Marchese M, Mascio LD, Pazzaglia UE. The surgical treatment of isolated mason type 2 fractures of the radial head in adults: comparison between radial head resection and open reduction and internal fixation. J Orthop Trauma. 2012;26(4):229–35.
21. Strauss EJ, Tejwani NC, Preston CF, Egol KA. The posterior Monteggia lesion with associated ulnohumeral instability. J Bone Joint Surg Br. 2006;88(1):84–9.
22. Guitton TG, Ring D, Kloen P. Long-term evaluation of surgically treated anterior monteggia fractures in skeletally mature patients. J Hand Surg Am. 2009;34(9):1618–24.

# Radial Head Fractures

Brenton P. Hill and Derek J. Cuff

## History

- Injury typically related to a fall on the outstretched arm.
- Important to assess for ipsilateral shoulder, forearm, wrist, and hand pain as possible concomitant injuries can occur.
- Patient will localize pain on the lateral aspect of the elbow joint and proximal forearm [1–4].
- Flexion/extension of the elbow and pronation/supination of forearm cause pain due to hemarthrosis or mechanical blocks in motion [3].
- Important to inquire about any neurologic symptoms to the wrist and hand.

## Physical Exam

1. *Inspection/Palpation.*
   - (a) Tender to palpation over the lateral aspect of the elbow joint, radial head [1–4].
   - (b) Varying degrees of swelling and/or ecchymosis may be present, which correlate with degree of ligamentous injury [3].
   - (c) Palpate lateral epicondyle for associated lateral collateral ligament injuries and medial epicondyle/sublime tubercle for associated medial collateral ligament injuries [1].
   - (d) Palpate forearm, interosseous membrane, distal radioulnar joint, and wrist for associated injuries, such as Essex-Lopresti injuries [1].

B. P. Hill (✉)
University of South Florida, Florida Orthopaedic Institute, Tampa, FL, USA
e-mail: bhill@usf.edu

D. J. Cuff
Suncoast Orthopedic Surgery and Sports Medicine, Venice, FL, USA

2. *Range of Motion.*
   (a) Passive and active flexion/extension of the elbow and pronation/supination of the forearm are painful due to intracapsular hematoma in acute injuries [2].
   (b) Note mechanical blocks to motion before and after hematoma aspiration and injection of local anesthetic [1–4]. If range of motion is still limited after this procedure, a mechanical block is more likely [1].
   (c) Small limitations in flexion/extension are common due to hemarthrosis and do not necessarily indicate a mechanical block to motion that needs surgical treatment [1].
3. *Strength Testing.*
   (a) Complete neurovascular exam of the extremity should be performed, although neurovascular injuries are rarely associated with isolated radial head fractures [1].
   (b) AIN: ask patient to flex the interphalangeal joint of the thumb (A-OK sign), assessing the flexor pollicis longus muscle.
   (c) PIN: ask patient to extend the metacarpophalangeal joint of the thumb (thumbs up), assessing the extensor pollicis longus muscle.
   (d) Ulnar nerve: ask the patient the cross their fingers, assessing the interosseous muscles of the hand.
   (e) Sensation should be tested in the median, radial, and ulnar nerve distributions.
4. *Directed Tests Based on History or Mechanism of Injury.*
   Aspiration of intracapsular hematoma and injection of local anesthetic:
   (a) Aids in diagnosis of mechanical blocks to motion [1, 2].
   (b) Using a sterile technique, a needle is inserted into the lateral "soft spot" of the elbow formed by a triangle between the lateral epicondyle, olecranon, and radial head, and hematoma is aspirated [1, 2] (Fig. 25.1).

**Fig. 25.1** Image demonstrating the "soft spot" of the elbow formed by a triangle between the lateral epicondyle, olecranon, and radial head

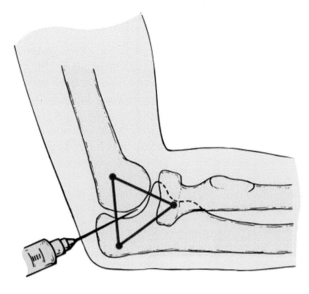

(c) Pronate forearm to avoid injury to the radial nerve [1].

(d) About 10 cc of 1% lidocaine is injected into the elbow joint, and elbow range of motion is assessed [2].

## Imaging (What to Order and When) (Need High Quality Imaging)

1. *X-rays (views).*
   (a) AP, lateral, and oblique radiographs of the injured elbow.
   (b) Oblique radiocapitellar view places the radial head in profile (lateral view with beam positioned 45 degrees cephalad) (Fig. 25.2) [1].
   (c) Postreduction films must be obtained after reduction of any elbow dislocation [2].
   (d) Bilateral PA wrist films in patients with wrist or forearm pain to evaluate ulnar variance to evaluate for interosseous membrane injury [1].

**Fig. 25.2** Oblique radiocapitellar

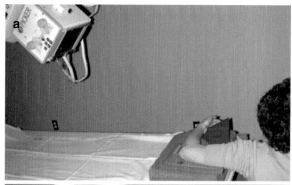
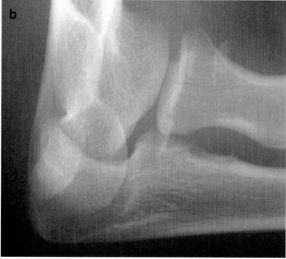

   (e) In nondisplaced fractures, anterior and/or posterior fat pads may be present
      (Fig. 25.3) [1].

   (f) Mason classification of radial head fractures (Fig. 25.4) [5]

2. *MRI.*

   (a) To evaluate for associated collateral ligament injury, rarely indicated

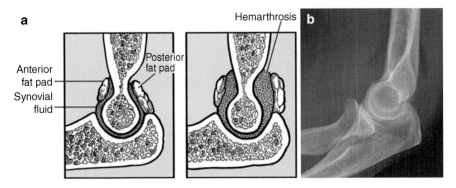

**Fig. 25.3** Anterior and posterior fat pad signs may indicate occult injuries to the elbow

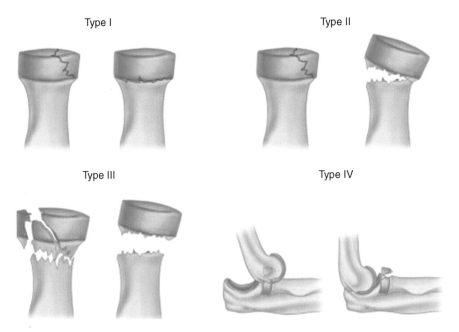

**Fig. 25.4** I: Minimally displaced (<2 mm), no mechanical block to motion. II: Displaced (>2 mm). III: Comminuted, multifragmented. IV: Associated with elbow dislocation

3. *CT scan*
   (a) May be useful to further delineate injury patterns, comminution, degree of displacement, and fragment size in cases where indications for surgery are less clear [1]
   (b) Preoperative planning
4. *Ultrasound.*
   (a) Rarely indicated view of the elbow. Image is obtained with a lateral view of the elbow with the beam positioned 45 degrees cephalad.

## Treatment

1. *Nonoperative treatment.*
   (a) Indicated in all type I and II fractures without mechanical blocks to motion [2]
   (b) Sling for comfort, early range mobilization within 1 week to avoid stiffness [1, 2]
   (c) Important to institute early range of motion as elbow stiffness a complication of prolonged immobilization.
2. *Operative treatment.*
   (a) *Surgical options* (Fig. 25.5).
      • Open reduction internal fixation (type II and type III able to obtain stable fixation) [1].

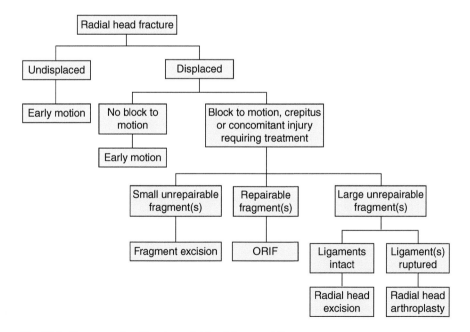

**Fig. 25.5** Treatment algorithm for radial head fractures [1]

- "Safe zone" for placement of hardware: region of radial head and neck that does not articulate with the proximal radioulnar joint [2]. Marked by 90 degree arc with the midpoint directly lateral with the arm in neutral [3]
- Radial head arthroplasty for non-reconstructable fractures.
- Radial head excision (can lead to wrist symptoms due to proximal migration of the radius and longitudinal instability).
- Fragment excision if <25% involvement and stable elbow after excision.

(b) *Surgical approaches* [2].
- Kocher (anconeus and ECU).
- Kaplan (ECRB and EDC).
- Medial approach to elbow if associated medial-sided injury.
- Direct posterior approach if need to address medial and lateral sides.
- Structures at risk:
- PIN: pronate forearm when performing lateral approaches to the elbow to avoid injury.
- Radial nerve.
- Lateral collateral ligament complex.
- Recurrent radial artery.
- Lateral antebrachial cutaneous nerve.
- Postoperative care: splint and sling for comfort, early gentle range of motion exercises after 1 week.

(c) *Risks and complications* [6].
- Malunion.
- Nonunion.
- Limited forearm rotation.
- Overlengthening/poor sizing (radial head arthroplasty).
- Infection.

## References

1. Wolfe SW, Hotchkiss RN, Pederson WC, et al. Fractures of the radial head. In: Green's operative hand surgery. Philadelphia, PA: Elsevier; 2017. p. 734–69.
2. Browner BD, Jupiter JB, Krettek C, Anderson P. Trauma to the adult elbow. In: Skeletal trauma: basic science, management, and reconstruction. Philadelphia, PA: Elsevier/Saunders; 2020. p. 1470–87.
3. Bucholz RW, MacQueen M, Rockwood CA, Green DP. Elbow fractures and dislocations. In: Rockwood and Green's fractures in adults. Philadelphia, PA: Wolters Kluwer/Lippincott Williams & Wilkins; 2010.
4. Morrey BF. Radial head fracture: general considerations, conservative treatment, and radial head resection. In: Morrey's the elbow and its disorders. New York, NY: Elsevier; 2018. p. 375–87.
5. Canale ST, Azar FM, Beaty JH, Campbell WC. Fractures of the shoulder, arm, and forearm. In: Campbell's operative orthopaedics. 13th ed. Philadelphia, PA: Elsevier, Inc.; 2017. p. 2927–3016.
6. Morrey BF. Radial head fracture: management of complications after treatment. In: Morrey's the elbow and its disorders. New York, NY: Elsevier; 2018. p. 403–9.

# Terrible Triad of the Elbow

# 26

Roman Ashmyan and Cyrus Lashgari

Essential Steps:

- Open reduction and internal fixation (ORIF) of coronoid.
- ORIF vs arthroplasty of the radial head.
- LUCL repair.

If still unstable, consider the following:

- MCL repair +/− repair of flexor origin.
- Possible external fixation.
- Internal joint stabilizer.

## Introduction

Elbow dislocations are characterized as simple or complex. A simple dislocation involves capsular and ligament injury only while a complex dislocation is associated with both soft tissue and bony injury. A terrible triad injury is used to describe a complex elbow dislocation specifically involving fractures of the radial head and coronoid with disruption of the lateral ulnar collateral ligament complex (LUCL).

R. Ashmyan
Piedmont Cartersville Medical Center, Cartersville, GA, USA

C. Lashgari (✉)
Orthopedic and Sports Medicine Center, Anne Arundel Medical Center, Annapolis, MD, USA

# History

- Typically involves a traumatic episode with a fall on an outstretched hand. Have the patient describe the event and beware of concurrent injuries. Always evaluate the wrist and shoulder in addition to the elbow.
- Patient will complain of pain and inability to move elbow.
- Ask about numbness, tingling, and pain level and is the level of pain and swelling worsening.
- Ask about history of prior injuries/dislocations involving that elbow.

# Physical Exam

- Begin with inspection and palpation evaluating for any obvious deformity concentrating on the elbow.
- Evaluate for areas of ecchymosis, abrasions, and swelling.
- Beware of compartment syndrome with higher energy injuries.
- Any open wounds must be carefully evaluated to rule out open fracture.
- Evaluate the shoulder and wrist joints for tenderness with palpation and range of motion.
  - NOTE: Tenderness and instability at the distal radial ulnar joint (DRUJ) may indicate an injury to the interosseous membrane (Essex-Lopresti injury).
- Evaluate the range of motion in flexion, extension, pronation, and supination. Note any obvious blocks to motion. Attempt varus/valgus stress testing. The patient will likely be very guarded during this initial evaluation.
- Perform a detailed neurologic examination to evaluate the axillary, musculocutaneous, median, ulnar, and radial nerves.
- Assess vascular status by checking distal capillary refill and pulses. Compare with the uninjured arm. If abnormal, further imaging and vascular consultation may be necessary.

# Imaging

- Initial imaging includes AP and lateral imaging of the involved elbow:
  - A line drawn through the radial head should intersect the center of the capitellum on all radiographs.
  - Evaluate concentricity of both the ulnohumeral and radiocapitellar joints.
  - Lateral X-rays are better for evaluation of coronoid fractures although it is difficult to sometimes differentiate displaced coronoid versus radial head fracture fragments.
- Must obtain postreduction films to confirm a concentric reduction.
- Obtain radiographs of ipsilateral humerus/forearm and shoulder/wrist as indicated based on the patient's history and physical exam.

- May obtain traction view during reduction if there is significant fracture comminution and elbow remains subluxated/dislocated after initial reduction attempt.
- A postreduction CT scan is routinely used to better evaluate fracture patterns for preoperative planning. May obtain sagittal, coronal, and 3-D reconstructions, as well as humeral subtraction images.
- MRI and ultrasound are not routinely needed for these injuries.

## Treatment Algorithm

Treatment of a terrible triad injury is based on understanding the mechanism and pathophysiology of this injury. This understanding guides the principles of nonoperative and operative treatment.

## Mechanism and Pathophysiology

- Posterolateral rotatory pattern.
  - Typically caused by a fall on the outstretched hand with the elbow in extension. The posterior force levers the ulna on the trochlea dislocating the ulnohumeral joint.
  - The forearm becomes fixed to the ground. The body then generates valgus stress, axial, and posterolateral rotatory forces across the elbow.
  - During the dislocation, the radial head and coronoid are frequently fractured.
  - Structures fail from lateral to medial. The LUCL is disrupted first, followed by the anterior capsule, and lastly disruption of the MCL.

## Anatomy

1. Primary Stabilizers of the Elbow.
   (a) Ulnohumeral joint.
      - The greater sigmoid notch of the ulna articulates with the trochlea of the distal humerus. The greater sigmoid notch is composed of the coronoid and olecranon.
      - The coronoid provides both an anterior and varus buttress. It resists posterior subluxation beyond 30° of flexion. It is made up of the coronoid tip, body, and anteromedial facet (sublime tubercle). The coronoid tip is an intra-articular structure.
   (b) Medial Collateral Ligament (MCL).
      - Anterior bundle.
        - Strongest and most significant stabilizer to valgus stress during functional range of motion (radial head is a secondary restraint).

   – Originates from the medial epicondyle, and inserts on sublime tubercle of the coronoid.
(c) Lateral Ulnar Collateral Ligament (LUCL).
   • Consists of the lateral ulnar collateral ligament (primary stabilizer), radial collateral ligament, annular ligament, and accessory collateral ligament.
   • LUCL originates at the isometric point on the lateral epicondyle and inserts on the supinator crest of the ulna.
   • Usually avulsed off the lateral epicondyle when injured.

## Secondary Stabilizers

1. Radial head.
   (a) Radial head is a restraint to posterolateral rotatory and valgus instability.
   (b) The anterolateral margin is nonarticulating with the sigmoid notch and therefore devoid of cartilage.
      • NOTE: This is described as a 90-degree arc between the radial styloid and lister's tubercle followed proximally. Termed the "safe zone" for plate placement. A plate placed distal to the bicipital tuberosity will endanger the posterior interosseous nerve.
2. Elbow capsule.
3. The flexor pronator mass originates from the medial epicondyle and provides valgus stability.
4. The common extensor mass originates from the lateral epicondyle and provides varus stability.
5. The biceps and brachialis anteriorly and the triceps and anconeus posteriorly compress the elbow joint to provide dynamic stability.

## Initial Management

• This consists of performing a closed reduction utilizing an intra-articular hematoma block, conscious sedation, or general anesthesia.
• Closed reduction is achieved by initial gentle extension and axial traction at the proximal forearm. The forearm should then be supinated followed by flexion of the elbow while providing direct pressure over the olecranon tip.
• Evaluate for stability, specifically at what degree of extension does the elbow begin to subluxate. Evaluate elbow range of motion looking for any mechanical blocks to motion.
• Repeat neurologic and vascular examination.
• Place extremity in a well-padded posterior splint at 90° of flexion.
• Obtain post reduction x-rays and CT scan.

## Treatment

### Nonoperative

- Rare indication—Most terrible triads are treated surgically.
- Criteria.
  - CT scan should be obtained to confirm both radial head and coronoid fractures do not meet surgical indications:

    Radial head- Mason type I and potentially type II without mechanical block.

    Coronoid Regan and Morrey type I.
- If the radial head and coronoid fractures are minimally displaced as noted above and if there is no mechanical block to motion, nonoperative treatment can be attempted.
- Patients should follow-up weekly for 6 weeks for clinical and radiographic evaluation to ensure these nonoperative criteria are still being met.
- Rehab protocol:
  - Day 0—7/10 days:

    Immobilization of elbow at 90° in a well-padded posterior splint.

    Encourage isometric biceps and triceps contracture to improve dynamic stability.
  - Week 1—week 4/6:

    Place into ROM elbow brace with extension block.

    Active motion initiated with avoidance of terminal extension (the point where recurrent instability was noted during closed reduction).

    Supination/pronation with arm at 90° of flexion.
  - Week 4/6—Week 12:

    Static progressive extension splinting at night time to aid in maximizing elbow extension.

    May initiate strengthening exercises.

### Operative

- Systematic approach.
- Must have all necessary equipment including an external fixator available.
- Ideally, elbow stability is restored allowing for early motion.
- If stability and fracture fixation is tenuous, protection of the repair and fracture healing is more important than early motion. It is easier to release a stiff, stable elbow then to salvage recurrent instability.

Essential steps:

- Open reduction and internal fixation (ORIF) of coronoid.
- ORIF vs arthroplasty of the radial head.
- LUCL repair.

If still unstable, consider the following:

- MCL repair ± repair of flexor origin.
- Possible external fixation.
- Internal joint stabilizer (Pasternack JB, Ciminero ML, Choue Kang, KK, JSES Vol 29, Issue 6, E238-E244, June, 2020).

## Patient Positioning

- Supine with the elbow on an arm table. This allows lateral and medial exposure. Posterior exposure can be achieved by placing the arm across the chest.
- Alternatively, the patient can be positioned in the lateral decubitus position. This is achieved with a bean bag and a well-padded arm holder placed under the anterior humerus.
- A tourniquet should be placed high in the axilla to avoid limiting exposure.
- Fluoroscopic images should always be attained prior to draping to ensure adequate visualization.

## Surgical Approaches

- Lateral, medial, and posterior approaches can be utilized depending on fracture pattern and stability [3–6].
- Posterior approach:
  - A posterior incision is the utilitarian approach to the elbow, which will allow for medial and lateral access. Additionally, this approach minimizes injury to cutaneous nerves and may be used for future complex revision surgeries. This approach is more cosmetic. Disadvantages include the increased risk for postop hematomas and seromas as well as flap necrosis.
- Lateral approach—most common in author's practice [3].
  - Kocher interval is identified between the anconeus posteriorly and the extensor carpi ulnaris.
  - NOTE: The majority of the deep dissection and approach will often already be accomplished by the traumatic event. The LUCL complex is disrupted and the extensor origin at the lateral epicondyle. LUCL will often leave a barespot where it avulsed off the distal humerus.
  - IMPORTANT CONSIDERATION: If the radial head is amenable to ORIF, the coronoid will likely need to be repaired via a medial approach as exposure may be difficult from the lateral aspect. If a radial head arthroplasty is indicated, the coronoid can be accessed laterally since the radial head will be resected in preparation for arthroplasty.
  - Careful anterior retraction and pronation of the forearm during the lateral approach reduces the risk of neurovascular injury.

- Medial approach [4].
  - Utilized when the coronoid cannot be adequately fixed through the lateral approach or when repair of the MCL/flexor mass is required for stability.
  - Incision is centered on medial epicondyle made along the supracondylar ridge curving distally just posterior to the medial epicondyle.
  - Ulnar nerve should be identified and protected.
  - Options for deep exposure.

    Flexor pronator split—minimal exposure; allows access to MCL.

    "Over-the-top" Hotchkiss approach—split and detachment of the anterior half of the flexor pronator mass of the medial epicondyle.

    Can also expose the coronoid for plate fixation by dissecting the ulnar nerve to its first motor branch distally. Retract the ulnar nerve posteriorly and split the flexor carpi ulnaris deep to the ulnar nerve lifting the flexor pronator group anteriorly. Start the deep dissection distally, and proceed proximally to expose the coronoid.

    Taylor Scham approach can be used for access to the coronoid base. After identification and protection of the ulnar nerve, elevate the entire flexor-pronator mass extraperiosteally using blunt dissection.

1. Hardware and Operative Considerations.
   (a) Coronoid Fracture.
      - *Large fragment* and *radial head not amenable to repair*—access the coronoid laterally after radial neck osteotomy and radial head removal. Use of one or two screws is preferred depending on the size of the fragment. Pass a guidewire from the subcutaneous border of the ulnar into the fracture bed of the coronoid fracture. An ACL guide may be used to help with placement. Pull back the wire until it is just buried beneath the fracture bed, reduce the coronoid fragment, and advance the wire. Place the screw(s) in a lag fashion.
      - *Small or comminuted fragment and radial head not amenable to repair* – access the coronoid laterally after the radial neck osteotomy and radial head removal. These smaller comminuted fragments require suture fixation. Nonabsorbable braided suture is passed through the anterior capsule on either side of the coronoid. These sutures are then passed through two bone tunnels in the fracture bed and tied on the subcutaneous border of the ulna. The suture is tied after the radial head replacement is completed.
      - NOTE: In situations where the radial head is not amenable to repair, the radial head can be used, if needed, as graft for coronoid fixation.
      - *Large fragment* and *radial head is amenable to repair*—must access coronoid medially as the radial head limits exposure. An anterior medial buttress plate [Fig. 1B] can be used or similar screw fixation as described earlier.

- *Small or comminuted fragment* (Fig. 26.1a) and *radial head is amenable to repair*—medial or lateral access depending upon initial lateral exposure with suture fixation as described above. Displacement of a large radial head fragment may provide enough exposure of the coronoid.
(b) Radial Head Fracture.
  - If amenable to fixation (usually <3 fragments):
    – After provisional fixation with k-wires or reduction clamps, 1.5 or 2.0 mm minifragment screws or similar sized variable compression screws are buried beneath the articular surface. A radial head plate placed in the safe zone may be necessary for radial neck involvement.

Above is 22 yo M 8 weeks s/p radial head fixation utilizing two crossing screws fixation (Fig. 26.2a–c). His motion at 8 weeks is demonstrated in Fig. 26.3a–d.

- If comminuted:
  – Remove the comminuted fragments, and resect any residual radial head at the level of the neck. Reassemble fragments on back table to judge radial head

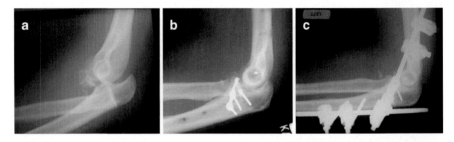

**Fig. 26.1** (**a–c**) (Lateral radiographs demonstrating terrible triad injury (**a**), anterior medial buttress plate for coronoid fixation (**b**), and external fixation placement for continued instability [**c**])

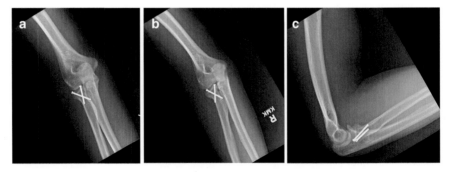

**Fig. 26.2** (**a–c**) (AP, oblique, and lateral radiographs of right elbow status post cross screw fixation of radial head)

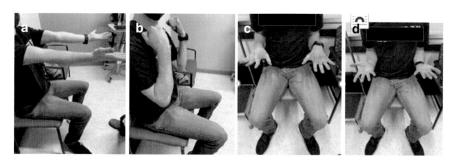

**Fig. 26.3** (**a–d**) (Clinical images demonstrating extension (**a**), flexion (**b**), pronation (**c**), and supination (**d**) at 8 weeks postoperatively)

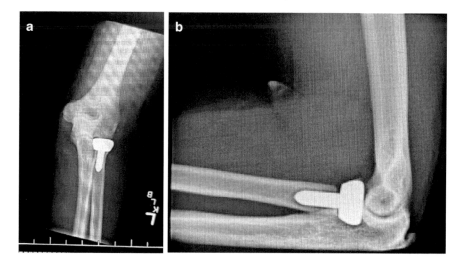

**Fig. 26.4** (**a, b**) (AP and lateral view demonstrating radial head replacement)

size. Err on the side of a smaller head if in between sizes. The radial head implant should articulate 1–2 mm distal to the coronoid process. Assess the medial ulnohumeral joint fluoroscopically as any widening suggests overstuffing of the joint. Overstuffing is a common mistake because of the associated ligament injury in this scenario.

- Do not resect the radial head without replacing it.
- Partial excision may be performed if the comminuted aspect of radial head fracture is <25%.
- Err on the side of replacement—tenuous fixation may lead to early failure and recurrent instability.

Above is a patient with a terrible trial who underwent radial head replacement, coronoid ORIF with suture and LCL repair through bone tunnel (Fig. 26.4a, b).

- Lateral collateral ligament (LCL) repair.
    - Fixation after radial head and coronoid has been addressed.
    - Usually avulsed off the humeral origin. May be reattached using suture anchors or through bone tunnels (author's preferred technique) with no. 2 braided nonabsorbable suture. A locking, grasping suture is passed through the deep surface of the anterior half of the LUCL from the lateral epicondyle to the supinator crest and then back proximally through the superficial fascial layer of the anterior common extensor. A second suture is passed in similar fashion through the posterior LUCL/common extensor tissue.
    - Mark the isometric point on the distal humerus. This is approximately at the geometric center of the capitellum. NOTE: The isometric point may be checked by grasping the avulsed LUCL tissue with a heavy forceps and advancing to the presumed isometric point. As the elbow is brought through a range of motion, the LUCL tension should remain constant. If visible slack is noted, the planned point of reattachment should be changed and rechecked.
    - Passing suture at proximal most portion of LUCL may leave graft loose. Advance suture just distal to the point of reattachment to ensure proper tensioning.
    - Tie sutures with elbow in 90° of flexion and full pronation with a valgus force placed on the elbow (if MCL torn and needs repair, repair in neutral).
- Medial collateral ligament (MCL) repair.
    - Elbow evaluated under fluoroscopy through all planes of ROM after fixation of the coronoid, radial head, and LUCL.
    - If continued instability with the elbow in greater than 30° of flexion, MCL will require repair.
    - If the ligament is avulsed off the humerus, similar repair to LCL utilizing bone anchors of tunnels.
- External fixation.
    - If all structures are repaired and there is continued instability, an external fixator may be applied (Fig. 26.1c).
    - Alternatively, an internal joint stabilizer of the elbow may be used [7].
    - NOTE: Must ensure proper pin placement along the axis of rotation so that joint congruity is maintained once ROM is initiated.
    - Protect the radial nerve during lateral humeral pin placement.

Above is patient with terrible triad. Radial head rim fracture piece was too small for fixation. Coronoid and LCL were fixed; however, the patient continued to be unstable. External fixator was then placed.

Below is a flowchart demonstrating treatment algorithm (Fig. 26.5).

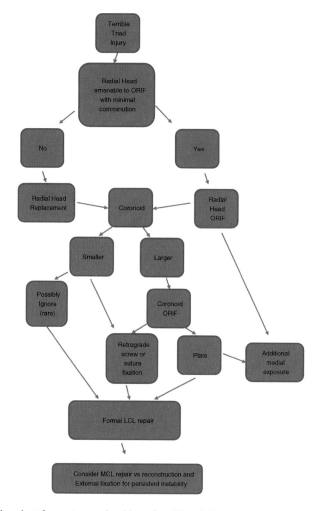

**Fig. 26.5** Flowchart for treatment algorithm of terrible triad

## Postoperative Care

- Upper extremity placed in well-padded posterior arm splint at 90° of flexion.
- If only LCL repaired, splint in full pronation (protects repair).
- If LCL and MCL repaired, splint in neutral rotation.
- Obtain radiographs in the PACU.
- Same day discharge is acceptable.
- Heterotopic ossification prophylaxis is controversial. Not routinely done at many institutions. Consider if there is concomitant brain injury. Indomethacin 25 mg three times daily for 3 weeks.

- Return to clinic at 5–7 days to remove splint and begin active and active-assisted ROM under therapy supervision. Limit motion from 30° to 130°. Avoid shoulder abduction as this creates a varus force stressing the LUCL repair. Initiate forearm rotation with the elbow at 90° of flexion only. Send for custom split, which may be removed for hygiene.
  - NOTE: If happy with fixation and stability at time of surgery, begin rehab after first postoperative visit. Do not wait past 10–14 days. It is better, however, to err on the side of some stiffness than to progress too quickly and have recurrent instability issues. Results of revision surgery for contracture release are better than for recurrent instability.
- At 4–6 weeks may advance ROM as tolerated. Progressive nighttime static extension splinting may be initiated.
- At 6–8 weeks may advance strengthening exercises.
- A static external fixator is typically removed around 3 weeks and an articulated external fixator around 6–8 weeks. A gentle manipulation should be done at this time to facilitate increased ROM postoperatively.

## Outcomes

- An acceptable outcome is considered a flexion extension arc of 30–130° and 50/50 for supination and pronation with minimal to no pain.
- Pugh et al. [1] reported on 36 elbows at a mean 34 month follow-up:
  - Average ulnohumeral arc of motion was 112° and 136° of rotation.
  - Utilizing the Mayo Elbow Performance Score, 15 patients rated as excellent, 13 as good, 7 as fair, and 1 as poor.
- Forthman et al. [2] reported 30 patients with mean follow-up of 32 months. Average arc of motion was reported at 117° and average rotation of 137°.
- Fitsgibbons et al. [8] reported on 11 patients with average follow-up of 38 months. Average arc of motion was reported at 112° and average VAS at 2.2.

## Complications

- Post-traumatic stiffness.
  - Most common complication. Initiate early ROM. Progress does not plateau for up to 1 year postoperatively. After 1 year, patients may consider revision surgery for hardware removal and contracture release.
- Heterotopic ossification and synostosis.
  - Consider prophylaxis in patient with concomitant head injury.
  - Obtain CT scan preoperatively for surgical planning.
- Persistent instability.
  - More common when type 1 or 2 coronoid fractures were not addressed. These cases may require formal ligament reconstruction and external fixation.

- Post-traumatic arthritis can result from chondral injury at the time of the initial trauma, malreduction of articular surfaces, poorly sized radial head replacement (overstuffed), and/or residual instability.
- Failure of fixation.
  - Most commonly at the radial head due to osteonecrosis after attempted ORIF.
- Superficial and deep wound infection.

## References

1. Pugh DMW, Wild LM, Schemitsch EH, King GJW, McKee MD. Standard surgical protocol to treat elbow dislocations with radial head and coronoid fractures. J Bone Joint Surg Am. 2004;86:1122–30.
2. Forthman C, Henket M, Ring DC. Elbow dislocation with intra-articular fracture: the results of operative treatment without repair of the medial collateral ligament. J Hand Surg [Am]. 2007;32:1200–9.
3. Stein JA, Murthi AM. Posterolateral rotatory instability of the elbow: our approach. Oper Tech Orthopaed. 2009;19(4):251–7.
4. Niloofar D, McKee M. Open reduction and internal fixation of fracture dislocations of the elbow with complex instability. In: Wiesel SW, editor. Operative techniques in orthopaedic surgery. Philadelphia, PA: Wolters Kluwer; 2016. p. 4041–50.
5. Mathew PK, et al. Terrible triad injuries of the elbow. In: Schemitsch EH, McKee MD, editors. Operative techniques: orthopaedic trauma surgery. Philadelphia, PA: Saunders; 2010. p. 131–54.
6. Mathew PK, et al. Terrible triad injury of the elbow: current concepts. J Am Acad Orthopaed Surg. 2009;17(3):137–51. https://doi.org/10.5435/00124635-200903000-00003.
7. Pasternack JB, et al. Patient outcomes for the internal joint stabilizer of the elbow (IJS-E). J Shoulder Elbow Surg. 2020;29(6):E238–44.
8. Fitzgibbons PG, et al. Functional outcomes after fixation of "terrible triad"™ elbow fracture dislocations. Orthopedics. 2014;37(4):e373–6. https://doi.org/10.3928/01477447-20140401-59.

# Pediatric Supracondylar Humerus Fracture

**27**

Kyle G. Achors and Gregory S. Bauer

---

## Introduction

1. Epidemiology.
    (a) Median age of injury is 6 years [1–3].
    (b) Equal distribution of males to females [4–6]:
        • Infantile supracondylar humerus fractures more common in females [7],
        • Adolescent supracondylar humerus fractures more common in males [8, 9].
    (c) Twelve to fifteen percent of all pediatric fractures [10, 11].
    (d) Sixty percent of all pediatric elbow injuries are supracondylar humerus fractures [12].
    (e) Most common reason for children to undergo elbow surgery [13].
    (f) Occur more often on school holidays and during sunny weather I [1, 14].
    (g) Nondominant extremity more frequently involved [5, 6, 15].
2. Pathomechanics.
    (a) Pediatric elbow.
    (b) Two columns.
        • Medial column.
            – Trochlea and medial epicondyle.
        • Lateral column.
            – Capitellum and lateral epicondyle.

K. G. Achors (✉)
University of South Florida, Tampa, FL, USA

G. S. Bauer
University of North Carolina Physicians Network, Durham, NC, USA

© The Author(s), under exclusive license to Springer Nature Switzerland AG 2022
C. M. Chebli, A. M. Murthi (eds.), *The Resident's Guide to Shoulder and Elbow Surgery*, https://doi.org/10.1007/978-3-031-12255-2_27

- Distal humerus thins in sagittal and coronal planes where these two columns join [16].
  - Area bordered by the olecranon fossa posterior, coronoid fossa anterior, and medial/lateral supracondylar ridges.
  - Creates a point of weakness and predisposes to fracture [17].
3. Divided into extension or flexion type.
   (a) Extension type.
       - Most common: >97% [3].
       - Fall onto outstretched arm with elbow in extension.
         - Olecranon engages the olecranon fossa, anterior capsule tensed.
           Leads to the distal humeral anterior cortex failing in tension [18].
   (b) Flexion type.
       - Less common: <3% [3].
       - Fall onto elbow in flexion.
         - Force directed through elbow causes posterior cortex to fail in tension [18].
   (c) Ligamentous laxity/elbow hyperextension.
       - Theorized to increase risk [19].
         - However, conflicting data on the subject [20].

## Initial Presentation

1. ED management.
   (a) History.
       - Usually due to a fall onto an outstretched upper extremity.
       - Assess other areas of pain.
         - Ipsilateral forearm and shoulder.
           Higher incidence of neurovascular injury/compartment syndrome with ipsilateral forearm injury [21, 22].
       - Locate any areas of paresthesia or numbness.
       - Determine associated head injury.
         - Fall from height.
         - Loss of consciousness.
         - General neurologic evaluation.
       - Must evaluate for nonaccidental injury (NAT).
         - One-third of all child abuse victims will visit an orthopedic surgeon [23].
         - Important history.
           Height of fall.
             Falls from the bed/couch in young should be suspicious [24].
           Was the injury witnessed?
           Are there any discrepancies in the reports from parents/guardians?
         - Typically will present with >1 fracture [25–27].

    – Risk factors.
        Young age child.
            Majority occur in children <1 year of age [28].
            Estimated that 10% of trauma cases in children <3 years are NAT [23].
            Young children are unable to defend themselves, communicate, or ambulate [29].
        Child with special needs.
            Disability, health issues.
        Parental factors.
            Young age, low education, socioeconomic status, transient non-biologic caregiver, and personal history of child abuse [30].
    – Physical signs of abuse.
        Note general hygiene and nutritional status.
            Both important in evaluating for a battered child [31].
        Bruising.
            Most common indication of child abuse [32].
            Bruising pattern.
            Multiple bruises, bruises of varying age, and bruises about the buttocks, perineum/genitals, trunk, and back of legs/head suggestive of NAT [32].
    – Diagnosis is made via team effort.
        Emergency medicine physician, pediatrician, social workers, law enforcement.
(b) Physical examination.
    • Thorough and complete general/orthopedic exam must be performed.
    • Soft tissue evaluation.
      – Integrity of soft tissues.
         "Puckering"
            Occurs when the proximal fragment button-holes through the brachialis [33].
            Indication for high energy.
            Oftentimes associated with vascular/nerve injury [34, 35].
            Suggestive of increased difficulty with reduction [36].
            Reduced via Milking maneuver.
            Gradual traction and massage of the brachialis muscle to reduce [37].
            Typically performed in the operating room while sedated.
         Open injury.
             Rare injury [38, 39].
            Bleeding wounds about the fracture should raise suspicion.
         Note forearm compartment turgor or antecubital ecchymosis.
    • Deformity.
      – Typical "S-shaped" deformity of Gartland types 3 and 4 [40].

(c) Distal neurovascular status.
- Neurovascular injury to be reported as high as 49% [41].
- Assess motor and sensory function of all distal nerves.
  - Nerve injury can occur in up to 10–20% of patients [41].
  - Typically a traction neuropraxia [42].
  - Anterior interosseous nerve.
      Most common nerve injury, [43, 44] predominantly motor branch of the median nerve.
        Innervates FDP to index/middle finger, FPL, and pronator quadratus.
        Tested by asking patient to make "OK" sign.
  - Median nerve.
      Posterolateral displacement associated with median nerve [41].
      Given proximity: there is a significant association between median and brachial artery injury [45].
        Associated injury strongly predicts need for exploration [46].
      Differentiate from AIN palsy via paresthesias in the volar thumb, thenar palm, index, and radial ½ middle finger.
  - Radial nerve.
      Posteromedial displacement associated with radial nerve/PIN [41].
      Radial nerve innervates anconeus, ECRL, ECRB, brachioradialis.
        Tested via wrist extension.
      PIN innervates EDC, supinator, EDM, ECU, APL, EPL, EPB, and EIP.
        Tested via digit extension.
  - Ulnar nerve.
      Flexion type associated with ulnar nerve [47].
      Innervates hand intrinsics, FCU, FDP to ring and small finger.
        Tested via finger abduction/adduction.
  - Inability to perform adequate neurologic exam.
      Due to child's age, pain, development, etc.
      Must document this from a medicolegal aspect.
      May assess via autonomic nerve function.
        Wrap the hand in a wet cloth and examining for normal skin wrinkling [48, 49].
        Absence indicates injured peripheral nerve
- Examine perfusion of the distal limb.
  - Vascular injury can occur in up 20% of patients [41, 50–53].
  - Document radial and ulnar pulses.
  - Note capillary refill, color, and temperature of the hand.
      Two second capillary refill is generally defined as normal [54].
      Compare findings to contralateral limb.

Even with brachial arterial injury collateral flow around the elbow can keep the hand perfused [40].

> Important distinction between: pink and perfused vs. pink and pulseless vs. pale and pulseless.

- Serial examinations should be performed if there is a delay to the OR. Note agitation, anxiety, pain level, analgesia required, changing vascular status.

> Progression may indicate worsening ischemia or impending compartment syndrome [55].

2. Radiographs.
   (a) Supracondylar humerus fractures are defined as an extra-articular fracture that passes about the metaphyseal portion of the distal humerus [56].
   (b) Obtain radiographs of ipsilateral humerus, elbow, and forearm.
   (c) Elbow radiographs to make the diagnosis.
      - Establish fracture characteristics.
         - Magnitude of displacement.
         - Malrotation.
         - Comminution.
   (d) AP radiograph of the distal humerus.
      - A transverse or short oblique fracture may be present just superior to the olecranon fossa.
      - Note direction of displacement.
      - Posterior fat pad sign.
         - Elevation of the posterior fat pad.
           Caused by bleeding from the fracture.
         - Important for occult/nondisplaced [57, 58].
   (e) Humerocapitellar angle.
      - Also known as Baumann's angle [59].
      - Angle formed at the intersection of the longitudinal axis of the humerus with the line drawn tangential to the capitellar physis.
         - Normal is 9–26 degrees.
         - Decreased Baumann's angle signifies varus angulation.
      - Difficult to assess in younger children [60].
      - Varies with rotation [61].
   (f) Ulnohumeral angle.
      - Radiographic carrying angle of the upper extremity.
      - Angle formed by long axis of the humerus and long axis of the ulna.
   (g) Lateral radiograph of the elbow.
      - Anterior humeral line.
         - Line drawn about the anterior cortex of the humerus should intersect the middle 1/3rd of the capitellum.
           In children <4 it will intersect the anterior 1/3rd [62].

- If the line is anterior to the capitellum, it is suggestive of an extension type supracondylar humerus fracture.

(h) Radiocapitellar line.
  - Line drawn about the long axis of the radius should intersect the capitellum and should be present on all views.
    - Suspect associated injury when not intact.

(i) Classification.
  - Described by Gartland in 1959 [63].
    - Initially described as nondisplaced, moderately displaced, and severely displaced.
    - Later modified by Wilkins in 1984 to make the classification more clinically relevant.
      Distinguishing posterior humeral cortical contact and malrotation for type II fractures [64, 65].
    - Modified again by DeBoeck in 1995 describing medial column comminution with loss of Baumann's angle [66].
    - Completely unstable injuries were suggested by Leitch in 2006 [67].
    - Shown to provide good inter and intraobserver reliability [68].
  - Modified Gartland classification.
    - Extension type.
      Type I: Minimally displaced (<2 mm) (Fig. 27.1).
      Type II: Moderately displaced (>2 mm) (Fig. 27.2).
        Type IIA: Displaced with intact posterior hinge.
        Type IIB: Displaced with intact posterior hinge and malrotation.

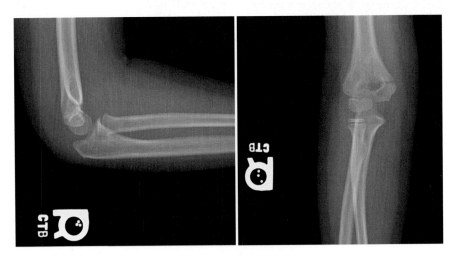

**Fig. 27.1** Type I fracture (Image Courtesy of Dr. Lee Phillips)

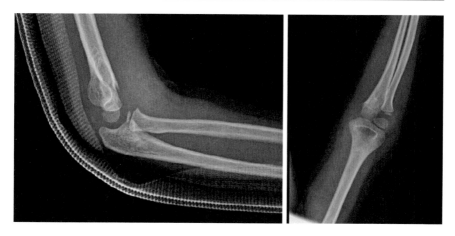

**Fig. 27.2**  Type II (Image Courtesy of Dr. Lee Phillips)

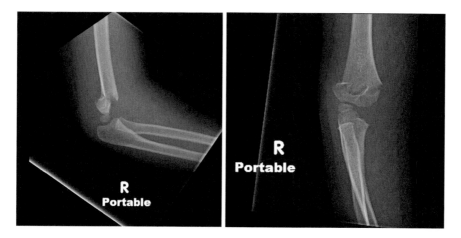

**Fig. 27.3**  Type III (Image Courtesy of Dr. Lee Phillips)

Type III: Completely displaced fracture with no posterior cortical contact (Fig. 27.3).

Type IV: Completely displaced with multidirectional instability.
  No periosteal hinge.
 – Flexion type (Fig. 27.4).
    Much more rare.
      Usually a more severe injury with higher complication rate [69].

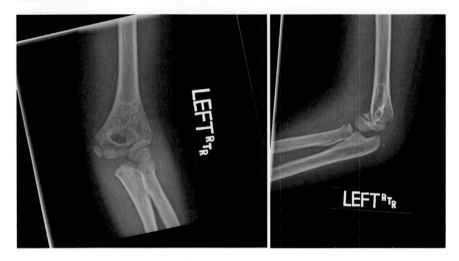

**Fig. 27.4** Flexion type (Image Courtesy of Dr. Lee Phillips)

## Management.

1. Historical definitive treatment options.
    (a) Nonoperative.
        • Cuff and collar [70, 71].
        • Blount's method.
            – Immobilization in hyperflexion of the elbow [72].
                Relies on intact posterior periosteum.
                Required careful patient selection.
                    Good results when indicated [73, 74].
                No longer widely utilized due to risk of ischemia/compartment syndrome [73].
        • Traction.
            – Skin or skeletal traction [75–77].
            – Requires prolonged hospital stay (2–3 weeks).
            – Later demonstrated to be inferior to percutaneous pinning [78].
            – No longer widely utilized in modernized healthcare systems.
    (b) Operative.
        • Open reduction was first described by Ramsey and Griz in 1973 [79].
        • Closed reduction and percutaneous pinning first described by Swenson.
            – Utilized cross pinning [80].
            – Early on this required a high degree of skill and had to be done blind via anatomic landmarks [81].
2. In Emergency Department.
    (a) Splint.
        • Well-padded posterior long arm splint with elbow in approximately 20–40 degrees of flexion [40].

- Do not splint in >90 degrees of flexion or in full extension.
  - Increases compartment pressures [82].
- No reduction required.
  - In situ splint demonstrate early access to OR and shorter hospitalization.
  - One less anesthesia event when reduction in ED is avoided [83].
3. Nonoperative management.
   (a) Most (76%) are able to be managed nonoperatively [38].
   (b) Indications.
   - All type I fractures [84].
   - Select type II fractures.
     - When there is marginal displacement of the anterior humeral line.
     - In children <3 years [85].
       Great remodeling potential in toddlers.
   (c) Immobilize in an above elbow cast.
   - Cast has been determined to provide better pain control [86, 87].
   - Cast in <90 degrees flexion.
     - Greater than 90 degrees increases compartment pressures [82, 88].
   - Type II fractures managed nonoperatively produce satisfactory outcomes [89].
4. Operative management.
   (a) Indications.
   - Most type II fractures.
     - Lessens risk of malreduction/loss of reduction [90, 91].
     - Obviates need for casting in flexion.
       Reduces risk of compartment syndrome [88].
   - Type III, IV [84].
   - Any medial comminution.
     - Prevents collapse and resultant cubitus varus [66].
   (b) Timing.
   - Delayed intervention.
     - Acceptable for well perfused hand without neurovascular injury [92].
       Surgical delay does not increase complication rate or necessitate opening the fracture [93–96].
       Surgery overnight with inexperienced team can potentially increase errors [97]
     - Significant swelling may require serial exams and earlier intervention.
   - Urgent intervention.
     - Well perfused hand with neurovascular injury, open fractures, floating elbow, and inability to communicate.
   - Emergent intervention required.
     - Compartment syndrome, dysvascular limb.
   (c) Techniques.
   - Closed reduction, percutaneous pinning (CRPP).
   - Vast majority of cases (87%) managed with CRPP [38].
   - Closed reduction.

- Goal is anatomic reduction with restoration of Baumann's angle.
- General principle to use intact periosteum on compression side of injury to aid in reduction [18].
- Traction with elbow in slight flexion.
  - Pulls the fracture out to length.
  - Triceps and posterior periosteum are stabilizing forces, flexion stabilizes but also potentially disrupts circulation [98].
  - Slight elbow flexion to avoid injury to neurovascular structures.
    - Extension of elbow can cause tethering of neurovascular structures.
- Supination for varus and pronation for valgus correction.
  - Posteromedial displacement.
    - Pronation will tension the intact medial periosteum and aid in reduction [98, 99].
  - Posterolateral displacement.
    - Supination will tension intact lateral periosteum and aid in reduction [98, 99].
- Elbow is flexed with direct pressure on the olecranon to correct sagittal plane.
  - Elbow held in flexion while percutaneous Kirschner wires (K-wires) placed.
- Joystick method can aid in difficult/unstable reductions.
  - Described by Leitch et al. [67, 100].
  - Passed medial to lateral to aid in maintaining reduction.
- Constructs.
  - Lateral only pins (Figs. 27.5 and 27.6).
    - Most utilized construct.
    - Less stable than cross pin constructs. [101–103]
      - However, some studies contradict this finding [104, 105].
        - Three lateral pins at least as stable as crossed pins [105].
    - Maximal stability.

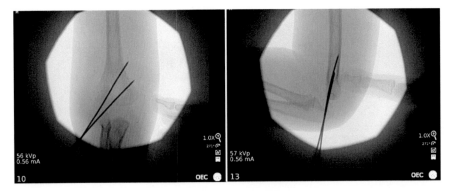

**Fig. 27.5** Two lateral pins (Image Courtesy of Dr. Lee Phillips)

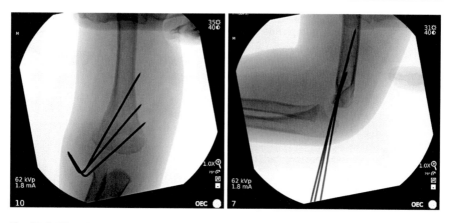

**Fig. 27.6** Three lateral pins (Image Courtesy of Dr. Lee Phillips)

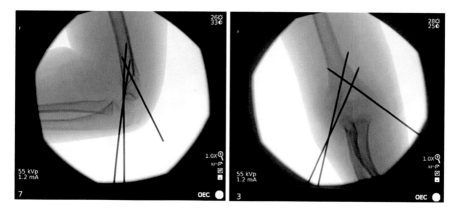

**Fig. 27.7** Medial pin (Image Courtesy of Dr. Lee Phillips)

Capitellar starting point [106].

Wide pin divergence at the fracture for rotational control [107].
2 mm vs 1.6 mm [106].

Trans-olecranon fossa quadricortical pin more stable than bicortical standard pin [108].

Advantage: Lateral only constructs provide stability with decreased risk of iatrogenic ulnar nerve injury [109, 110].

- Medial pin (Fig. 27.7).
  - Biomechanically stronger [103, 111].

    Less reported loss of reduction when compared with lateral only [112].
  - Higher risk of ulnar nerve injury [113–118].

    Can be due to direct injury or compression due to close proximity [119].

Nerve injury can be decreased with technique change [120].

Extending elbow, direct palpation, pin anterior side of medial epicondyle, mini open technique [101, 120–122].

Ultrasound and nerve monitoring have been proposed as well [123, 124].

- When is cross pinning useful [120] (Fig. 27.8).

High metadiaphyseal fxs where two lateral pins are unable to be performed.

Medial cortical comminution.

Initial cubitus varus and medial instability.

Concern for instability after two lateral pins.

- Common errors in pinning [125]:
  - Failure to engage the two fragments with at least two pins.
  - Failure to achieve bicortical fixation with at least two pins.
  - Failure of adequate pin spread at the fracture.
- Open reduction, percutaneous pinning:
  - Indications.

Open fracture.

Dysvascular limb.

  - When perfusion not reinstated with closed reduction in dysvascular limb.

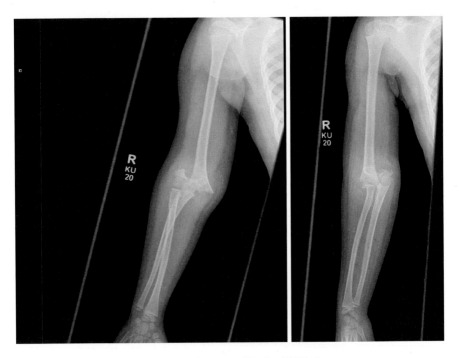

**Fig. 27.8** Medial comminution (Image Courtesy of Dr. Lee Phillips)

Failed closed reduction.
Likely soft tissue interposition.
– Typically performed via a direct anterior approach [126].
Easier access to brachial artery, median nerve, and the fracture [127].
– No difference in complication rates compared with percutaneous techniques [128–130].
• Postop management:
– Cast.
Water proof or standard cotton.
Higher satisfaction with water proof liner [131].
Cast in less than 90 degrees of flexion.
Decreases volume of antecubital fossa and increases compartment pressures [71, 82].
Bivalve vs univalve.
Recommend in all cases postop.
Spacer use decreases compartment pressures even further [132].
Univalve with spacer equivalent to bivalve with Ace wrap [133].
Immobilize typically for 3–4 weeks.
For nonoperatively treated fractures.
Recommend follow-up at 1 and 2 weeks post cast application for radiographic surveillance.
Cast removal at 3 weeks.
For operatively treated fractures.
Dependent upon fracture pattern.
No gold standard for timing of pin removal or return to activity [84].
– Physical therapy shown to provide no benefit [134].

## Vascular Status

1. Vascular injury.
   (a) Typically artery is draped over the proximal fragment. [34]
   (b) Intimal injury can cause thrombus or aneurysm. [135]
   (c) Laceration can occur as well [41].
   (d) Missed injuries associated with high rates of ischemic contracture [135].
2. Management.
   (a) Pulseless, well perfused hand.
       • Urgent fracture reduction/stabilization alone often times is sufficient treatment [51, 52].
       • Frequently after reduction/stabilization the pulse will remain absent [52].
         – Controversy exists regarding exploration for this scenario.

Most recommend observation with frequent vascular checks. [136–138]

> Monitor for 24–48 h [52, 139, 140].
>> Low threshold for return to OR for compartment release/vascular exploration.
>> Good waveform on pulse ox predicts good results [141].
>> Early repair associated with high rate of reocclusion/stenosis [136].
> However, some recommend early exploration to prevent late sequelae [142, 143].
>> Sequelae include: vascular abnormalities, contracture, cold intolerance, and exercise induced ischemia [135, 144, 145].

- If anatomic reduction cannot be attained with closed reduction.
  - Anterior approach is indicated to free incarcerated structures in the fracture [146].
    > If arterial vasospasm is noted: warming and lidocaine/papaverine [85, 147].
    > If after 10–15 min the artery is still stenosed, open revascularization is indicated [85].

(b) Poorly perfused, pulseless.
- Emergent situation.
  - No delays toward fracture reduction and stabilization in OR.
    > Return of pulses usually in ~50% of patients after closed reduction [50, 52, 55, 145].
    > If pulses do not return.
    >> Immediate open vascular exploration [148].
    >>> Recommend vascular surgery assistance.
    >>> Anterior transverse incision about the antecubital fossa crease.
    >>> Artery is usually tethered anterior to the fracture site [34].
    >> High incidence of brachial artery injury and need for repair [52, 145].

(c) When a well perfused arm with pulses loses pulses after reduction.
- Remove K wires, reassess, and then open exploration if pulses do not return.

(d) Role of angiography.
- Preoperative use should not delay treatment as reduction is typically sufficient to restore pulse [52].
- Defining site of injury is not indicated given the fracture site is the assumed site of injury [148].
- Many authors argue against use as it does not alter course [50, 149].
- Postreduction angiography may assist in diagnosis of intimal tears [45].

## Complications

1. Pin migration/infection.
   (a) Less than one in ten obtain a pin tract infection [93, 95, 150].
   (b) Low risk of severe infection 0.2% [150, 151].
   (c) Does not correlate with length of fixation.
   (d) Most resolve with pin removal and oral antibiotics [150].
   (e) Limited sterile prep and towel draping shown to be safe [151].
2. Malunion.
   (a) Susceptible due to distal humerus' lesser potential to remodel.
   - Twenty percent of longitudinal growth of the humerus is via the distal humeral physeal [152].
   - Children <5 years have greater remodeling potential [85].
   (b) Typically due to inadequate reduction or loss of fixation.
   (c) Recurvatum deformity.
   - Causes increase in extension and lack of flexion.
   - Treat with supracondylar osteotomy if functional deficit present [153].
   (d) Cubitus varus.
   - Higher risk with medial column comminution [154].
   - May be due to internal rotation malunion [155].
   - Traditionally thought of as only a cosmetic deformity.
     - However, posterolateral rotatory instability, recurrent radial head instability, tardy ulnar nerve palsy, and increase risk for fracture have been reported [156–159].
   - Treat with corrective osteotomy [160, 161].
3. Compartment syndrome.
   (a) Rare: 0.1–0.3% incidence [22, 82].
   (b) Presence of ecchymosis and severe swelling should raise suspicion [162].
   (c) Elbow should be immobilized in less than 90 degrees of flexion at all times.
   (d) Prolonged ischemia time (>6 h) should be treated with compartment release [148].
   (e) Missed compartment syndrome causes Volkman's ischemic contracture [135].
4. Neurovascular injury.
   (a) See above.
5. Stiffness.
   (a) Usually acute post cast removal.
   (b) Ninety-eight percent of motion returns within first year [163].
6. Saw burns.
   (a) Increased risk with inexperienced users and dull saw blades [164, 165].
   (b) Well-padded casts prevent saw burn injuries [166].

# References

1. Barr LV. Paediatric supracondylar humeral fractures: epidemiology, mechanisms and incidence during school holidays. J Child Orthop. 2014;8(2):167–70. https://doi.org/10.1007/s11832-014-0577-0.
2. Holt JB, Glass NA, Shah AS. Understanding the epidemiology of pediatric supracondylar humeral fractures in the United States: identifying opportunities for intervention. J Pediatr Orthop. 2018;38(5):e245–51. https://doi.org/10.1097/BPO.0000000000001154.
3. Cheng JCY, Lam TP, Maffulli N. Epidemiological features of supracondylar fractures of the humerus in Chinese children. J Pediatr Orthop B. 2001;10(1):63–7. https://doi.org/10.1097/00009957-200101000-00011.
4. Houshian S, Mehdi B, Larsen MS. The epidemiology of elbow fracture in children: analysis of 355 fractures, with special reference to supracondylar humerus fractures. J Orthop Sci. 2001;6(4):312–5. https://doi.org/10.1007/s007760100024.
5. Landin LA. Fracture patterns in children. Analysis of 8,682 fractures with special reference to incidence, etiology and secular changes in Swedish urban population 1950-1979. Acta Orthop Scand. 1983;202:1–109.
6. Farnsworth CL, Silva PD, Mubarak SJ. Etiology of supracondylar humerus fractures. J Pediatr Orthop. 1998;18(1):38–42. https://doi.org/10.1097/01241398-199801000-00008.
7. Mehlman CT, Denning JR, McCarthy JJ, Fisher ML. Infantile supracondylar humeral fractures (patients less than two years of age). J Bone Joint Surg Am. 2019;101(1):25–34. https://doi.org/10.2106/jbjs.18.00391.
8. Fletcher ND, Schiller JR, Garg S, et al. Increased severity of type III supracondylar humerus fractures in the preteen population. J Pediatr Orthop. 2012;32(6):567–72. https://doi.org/10.1097/BPO.0b013e31824b542d.
9. Bell P, Scannell BP, Loeffler BJ, et al. Adolescent distal humerus fractures: ORIF versus CRPP. J Pediatr Orthop. 2017;37(8):511–20. https://doi.org/10.1097/BPO.0000000000000715.
10. Mangwani J, Nadarajah R, Paterson JMH. Supracondylar humeral fractures in children. Ten years' experience in a teaching hospital. J Bone Joint Surg Br. 2006;88(3):362–5. https://doi.org/10.1302/0301-620X.88B3.16425.
11. Landin LA. Epidemiology of children's fractures. J Pediatr Orthop B. 1997;88(3):362–5. https://doi.org/10.1097/01202412-199704000-00002.
12. Saroff DA, Mehlman CT, Strub WM, et al. Time to treatment: the question of beneficial surgical delays [2] (multiple letters). J Bone Joint Surg Am. 2001;83(11):1755–6. https://doi.org/10.2106/00004623-200111000-00023.
13. Vallila N, Sommarhem A, Paavola M, Nietosvaara Y. Pediatric distal humeral fractures and complications of treatment in Finland: a review of compensation claims from 1990 through 2010. J Bone Joint Surg Am. 2015;97(6):494–9. https://doi.org/10.2106/JBJS.N.00758.
14. Masterson E, Borton D, O'Brien T. Victims of our climate. Injury. 1993;24(4):247–8. https://doi.org/10.1016/0020-1383(93)90179-A.
15. Anjum R, Sharma V, Jindal R, Singh TP, Rathee N. Epidemiologic pattern of paediatric supracondylar fractures of humerus in a teaching hospital of rural India: a prospective study of 263 cases. Chin J Traumatol. 2017;20(3):158–60. https://doi.org/10.1016/j.cjtee.2016.10.007.
16. Mencio GA. Fractures and dislocations about the elbow. In: Green's skeletal trauma in children. 5th ed. Philadelphia, PA: Elsevier/Saunders; 2015. https://doi.org/10.1016/B978-0-323-18773-2.00010-X.
17. Hammond WA, Kay RM, Skaggs DL. Supracondylar humerus fractures in children. AORN J. 1998;68(2):186–99. https://doi.org/10.1016/s0001-2092(06)62513-1.
18. Catterall A. Rockwood and Wilkins' fractures in children. J Bone Joint Surg Br. 2002; https://doi.org/10.1302/0301-620x.84b3.0840465b.

19. Nork SE, Hennrikus WL, Loncarich DP, Gillingham BL, Lapinsky AS. Relationship between ligamentous laxity and the site of upper extremity fractures in children: extension supracondylar fracture versus distal forearm fracture. J Pediatr Orthop B. 1999;8(2):90–2. https://doi.org/10.1097/01202412-199904000-00005.

20. McLauchlan GJ, Walker CRC, Cowan B, Robb JE, Prescott RJ. Extension of the elbow and supracondylar fractures in children. J Bone Joint Surg Br. 1999;81(3):402–5. https://doi.org/10.1302/0301-620X.81B3.9194.

21. Muchow RD, Riccio AI, Garg S, Ho CA, Wimberly RL. Neurological and vascular injury associated with supracondylar humerus fractures and ipsilateral forearm fractures in children. J Pediatr Orthop. 2015;35(2):121–5. https://doi.org/10.1097/BPO.0000000000000230.

22. Blakemore LC, Cooperman DR, Thompson GH, Wathey C, Ballock RT. Compartment syndrome in ipsilateral humerus and forearm fractures in children. Clin Orthop Relat Res. 2000;376:32–8. https://doi.org/10.1097/00003086-200007000-00006.

23. Akbarnia BA, Akbarnia NO. The role of the orthopedist in child abuse and neglect. Orthop Clin North Am. 1976;7(3):733–42.

24. Nimityongskul P, Anderson LD. The likelihood of injuries when children fall out of bed. J Pediatr Orthop. 1987;7(2):184–6. https://doi.org/10.1097/01241398-198703000-00014.

25. Leventhal JM, Thomas SA, Rosenfield NS, Markowitz RI. Fractures in young children: distinguishing child abuse from unintentional injuries. Am J Dis Child. 1993;147(1):87–92. https://doi.org/10.1001/archpedi.1993.02160250089028.

26. Worlock P, Stower M, Barbor P. Patterns of fractures in accidental and non-accidental injury in children: a comparative study. Br Med J (Clin Res Ed). 1986;293(6539):100–2. https://doi.org/10.1136/bmj.293.6539.100.

27. King J, Diefendorf D, Apthorp J, Negrete VF, Carlson M. Analysis of 429 fractures in 189 battered children. J Pediatr Orthop. 1988;8(5):585–9. https://doi.org/10.1016/s0022-3468(89)80783-3.

28. Clarke NMP, Shelton FRM, Taylor CC, Khan T, Needhirajan S. The incidence of fractures in children under the age of 24 months - in relation to non-accidental injury. Injury. 2012;43(6):762–5. https://doi.org/10.1016/j.injury.2011.08.024.

29. Kocher MS, Kasser JR. Orthopaedic aspects of child abuse. J Am Acad Orthop Surg. 2000;8(1):10–20. https://doi.org/10.5435/00124635-200001000-00002.

30. Mersky JP, Berger LM, Reynolds AJ, Gromoske AN. Risk factors for child and adolescent maltreatment: a longitudinal investigation of a cohort of inner-city youth. Child Maltreat. 2009;14(1):73–88. https://doi.org/10.1177/1077559508318399.

31. Kempe CH, Silverman FN, Steele BF, Droegemueller W, Silver HK. The battered-child syndrome. Child Abus Negl. 1985;9(2):143–54. https://doi.org/10.1016/0145-2134(85)90005-5.

32. McMahon P, Grossman W, Gaffney M, Stanitski C. Soft-tissue injury as an indication of child abuse. J Bone Joint Surg A. 1995;77(8):1179–83. https://doi.org/10.2106/00004623-199508000-00006.

33. Archibeck MJ, Scott SM, Peters CL. Brachialis muscle entrapment in displaced supracondylar humerus fractures: a technique of closed reduction and report of initial results. J Pediatr Orthop. 1997;17(3):298–302. https://doi.org/10.1097/00004694-199705000-00006.

34. Rasool MN, Naidoo KS. Supracondylar fractures: posterolateral type with brachialis muscle penetration and neurovascular injury. J Pediatr Orthop. 1999;19(4):518–22. https://doi.org/10.1097/00004694-199907000-00019.

35. Smuin DM, Hennrikus WL. The effect of the pucker sign on outcomes of type III extension supracondylar fractures in children. J Pediatr Orthop. 2017;37(4):e229–32. https://doi.org/10.1097/BPO.0000000000000893.

36. Aksakal M, Ermutlu C, Sarisözen B, Akesen B. Approach to supracondylar humerus fractures with neurovascular compromise in children. Acta Orthop Traumatol Turc. 2013;47(4):244–9. https://doi.org/10.3944/AOTT.2013.3012.

37. Davey J. Milking maneuver for supracondylar fractures of the humerus in children. AAOS OrthoPortal.
38. Holt JB, Glass NA, Bedard NA, Weinstein SL, Shah AS. Emerging U.S. national trends in the treatment of pediatric supracondylar humeral fractures. J Bone Joint Surg Am. 2017;99(8):681–7. https://doi.org/10.2106/JBJS.16.01209.
39. Khoshbin A, Leroux T, Wasserstein D, et al. The epidemiology of paediatric supracondylar fracture fixation: a population-based study. Injury. 2014;45(4):701–8. https://doi.org/10.1016/j.injury.2013.10.004.
40. Kasser JR, Beaty JH. Supracondylar fractures of the distal humerus. In: Rockwood and Wilkins; fractures in children. Philadelphia, PA: Wolters Kluwer; 2001.
41. Campbell CC, Waters PM, Emans JB, Kasser JR, Millis MB. Neurovascular injury and displacement in type III supracondylar humerus fractures. J Pediatr Orthop. 1995;15(1):47–52. https://doi.org/10.1097/01241398-199501000-00011.
42. Guner S, Guven N, Karadas S, et al. Iatrogenic or fracture-related nerve injuries in supracondylar humerus fracture: is treatment necessary for nerve injury? Eur Rev Med Pharmacol Sci. 2013;17(6):815–9.
43. Spinner M, Schreiber SN. Anterior interosseous-nerve paralysis as a complication of supracondylar fractures of the humerus in children. J Bone Joint Surg Am. 1969;51(8):1584–90. https://doi.org/10.2106/00004623-196951080-00008.
44. Cramer KE, Green NE, Devito DP. Incidence of anterior interosseous nerve palsy in supracondylar humerus fractures in children. J Pediatr Orthop. 1993; https://doi.org/10.1097/01241398-199307000-00015.
45. Luria S, Sucar A, Eylon S, et al. Vascular complications of supracondylar humeral fractures in children. J Pediatr Orthop B. 2007;13(4):502–5. https://doi.org/10.1097/01.bpb.0000236236.49646.03.
46. Mangat KS, Martin AG, Bache CE. The "pulseless pink" hand after supracondylar fracture of the humerus in children: the predictive value of nerve palsy. J Bone Joint Surg Br. 2009;91(11):1521–5. https://doi.org/10.1302/0301-620X.91B11.22486.
47. Fowles JV, Kassab MT. Displaced supracondylar fractures of the elbow in children. A report on the fixation and extension and flexion fractures by two lateral percutaneous pins. J Bone Joint Surg Br. 1974;56B(3):490–500. https://doi.org/10.1302/0301-620x.56b3.490.
48. Phelps PE, Walker E. Comparison of the finger wrinkling test results to established sensory tests in peripheral nerve injury. Am J Occup Ther. 1977;31(9):565–72.
49. Tsai N, Kirkham S. Fingertip skin wrinkling - the effect of varying tonicity. J Hand Surg Am. 2005;30(3):273–5. https://doi.org/10.1016/j.jhsa.2004.12.010.
50. Shaw BA, Kasser JR, Emans JB, Rand FF. Management of vascular injuries in displaced supracondylar humerus fractures without arteriography. J Orthop Trauma. 1990;4(1):25–9. https://doi.org/10.1097/00005131-199003000-00004.
51. Gosens T, Bongers KJ. Neurovascular complications and functional outcome in displaced supracondylar fractures of the humerus in children. Injury. 2003;34(4):267–73. https://doi.org/10.1016/S0020-1383(02)00312-1.
52. Choi PD, Melikian R, Skaggs DL. Risk factors for vascular repair and compartment syndrome in the pulseless supracondylar humerus fracture in children. J Pediatr Orthop. 2010;30(1):50–6. https://doi.org/10.1097/BPO.0b013e3181c6b3a8.
53. Louahem D, Cottalorda J. Acute ischemia and pink pulseless hand in 68 of 404 gartland type III supracondylar humeral fractures in children: urgent management and therapeutic consensus. Injury. 2016;47(4):848–52. https://doi.org/10.1016/j.injury.2016.01.010.
54. Schriger DL, Baraff L. Defining normal capillary refill: variation with age, sex, and temperature. Ann Emerg Med. 1988;17(9):932–5. https://doi.org/10.1016/S0196-0644(88)80675-9.
55. Shah AS, Waters PM, Bae DS. Treatment of the "pink pulseless hand" in pediatric supracondylar humerus fractures. J Hand Surg Am. 2013;38(7):1399–403. https://doi.org/10.1016/j.jhsa.2013.03.047.

56. Bahk MS, Srikumaran U, Ain MC, et al. Patterns of pediatric supracondylar humerus fractures. J Pediatr Orthop. 2008;28(5):493–9. https://doi.org/10.1097/BPO.0b013e31817bb860.
57. Samelis PV, Papagrigorakis E, Ellinas S. Role of the posterior fat pad sign in treating displaced extension type supracondylar fractures of the pediatric elbow using the Blount method. Cureus. 2019;11(10):e6024. https://doi.org/10.7759/cureus.6024.
58. Skaggs DL, Mirzayan R. The posterior fat pad sign in association with occult fracture of the elbow in children. J Bone Joint Surg Am. 1999;81(10):1429–33. https://doi.org/10.2106/00004623-199910000-00007.
59. Dodge HS. Displaced supracondylar fractures of the humerus in children--treatment by Dunlop's traction. J Bone Joint Surg Am. 1972;54(7):1408–18. https://doi.org/10.2106/00004623-197254070-00003.
60. Nacht JL, Ecker ML, Chung SMK, Lotke PADM. Supracondylar fractures of the humerus in children treated by closed reduction and percutaneous pinning. Clin Orthop. 1983;177:203–9.
61. Camp J, Ishizue K, Gomez M, Gelberman R, Akeson W. Alteration of baumann's angle by humeral position: implications for treatment of supracondylar humerus fractures. J Pediatr Orthop. 1993;13(4):521–5. https://doi.org/10.1097/01241398-199307000-00019.
62. Herman MJ, Boardman MJ, Hoover JR, Chafetz RS. Relationship of the anterior humeral line to the capitellar ossific nucleus: variability with age. J Bone Joint Surg Am. 2009;91(9):2188–93. https://doi.org/10.2106/JBJS.H.01316.
63. GARTLAND JJ. Management of supracondylar fractures of the humerus in children. Surg Gynecol Obstet. 1959;109(2):145–54.
64. Alton TB, Werner SE, Gee AO. Classifications in brief: the Gartland classification of supracondylar Humerus fractures. Clin Orthop Relat Res. 2015;473(2):738–41. https://doi.org/10.1007/s11999-014-4033-8.
65. Wilkins K. Fractures and dislocations of the elbow region. Philadelphia: JB Lippincott; 1984. p. 363–575.
66. De Boeck H, De Smet P, Penders W, De Rydt D. Supracondylar elbow fractures with impaction of the medial condyle in children. J Pediatr Orthop. 1995;15(4):444–8. https://doi.org/10.1097/01241398-199507000-00006.
67. Leitch KK, Kay RM, Femino JD, Tolo VT, Storer SK, Skaggs DL. Treatment of multidirectionally unstable supracondylar humeral fractures in children: a modified Gartland type-IV fracture. J Bone Joint Surg Am. 2006;88(5):980–5. https://doi.org/10.2106/JBJS.D.02956.
68. Barton KL, Kaminsky CK, Green DW, Shean CJ, Kautz SM, Skaggs DL. Reliability of a modified Gartland classification of supracondylar humerus fractures. J Pediatr Orthop. 2001;21(1):27–30. https://doi.org/10.1097/00004694-200101000-00007.
69. Kuoppala E, Parviainen R, Pokka T, Sirviö M, Serlo W, Sinikumpu J-J. Low incidence of flexion-type supracondylar humerus fractures but high rate of complications. Acta Orthop. 2016;87(4):406–11. https://doi.org/10.1080/17453674.2016.1176825.
70. Cooper SA. A treatise on dislocations and fractures of the joints. 5th ed. London: Longman; 1826. https://doi.org/10.1136/bmj.s1-3.21.415.
71. Charnley J. Closed treatment of common fractures. 3rd ed. E & S Livingstone: Edinburgh; 1961.
72. Blount WP. Fractures in children. Postgrad Med. 1954;16(3):209–16. https://doi.org/10.1080/00325481.1954.11711663.
73. Pham TT, Accadbled F, Abid A, et al. Gartland types IIB and III supracondylar fractures of the humerus in children: is Blount's method effective and safe? J Shoulder Elb Surg. 2017;26(12):2226–31. https://doi.org/10.1016/j.jse.2017.05.018.
74. Muccioli C, ElBatti S, Oborocianu I, et al. Outcomes of Gartland type III supracondylar fractures treated using Blount's method. Orthop Traumatol Surg Res. 2017;103(7):1121–5. https://doi.org/10.1016/j.otsr.2017.06.011.
75. Dunlop J. Transcondylar fractures of the humerus. J Bone Joint Surg Am. 1939;21(59):73.
76. Palmer E, Niemann K, Vesely D, Armstrong J. Supracondylar fracture of the Humerus in children. J Bone Joint Surg Am. 1978;60:653–5.

77. Smith FM. Kirschner wire traction in elbow and upper arm injuries. Am J Surg. 1947;74(5):770–87. https://doi.org/10.1016/0002-9610(47)90235-3.
78. Prietto CA. Supracondylar fractures of the humerus. A comparative study of Dunlop's traction versus percutaneous pinning. J Bone Joint Surg Am. 1979;61(3):425–8. https://doi.org/10.2106/00004623-197961030-00019.
79. Ramsey RH, Griz J. Immediate open reduction and internal fixation of severely displaced supracondylar fractures of the humerus in children. Clin Orthop Relat Res. 1973;90:131–2.
80. Swenson AL. The treatment of supracondylar fractures of the humerus by Kirschner-wire transfixion. J Bone Joint Surg Am. 1948;30A(4):993–7. https://doi.org/10.2106/00004623-194830040-00023.
81. Flynn JC, Matthews JG, Benoit RL. Blind pinning of displaced supracondylar fractures of the Humerus in children. J Bone Jt Surg. 1974;56(2):263–72. https://doi.org/10.2106/00004623-197456020-00004.
82. Battaglia TC, Armstrong DG, Schwend RM. Factors affecting forearm compartment pressures in children with supracondylar fractures of the humerus. J Pediatr Orthop. 2002;22(4):431–9. https://doi.org/10.1097/01241398-200207000-00004.
83. Sylvia SM, Maguire KJ, Molho DA, et al. Emergency room closed reduction versus in situ splinting in the treatment of paediatric supracondylar humerus fractures. J Child Orthop. 2019;13(3):334–9. https://doi.org/10.1302/1863-2548.13.190018.
84. Mulpuri K, Hosalkar H, Howard A. AAOS clinical practice guideline: the treatment of pediatric supracondylar humerus fractures. J Am Acad Orthop Surg. 2012;20(5):328–30. https://doi.org/10.5435/JAAOS-20-05-328.
85. Omid R, Choi PD, Skaggs DL. Supracondylar humeral fractures in children. J Bone Joint Surg Am. 2008;90(5):1121–32. https://doi.org/10.2106/JBJS.G.01354.
86. Ballal MS, Garg NK, Bass A, Bruce CE. Comparison between collar and cuffs and above elbow back slabs in the initial treatment of Gartland type i supracondylar humerus fractures. J Pediatr Orthop B. 2008;17(2):57–60. https://doi.org/10.1097/BPB.0b013e3282f3d162.
87. Oakley E, Barnett P, Babl FE. Backslab versus nonbackslab for immobilization of undisplaced supracondylar fractures a randomized trial. Pediatr Emerg Care. 2009;25(7):452–6. https://doi.org/10.1097/PEC.0b013e3181ab7898.
88. Mapes RC, Hennrikus WL. The effect of elbow position on the radial pulse measured by Doppler ultrasonography after surgical treatment of supracondylar elbow fractures in children. J Pediatr Orthop. 1998;18(4):441–4. https://doi.org/10.1097/00004694-199807000-00006.
89. Moraleda L, Valencia M, Barco R, González-Moran G. Natural history of unreduced Gartland type-II supracondylar fractures of the humerus in children: a two to thirteen-year follow-up study. J Bone Joint Surg Am. 2013;95(1):28–34. https://doi.org/10.2106/JBJS.L.00132.
90. Parikh SN, Wall EJ, Foad S, Wiersema B, Nolte B. Displaced type II extension supracondylar humerus fractures: do they all need pinning? J Pediatr Orthop. 2004;24(4):380–4. https://doi.org/10.1097/01241398-200407000-00007.
91. Hadlow AT, Devane P, Nicol RO. A selective treatment approach to supracondylar fracture of the humerus in children. J Pediatr Orthop. 1996;16(1):104–6. https://doi.org/10.1097/00004694-199601000-00021.
92. Prabhakar P, Ho CA. Delaying surgery in type III supracondylar humerus fractures does not Lead to longer surgical times or more difficult reduction. J Orthop Trauma. 2019;33(8):e285–90. https://doi.org/10.1097/BOT.0000000000001491.
93. Mehlman CT, Strub WM, Roy DR, Wall EJ, Crawford AH. The effect of surgical timing on the perioperative complications of treatment of supracondylar humeral fractures in children. J Bone Joint Surg Am. 2001;83(3):323–7. https://doi.org/10.2106/00004623-200103000-00002.
94. Lyengar SR. Early versus delayed reduction and pinning of type III displaced supracondylar fractures of the humerus in children: a comparative study. J Orthop Trauma. 1999;13(1):51–5. https://doi.org/10.1097/00005131-199901000-00012.

95. Gupta N, Kay RM, Leitch K, Femino JD, Tolo VT, Skaggs DL. Effect of surgical delay on perioperative complications and need for open reduction in supracondylar humerus fractures in children. J Pediatr Orthop. 2004;24(3):245–8. https://doi.org/10.1097/01241398-200405000-00001.
96. Walmsley PJ, Kelly MB, Robb JE, Annan IH, Porter DE. Delay increases the need for open reduction of type-III supracondylar fractures of the humerus. J Bone Joint Surg Br. 2006;88(4):528–30. https://doi.org/10.1302/0301-620X.88B4.17491.
97. Scherl SA, Schmidt AH. Pediatric trauma: getting through the night. Instr Course Lect. 2010;59:455–63.
98. Rang M. Children's fractures. 2nd ed. Lippincott; 1974.
99. Smuin D, Hatch M, Winthrop Z, Gidvani S, Hennrikus W. The reduction maneuver for pediatric extension type 3 supracondylar humerus fractures. Cureus. 2020;12(7):e9213. https://doi.org/10.7759/cureus.9213.
100. Novais EN, Andrade MAP, Gomes DC. The use of a joystick technique facilitates closed reduction and percutaneous fixation of multidirectionally unstable supracondylar humeral fractures in children. J Pediatr Orthop. 2013;33(1):14–9. https://doi.org/10.1097/BPO.0b013e3182724d07.
101. Gordon JE, Patton CM, Luhmann SJ, Bassett GS, Schoenecker PL. Fracture stability after pinning of displaced supracondylar distal humerus fractures in children. J Pediatr Orthop. 2001;22(5):697. https://doi.org/10.1097/00004694-200105000-00010.
102. Lee SS, Mahar AT, Miesen D, Newton PO. Displaced pediatric supracondylar humerus fractures: biomechanical analysis of percutaneous pinning techniques. J Pediatr Orthop. 2002;22(4):440–3. https://doi.org/10.1097/00004694-200207000-00005.
103. Zionts LE, McKellop HA, Hathaway R. Torsional strength of pin configurations used to fix supracondylar fractures of the humerus in children. J Bone Joint Surg Am. 1994;76(2):253–6. https://doi.org/10.2106/00004623-199402000-00013.
104. Bloom T, Robertson C, Mahar AT, Newton P. Biomechanical analysis of supracondylar humerus fracture pinning for slightly malreduced fractures. J Pediatr Orthop. 2008;28(7):766–72. https://doi.org/10.1097/BPO.0b013e318186bdcd.
105. Larson L, Firoozbakhsh K, Passarelli R, Bosch P. Biomechanical analysis of pinning techniques for pediatric supracondylar humerus fractures. J Pediatr Orthop. 2006;26(5):573–8. https://doi.org/10.1097/01.bpo.0000230336.26652.1c.
106. Gottschalk HP, Sagoo D, Glaser D, Doan J, Edmonds EW, Schlechter J. Biomechanical analysis of pin placement for pediatric supracondylar humerus fractures: does starting point, pin size, and number matter? J Pediatr Orthop. 2012;32(5):445–51. https://doi.org/10.1097/BPO.0b013e318257d1cd.
107. Hamdi A, Poitras P, Louati H, Dagenais S, Masquijo JJ, Kontio K. Biomechanical analysis of lateral pin placements for pediatric supracondylar humerus fractures. J Pediatr Orthop. 2010;30(2):135–9. https://doi.org/10.1097/BPO.0b013e3181cfcd14.
108. Kasirajan S, Govindasamy R, Sathish BRJ, Meleppuram JJ. Trans-olecranon fossa four-cortex purchase lateral pinning in displaced supracondylar fracture of the humerus – a prospective analysis in 48 children. Rev Bras Ortop. 2018;53(3):342–9. https://doi.org/10.1016/j.rboe.2017.03.014.
109. Skaggs DL, Cluck MW, Mostofi A, Flynn JM, Kay RM. Lateral-entry pin fixation in the management of supracondylar fractures in children. J Bone Joint Surg Am. 2004;86(4):702–7. https://doi.org/10.2106/00004623-200404000-00006.
110. Yen YM, Kocher MS. Lateral entry compared with medial and lateral entry pin fixation for completely displaced supracondylar humeral fractures in children. J Bone Joint Surg Am. 2008;90(Suppl 2 Pt 1):20–30. https://doi.org/10.2106/JBJS.G.01337.
111. Brauer CA, Lee BM, Bae DS, Waters PM, Kocher MS. A systematic review of medial and lateral entry pinning versus lateral entry pinning for supracondylar fractures of the humerus. J Pediatr Orthop. 2007;27(2):181–6. https://doi.org/10.1097/bpo.0b013e3180316cf1.

112. Kocher MS, Kasser JR, Waters PM, et al. Lateral entry compared with medial and lateral entry pin fixation for completely displaced supracondylar humeral fractures in children: a randomized clinical trial. J Bone Joint Surg Am. 2007;89(4):706–12. https://doi.org/10.2106/JBJS.F.00379.

113. Zhao JG, Wang J, Zhang P. Is lateral pin fixation for displaced supracondylar fractures of the humerus better than crossed pins in children? Clin Orthop Relat Res. 2013;471(9):2942–53. https://doi.org/10.1007/s11999-013-3025-4.

114. Woratanarat P, Angsanuntsukh C, Rattanasiri S, Attia J, Woratanarat T, Thakkinstian A. Meta-analysis of pinning in supracondylar fracture of the humerus in children. J Orthop Trauma. 2012;26(1):48–53. https://doi.org/10.1097/BOT.0b013e3182143de0.

115. Lee KM, Chung CY, Gwon DK, et al. Medial and lateral crossed pinning versus lateral pinning for supracondylar fractures of the humerus in children: decision analysis. J Pediatr Orthop. 2012;32(2):131–8. https://doi.org/10.1097/BPO.0b013e3182471931.

116. Skaggs DL, Hale JM, Bassett J, Kaminsky C, Kay RM, Tolo VT. Operative treatment of supracondylar fractures of the humerus in children: the consequences of pin placement. J Bone Joint Surg Am. 2001;83(5):735–40. https://doi.org/10.2106/00004623-200105000-00013.

117. Lyons JP, Ashley E, Hoffer MM. Ulnar nerve palsies after percutaneous cross-pinning of supracondylar fractures in children's elbows. J Pediatr Orthop. 1998;18(1):43–5. https://doi.org/10.1097/00004694-199801000-00009.

118. Babal JC, Mehlman CT, Klein G. Nerve injuries associated with pediatric supracondylar humeral fractures: a meta-analysis. J Pediatr Orthop. 2010;30(3):253–63. https://doi.org/10.1097/BPO.0b013e3181d213a6.

119. Rasool MN. Ulnar nerve injury after K-wire fixation of supracondylar humerus fractures in children. J Pediatr Orthop. 1998;18(5):686–90. https://doi.org/10.1097/01241398-199809000-00027.

120. Edmonds EW, Roocroft JH, Mubarak SJ. Treatment of displaced pediatric supracondylar humerus fracture patterns requiring medial fixation: a reliable and safer cross-pinning technique. J Pediatr Orthop. 2012;32(4):346–51. https://doi.org/10.1097/BPO.0b013e318255e3b1.

121. Green DW, Widmann RF, Frank JS, Gardner MJ. Low incidence of ulnar nerve injury with crossed pin placement for pediatric supracondylar humerus fractures using a mini-open technique. J Orthop Trauma. 2005;19(3):158–63. https://doi.org/10.1097/00005131-200503000-00002.

122. Wind WM, Schwend RM, Armstrong DG. Predicting ulnar nerve location in pinning of supracondylar humerus fractures. J Pediatr Orthop. 2002;22(4):444–7. https://doi.org/10.1097/00004694-200207000-00006.

123. Shtarker H, Elboim-Gabyzon M, Bathish E, Laufer Y, Rahamimov N, Volpin G. Ulnar nerve monitoring during percutaneous pinning of supracondylar fractures in children. J Pediatr Orthop. 2014;34(2):161–5. https://doi.org/10.1097/BPO.0000000000000084.

124. Soldado F, Knorr J, Haddad S, et al. Ultrasound-guided percutaneous medial pinning of pediatric supracondylar humeral fractures to avoid ulnar nerve injury. Arch Bone Jt Surg. 2015;3(3):169–72. https://doi.org/10.22038/abjs.2015.4274.

125. Sankar WN, Hebela NM, Skaggs DL, Flynn JM. Loss of pin fixation in displaced supracondylar humeral fractures in children: causes and prevention. J Bone Joint Surg Am. 2007;89(4):713–7. https://doi.org/10.2106/JBJS.F.00076.

126. Koudstaal MJ, De Ridder VA, De Lange S, Ulrich C. Pediatric supracondylar humerus fractures: the anterior approach. J Orthop Trauma. 2002;16(6):409–12. https://doi.org/10.1097/00005131-200207000-00007.

127. Ersan O, Gonen E, Ilhan RD, Boysan E, Ates Y. Comparison of anterior and lateral approaches in the treatment of extension-type supracondylar humerus fractures in children. J Pediatr Orthop B. 2012;21(2):121–6. https://doi.org/10.1097/BPB.0b013e32834dd1b2.

128. Cramer KE, Devito DP, Green NE. Comparison of closed reduction and percutaneous pinning versus open reduction and percutaneous pinning in displaced supracondylar fractures of the humerus in children. J Orthop Trauma. 1992;6(4):407–12. https://doi.org/10.1097/00005131-199212000-00002.

129. Kaewpornsawan K. Comparison between closed reduction with percutaneous pinning and open reduction with pinning in children with closed totally displaced supracondylar humeral fractures: a randomized controlled trial. J Pediatr Orthop B. 2001;10(2):131–7. https://doi.org/10.1097/00009957-200104000-00010.

130. Weiland AJ, Meyer S, Tolo VT, Berg HL, Mueller J. Surgical treatment of displaced supracondylar fractures of the humerus in children. Analysis of fifty-two cases followed for five to fifteen years. J Bone Joint Surg Am. 1978;60(5):657–61. https://doi.org/10.2106/00004623-197860050-00012.

131. Guillen PT, Fuller CB, Riedel BB, Wongworawat MD. A prospective randomized crossover study on the comparison of cotton versus waterproof cast liners. Hand. 2016;11(1):50–3. https://doi.org/10.1177/1558944715614853.

132. Kleis K, Schlechter JA, Doan JD, Farnsworth CL, Edmonds EW. Under pressure: the utility of spacers in univalved fiberglass casts. J Pediatr Orthop. 2019;39(6):302–5. https://doi.org/10.1097/BPO.0000000000000961.

133. Shaw KA, Moreland C, Boomsma SE, Hire JM, Topolski R, Cameron CD. Volumetric considerations for Valving long-arm casts: the utility of the cast spacer. Am J Orthop (Belle Mead NJ). 2018;47(7):10.12788/ajo.2018.0061.

134. Schmale GA, Mazor S, Mercer LD, Bompadre V. Lack of benefit of physical therapy on function following supracondylar humeral fracture: a randomized controlled trial. J Bone Joint Surg Am. 2014;96(11):944–50. https://doi.org/10.2106/JBJS.L.01696.

135. Blakey CM, Biant LC, Birch R. Ischaemia and the pink, pulseless hand complicating supracondylar fractures of the humerus in childhood: long-term follow-up. J Bone Joint Surg Br. 2009;91(11):1487–92. https://doi.org/10.1302/0301-620X.91B11.22170.

136. Sabharwal S, Tredwell SJ, Beauchamp RD, et al. Management of pulseless pink hand in pediatric supracondylar fractures of humerus. J Pediatr Orthop. 1997;17(3):303–10. https://doi.org/10.1097/01241398-199705000-00007.

137. Ramisetty N. Pink pulseless hand following supra-condylar fractures: an audit of British practice. J Pediatr Orthop B. 2006;15(1):62–4. https://doi.org/10.1097/01202412-200609000-00015.

138. Malviya A, Simmons D, Vallamshetla R, Bache CE. Pink pulseless hand following supracondylar fractures: an audit of British practice. J Pediatr Orthop B. 2006;15(1):62–4. https://doi.org/10.1097/01202412-200601000-00013.

139. Griffin KJ, Walsh SR, Markar S, Tang TY, Boyle JR, Hayes PD. The pink pulseless hand: a review of the literature regarding Management of Vascular Complications of supracondylar humeral fractures in children. Eur J Vasc Endovasc Surg. 2008;36(6):697–702. https://doi.org/10.1016/j.ejvs.2008.08.013.

140. Weller A, Garg S, Larson AN, et al. Management of the pediatric pulseless supracondylar humeral fracture: is vascular exploration necessary? J Bone Joint Surg Am. 2013;95(21):1906–12. https://doi.org/10.2106/JBJS.L.01580.

141. Soh RCC, Tawng DK, Mahadev A. Pulse oximetry for the diagnosis and prediction for surgical exploration in the pulseless perfused hand as a result of supracondylar fractures of the distal humerus. Clin Orthop Surg. 2013;5(1):74–81. https://doi.org/10.4055/cios.2013.5.1.74.

142. Reigstad O, Thorkildsen R, Grimsgaard C, Reigstad A, Røkkum M. Supracondylar fractures with circulatory failure after reduction, pinning, and entrapment of the brachial artery: excellent results more than 1 year after open exploration and revascularization. J Orthop Trauma. 2011;25(1):26–30. https://doi.org/10.1097/BOT.0b013e3181db276a.

143. Schoenecker PL, Delgado E, Rotman M, Sicard GA, Capelli AM. Pulseless arm in association with totally displaced supracondylar fracture. J Orthop Trauma. 1996;10(6):410–5. https://doi.org/10.1097/00005131-199608000-00008.

144. Marck KW, Kooiman AM, Binnendijk B. Brachial artery rupture following supracondylar fracture of the humerus. Neth J Surg. 1986;38(3):81–4.

145. White L, Mehlman CT, Crawford AH. Perfused, pulseless, and puzzling: a systematic review of vascular injuries in pediatric supracondylar humerus fractures and results of a POSNA questionnaire. J Pediatr Orthop. 2010;30(4):328–35. https://doi.org/10.1097/BPO.0b013e3181da0452.

146. Fleuriau-Chateau P, McIntyre W, Letts M. An analysis of open reduction of irreducible supracondylar fractures of the humerus in children. Can J Surg. 1998;41(2):112–8.

147. Yokoyama T, Tosa Y, Kadomatsu K, Sato K, Hosaka Y. A novel approach for preventing the development of persistent vasospasms after microsurgery for the extremities: intermittent topical lidocaine application. J Reconstr Microsurg. 2010;26(2):79–85. https://doi.org/10.1055/s-0029-1243291.

148. Badkoobehi H, Choi PD, Skaggs DL, Bae DS. Current concepts review: management of the pulseless pediatric supracondylar humeral fracture. J Bone Joint Surg Am. 2014;97(11):937–43. https://doi.org/10.2106/JBJS.N.00983.

149. Copley LA, Dormans JP, Davidson RS. Vascular injuries and their sequelae in pediatric supracondylar humeral fractures: toward a goal of prevention. J Pediatr Orthop. 1996;97(11):937–43. https://doi.org/10.1097/00004694-199601000-00020.

150. Battle J, Carmichael KD. Incidence of pin track infections in children's fractures treated with kirschner wire fixation. J Pediatr Orthop. 2007;27(2):154–7. https://doi.org/10.1097/bpo.0b013e3180317a22.

151. Bashyal RK, Chu JY, Schoenecker PL, Dobbs MB, Luhmann SJ, Gordon JE. Complications after pinning of supracondylar distal humerus fractures. J Pediatr Orthop. 2009;29(7):704–8. https://doi.org/10.1097/BPO.0b013e3181b768ac.

152. Eastwood DM. Lovell and Winter's pediatric orthopaedics, 6th edition. J Bone Joint Surg Br. 2007; https://doi.org/10.1302/0301-620x.89b3.19281.

153. Vaquero-Picado A, González-Morán G, Moraleda L. Management of supracondylar fractures of the humerus in children. EFORT Open Rev. 2018;3(10):526–40. https://doi.org/10.1302/2058-5241.3.170049.

154. Labelle H, Bunnell WP, Duhaime M, Poitras B. Cubitus varus deformity following supracondylar fractures of the humerus in children. J Pediatr Orthop. 1982;3(5):622. https://doi.org/10.1097/01241398-198212000-00014.

155. Bender J, Busch CA. Results of treatment of supracondylar fractures of the humerus in children with special reference to the cause and prevention of cubitus varus. Arch Chir Neerl. 1978;30(1):29–41.

156. Abe M, Ishizu T, Morikawa J. Posterolateral rotatory instability of the elbow after post-traumatic cubitus varus. J Shoulder Elb Surg. 1997;6(4):405–9. https://doi.org/10.1016/S1058-2746(97)90011-2.

157. Davids JR, Maguire MF, Mubarak SJ, Wenger DR. Lateral condylar fracture of the humerus following posttraumatic cubitus varus. J Pediatr Orthop. 1994;14(4):466–70. https://doi.org/10.1097/01241398-199407000-00009.

158. Abe M, Ishizu T, Shirai H, Okamoto M, Onomura T. Tardy ulnar nerve palsy caused by cubitus varus deformity. J Hand Surg Am. 1995;20(1):5–9. https://doi.org/10.1016/S0363-5023(05)80047-4.

159. Abe M, Ishizu T, Nagaoka T, Onomura T. Recurrent posterior dislocation of the head of the radius in post-traumatic cubitus varus. J Bone Joint Surg Br. 1995;77(4):582–5. https://doi.org/10.1302/0301-620x.77b4.7615602.

160. Pankaj A, Dua A, Malhotra R, Bhan S. Dome osteotomy for posttraumatic cubitus varus: a surgical technique to avoid lateral condylar prominence. J Pediatr Orthop. 2006;26(1):61–6. https://doi.org/10.1097/01.bpo.0000189008.62798.70.

161. Greenhill DA, Kozin SH, Kwon M, Herman MJ. Oblique lateral closing-wedge osteotomy for cubitus varus in skeletally immature patients. JBJS Essent Surg Tech. 2019;9(4):e40.1–8. https://doi.org/10.2106/JBJS.ST.18.00107.

162. Ramachandran M, Skaggs DL, Crawford HA, et al. Delaying treatment of supracondylar fractures in children: has the pendulum swung too far? J Bone Joint Surg Br. 2008;90(9):1228–33. https://doi.org/10.1302/0301-620X.90B9.20728.

163. Zionts LE, Woodson CJ, Manjra N, Zalavras C. Time of return of elbow motion after percutaneous pinning of pediatric supracondylar humerus fractures. Clin Orthop Relat Res. 2009;467(8):2007–10. https://doi.org/10.1007/s11999-009-0724-y.

164. Killian JT, White S, Lenning L. Cast-saw bums: comparison of technique versus material versus saws. J Pediatr Orthop. 1999;19(5):683–7. https://doi.org/10.1097/00004694-199909000-00026.
165. Ansari MZ, Swarup S, Ghani R, Tovey P. Oscillating saw injuries during removal of plaster. Eur J Emerg Med. 1998;5(1):37–9. https://doi.org/10.1097/00063110-199803000-00009.
166. Shuler FD, Grisafi FN. Cast-saw burns: evaluation of skin, cast, and blade temperatures generated during cast removal. J Bone Joint Surg Am. 2008;90(12):2626–30. https://doi.org/10.2106/JBJS.H.00119.

# Index

Printed by Printforce, the Netherlands